Current Topics in Microbiology and Immunology

Volume 355

Series Editors

Klaus Aktories
Medizinische Fakultät, Institut für Experimentelle und Klinische Pharmakologie und Toxikologie, Albert-Ludwigs-Universität Freiburg, Abt. I, Albertstr. 25, 79104 Freiburg, Germany

Richard W. Compans
Influenza Pathogenesis and Immunology Research Center, Emory University, School of Medicine, Atlanta, GA 30322, USA

Max D. Cooper
Department of Pathology and Laboratory Medicine, Georgia Research Alliance, Emory University, 1462 Clifton Road, Atlanta, GA 30322, USA

Yuri Y. Gleba
ICON Genetics AG, Biozentrum Halle, Weinbergweg 22, 06120 Halle, Germany

Tasuku Honjo
Department of Medical Chemistry, Faculty of Medicine, Kyoto University, Sakyo-ku, Yoshida, Kyoto, 606-8501, Japan

Hilary Koprowski
Biotechnology Foundation, Inc., 119 Sibley Avenue, Ardmore, PA 19003, USA

Bernard Malissen
Centre d'Immunologie de Marseille-Luminy, Parc Scientifique de Luminy, Case 906, 13288, Marseille Cedex 9, 13288, France

Fritz Melchers
Max Planck Institute for Infection Biology, Charitéplatz 1, 10117 Berlin, Germany

Michael B. A. Oldstone
Department of Neuropharmacology, Division of Virology, The Scripps Research Institute, 10550 North Torrey Pines Road, La Jolla, CA 92037, USA

Peter K. Vogt
Department of Molecular and Experimental Medicine, The Scripps Research Institute, 10550 North Torrey Pines Road, BCC-239, La Jolla, CA 92037, USA

Current Topics in Microbiology and Immunology

Previously published volumes

Further volumes can be found at www.springer.com

Vol. 329: **Griffin, Diane E.;**
Oldstone, Michael B. A. (Eds.): Measles. 2009
ISBN 978-3-540-70522-2

Vol. 330: **Griffin, Diane E.;**
Oldstone, Michael B. A. (Eds.):
Measles. 2009.
ISBN 978-3-540-70616-8

Vol. 331: **Villiers, E. M. de (Ed.):**
TT Viruses. 2009.
ISBN 978-3-540-70917-8

Vol. 332: **Karasev A. (Ed.):**
Plant produced Microbial Vaccines. 2009.
ISBN 978-3-540-70857-5

Vol. 333: **Compans, Richard W.;**
Orenstein, Walter A. (Eds.):
Vaccines for Pandemic Influenza. 2009.
ISBN 978-3-540-92164-6

Vol. 334: **McGavern, Dorian; Dustin, Micheal (Eds.):**
Visualizing Immunity. 2009.
ISBN 978-3-540-93862-0

Vol. 335: **Levine, Beth; Yoshimori, Tamotsu;**
Deretic, Vojo (Eds.):
Autophagy in Infection and Immunity. 2009.
ISBN 978-3-642-00301-1

Vol. 336: **Kielian, Tammy (Ed.):**
Toll-like Receptors: Roles in Infection and
Neuropathology. 2009.
ISBN 978-3-642-00548-0

Vol. 337: **Sasakawa, Chihiro (Ed.):**
Molecular Mechanisms of Bacterial Infection via the Gut.
2009.
ISBN 978-3-642-01845-9

Vol. 338: **Rothman, Alan L. (Ed.):**
Dengue Virus. 2009.
ISBN 978-3-642-02214-2

Vol. 339: **Spearman, Paul; Freed, Eric O. (Eds.):**
HIV Interactions with Host Cell Proteins. 2009.
ISBN 978-3-642-02174-9

Vol. 340: **Saito, Takashi; Batista, Facundo D. (Eds.):**
Immunological Synapse. 2010.
ISBN 978-3-642-03857-0

Vol. 341: **Bruserud, Øystein (Ed.):**
The Chemokine System in Clinical
and Experimental Hematology. 2010.
ISBN 978-3-642-12638-3

Vol. 342: **Arvin, Ann M. (Ed.):**
Varicella-zoster Virus. 2010.
ISBN 978-3-642-12727-4

Vol. 343: **Johnson, John E. (Ed.):**
Cell Entry by Non-Enveloped Viruses. 2010.
ISBN 978-3-642-13331-2

Vol. 344: **Dranoff, Glenn (Ed.):**
Cancer Immunology and Immunotherapy. 2011.
ISBN 978-3-642-14135-5

Vol. 345: **Simon, M. Celeste (Ed.):**
Diverse Effects of Hypoxia on Tumor Progression. 2010.
ISBN 978-3-642-13328-2

Vol. 346: **Christian Rommel; Bart Vanhaesebroeck;**
Peter K. Vogt (Ed.):
Phosphoinositide 3-kinase in Health and Disease. 2010.
ISBN 978-3-642-13662-7

Vol. 347: **Christian Rommel; Bart Vanhaesebroeck;**
Peter K. Vogt (Ed.):
Phosphoinositide 3-kinase in Health and Disease. 2010.
ISBN 978-3-642-14815-6

Vol. 348: **Lyubomir Vassilev; David Fry (Eds.):**
Small-Molecule Inhibitors of Protein-Protein
Interactions. 2011.
ISBN 978-3-642-17082-9

Vol. 349: **Michael Kartin (Ed.):**
NF-kB in Health and Disease. 2011.
ISBN: 978-3-642-16017-2

Vol. 350: **Rafi Ahmed; Tasuku Honjo (Eds.):**
Negative Co-receptors and Ligands. 2011.
ISBN: 978-3-642-19545-7

Vol. 351: **Marcel, B. M. Teunissen (Ed.):**
Intradermal Immunization. 2011.
ISBN: 978-3-642-23689-1

Vol. 352: **Rudolf Valenta; Robert L. Coffman (Eds.):**
Vaccines against Allergies. 2011.
ISBN 978-3-642-20054-0

Vol. 353: **Charles E. Samuel (Ed.):**
Adenosine Deaminases Acting on RNA (ADARs)
and A-to-I Editing. 2011.
ISBN 978-3-642-22800-1

Vol. 354: **Pamela A. Kozlowski (Ed.):**
Mucosal Vaccines. 2012.
ISBN 978-3-642-23692-1

Ingo K. Mellinghoff · Charles L. Sawyers
Editors

Therapeutic Kinase Inhibitors

Responsible series editor: Peter K. Vogt

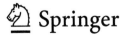 Springer

Ingo K. Mellinghoff
Human Oncology and Pathogenesis
Program
Memorial Sloan-Kettering
Cancer Center
1275 York Avenue
New York, NY 10065
USA

Charles L. Sawyers
Human Oncology and Pathogenesis
Program
Memorial Sloan-Kettering
Cancer Center
1275 York Avenue
New York, NY 10065
USA

The cover image shows PLX4032 inside the BRAF kinase and separately. Figure provided by G. Bollag.

ISSN 0070-217X
ISBN 978-3-642-28295-9   e-ISBN 978-3-642-28296-6
DOI 10.1007/978-3-642-28296-6
Springer Heidelberg New York Dordrecht London

Library of Congress Control Number: 2011945111

© Springer-Verlag Berlin Heidelberg 2012
This work is subject to copyright. All rights are reserved by the Publisher, whether the whole or part of the material is concerned, specifically the rights of translation, reprinting, reuse of illustrations, recitation, broadcasting, reproduction on microfilms or in any other physical way, and transmission or information storage and retrieval, electronic adaptation, computer software, or by similar or dissimilar methodology now known or hereafter developed. Exempted from this legal reservation are brief excerpts in connection with reviews or scholarly analysis or material supplied specifically for the purpose of being entered and executed on a computer system, for exclusive use by the purchaser of the work. Duplication of this publication or parts thereof is permitted only under the provisions of the Copyright Law of the Publisher's location, in its current version, and permission for use must always be obtained from Springer. Permissions for use may be obtained through RightsLink at the Copyright Clearance Center. Violations are liable to prosecution under the respective Copyright Law.
The use of general descriptive names, registered names, trademarks, service marks, etc. in this publication does not imply , even in the absence of a specific statement, that such names are exempt from the relevant protective laws and regulations and therefore free for general use.
While the advice and information in this book are believed to be true and accurate at the date of publication, neither the authors nor the editors nor the publisher can accept any legal responsibility for any errors or omissions that may be made. The publisher makes no warranty, express or implied, with respect to the material contained herein.

Printed on acid-free paper

Springer is part of Springer Science+Business Media (www.springer.com)

Preface

Cancer drug development is currently undergoing a profound shift. Drugs targeting fundamental cellular processes such as DNA–replication and microtubule function, often referred to as "chemotherapy" and still the backbone of most cancer treatment regimens, are increasingly being complemented by or replaced with kinase inhibitors. This new class of drugs targets enzymes which provide growth and survival signals to cancer cells by transferring phosphate groups from Adenosine-5'-triphosphate (ATP) to other proteins, lipids, nucleotides, and carbohydrates.

The earliest roots of kinase inhibitor therapy for cancer can be found in observations several decades ago that mutant kinases are often responsible for tumor inducing properties of certain animal viruses. The idea to develop drugs against these kinases was initially not pursued due to the important physiological functions of many of these enzymes and the concern that kinase inhibitors would be selective enough to provide a sufficiently wide "therapeutic window" between drug activity and drug toxicity. This concern was largely alleviated by the discovery that mutations in kinase encoding genes can render cancer cells uniquely "addicted" to signals provided by the mutant kinase. An early dramatic example for the paradigm of oncogene addiction was the durable remissions of BCR-ABL positive leukemias in response to the ABL kinase inhibitor imatinib (gleevec).

Since the first publication of the gleevec trials in the year 2001, much has happened. Pharmaceutical companies have designed and synthesized inhibitors against virtually all known human kinases and the genomes of many human cancer types have been surveyed for mutations that might result in oncogene addiction. These efforts have been rewarded by the development and regulatory approval of inhibitors against the ABL kinase (chronic myeloid leukemia), EGFR kinase (lung cancer), ALK kinase (lung cancer), PDGFR and KIT kinase (gastrointestinal stromal tumors), VEGFR (kidney cancer) and most recently the BRAF kinase (melanoma). As with any other cancer drug, responses to therapy are often not durable and acquired drug resistance has become a major challenge.

This book summarizes the current state of kinase inhibitor therapy for cancer. Successful drug development relies on the expertise and dedication of many experts. To reflect this team approach to finding new kinase inhibitors and defining their optimal use for cancer treatment, we invited experts in academia and pharmaceutical industry to share their insights into various aspects of this process, ranging from the first chemical screens, to preclinical testing and disease-focused clinical drug development. We hope these lessons will be instructive for the novice as well as the expert.

Charles L. Sawyers
Ingo K. Mellinghoff
Memorial Sloan-Kettering Cancer Center

Contents

Part I Fundamentals

Setting up a Kinase Discovery and Development Project 3
Gideon Bollag

Drug Efficacy Testing in Mice 19
William Y. Kim and Norman E. Sharpless

Part II Kinase Targets and Disease

Gastrointestinal Stromal Tumors 41
Cristina Antonescu

EGFR Mutant Lung Cancer 59
Yixuan Gong and William Pao

Targeting Oncogenic BRAF in Human Cancer 83
Christine A. Pratilas, Feng Xing and David B. Solit

Beyond BRAF in Melanoma 99
Adil Daud and Boris C. Bastian

JAK-Mutant Myeloproliferative Neoplasms 119
Ross L. Levine

Will Kinase Inhibitors Make it as Glioblastoma Drugs? 135
Ingo K. Mellinghoff, Nikolaus Schultz, Paul S. Mischel and
Timothy F. Cloughesy

Part III Perspectives

Predictive Genomic Biomarkers. 173
Rakesh Kumar and Rafael G. Amado

Epigenetic Biomarkers 189
Timothy A. Chan and Stephen B. Baylin

Adjuvant Trials of Targeted Agents: The Newest Battleground in the War on Cancer 217
Robert L. Cohen

Index 233

Contributors

Rafael G. Amado Oncology Research and Development, GlaxoSmithKline, Collegeville, PA 19426, USA, e-mail: rafael.g.amado@gsk.com

Cristina Antonescu Memorial Sloan-Kettering Cancer Center, New York, NY 10021, USA, e-mail: antonesc@mskcc.org

Boris C. Bastian Dermatopathology Section,Departments of Dermatology and Pathology, University of California San Francisco, San Francisco, CA 94143, USA, e-mail: Boris.Bastian@ucsf.edu

Stephen B. Baylin Johns Hopkins School of Medicine, Sidney Kimmel Comprehensive Cancer Center, Baltimore, MD 21231, USA

Gideon Bollag Plexxikon Inc, Berkeley, CA 94710, USA, e-mail: gbollag@plexxikon.com, e-mail: gbollag@plexxikon.com

Timothy A. Chan Memorial Sloan Kettering Cancer Center, New York, NY 10065, USA, e-mail: chant@mskcc.org

Timothy F. Cloughesy Department of Neurology, University of California Los Angeles, Los Angeles, CA, USA

Robert L. Cohen Genentech Inc, 1 DNA Way, South San Francisco, CA 94080, USA, e-mail: cohen.robert@gene.com

Adil Daud University of California, San Francisco, CA 94143, USA

Yixuan Gong Memorial Sloan-Kettering Cancer Center, New York, NY 10065, USA

William Y. Kim The Lineberger Comprehensive Cancer Center, The University of North Carolina, CB# 7295, Chapel Hill, NC 27599-7295, USA, e-mail: wykim@med.unc.edu

Rakesh Kumar Oncology Research and Development, GlaxoSmithKline, Collegeville, PA 19426, USA

Ross L. Levine Memorial Sloan Kettering Cancer Center, New York, NY 10021, USA, e-mail: leviner@mskcc.org

Ingo K. Mellinghoff Human Oncology and Pathogenesis Program, Department and Neurology, Memorial Sloan-Kettering Cancer Center, New York, NY, USA, e-mail: mellingi@mskcc.org

Paul S. Mischel Department of Pathology, University of California Los Angeles, Los Angeles, CA, USA

William Pao Vanderbilt University Medical Center, Nashville, TN 37232, USA, e-mail: william.pao@Vanderbilt.Edu

Christine A. Pratilas Memorial Sloan-Kettering Cancer Center, New York, NY 10065, USA

Nikolaus Schultz Computational Biology Program, Memorial Sloan-Kettering Cancer Center, New York, NY, USA

Norman E. Sharpless The Lineberger Comprehensive Cancer Center, The University of North Carolina, CB# 7295, Chapel Hill, NC 27599-7295, USA, e-mail: nes@med.unc.edu

David B. Solit Memorial Sloan-Kettering Cancer Center, New York, NY 10065, USA, e-mail: solitd@mskcc.org

Feng Xing Memorial Sloan-Kettering Cancer Center, New York, NY 10065, USA

Part I
Fundamentals

Setting up a Kinase Discovery and Development Project

Gideon Bollag

Abstract Discovery of novel kinase inhibitors has matured rapidly over the last decade. Paramount to the successful development of kinase inhibitors is appropriate selectivity for validated targets. Many different approaches have been applied over the years, with varied results. There are currently thirteen different small molecule protein kinase inhibitors on the marketplace. Interestingly, a majority of these compounds lack precise selectivity for specific targets. This will change in the coming years, as technology for achieving improved selectivity becomes more widely applied. This chapter will focus on some of the critical considerations in setting up a kinase discovery and development project, citing examples particularly targeting the Raf kinases.

Contents

1 Introduction 4
2 Choosing the Drug Target 4
3 Biochemical Assays for Screening and Counter Screening 7
4 Lead Optimization Using Crystallography and Cellular Assays 8
5 Improving Pharmaceutical Properties 11
6 Efficacy Studies in Mice 13
7 Toxicology and Safety Studies 14
8 Future Perspectives 14
References 15

G. Bollag (✉)
Plexxikon Inc, Berkeley, CA 94710, USA
e-mail: gbollag@plexxikon.com

Current Topics in Microbiology and Immunology (2012) 355: 3–18
DOI: 10.1007/82_2011_159
© Springer-Verlag Berlin Heidelberg 2011
Published Online: 2 August 2011

1 Introduction

It should first be noted that drug discovery and development, like other research, cannot be distilled to a simple recipe. Therefore, the considerations presented in this chapter provide just a few among infinite alternative approaches. Furthermore, the discussion is restricted to small molecule kinase inhibitors dosed orally on a daily schedule. In order to help illustrate the different steps in drug discovery, I will refer to the quite different approaches used to discover two quite different compounds: sorafenib (also known as BAY 43-9006 and marketed as Nexavar) and PLX4720. Both are Raf inhibitors, but sorafenib preferentially targets C-Raf (Wilhelm et al. 2004) while PLX4720 preferentially targets activated Raf enzymes typified by the oncogenic B-Raf^{V600E} kinase (Tsai et al. 2008). PLX4720 is a structurally related analog of vemurafenib (PLX4032), a compound currently undergoing clinical testing in patients with metastatic melanoma. It should be noted that sorafenib was identified and advanced into preclinical studies 3 years before the discovery of the *BRAF* oncogene (Davies et al. 2002; Lyons et al. 2001; Wilhelm et al. 2006). Therefore, the drug discovery effort culminating in sorafenib sought to identify C-Raf inhibitors, while the effort that produced PLX4720 and vemurafenib sought to identify inhibitors of B-Raf^{V600E} kinase activity.

2 Choosing the Drug Target

One of the key considerations to enable a successful drug discovery project involves choosing a good target. There are no standard principles for target selection, but validation in humans is probably the most compelling criterion. In that sense, improving on a currently marketed drug would be a lower risk project, especially if clear limitations exist to the predecessor. One example of this sort of approach involves the development of compounds that target resistant kinase mutations, such as dasatanib (Sprycel) and nilotinib (Tasigna), which show efficacy in cells that are resistant to imatinib (Gleevec) (Quintas-Cardama et al. 2007) (see "JAK-mutant Myeloproliferative Neoplasms"). Targets without pre-existing clinical validation pose a bigger risk, but may provide a more novel therapeutic entry. Sorafenib was discovered as an inhibitor of C-Raf because at the time (in the early 1990s) it was believed that C-Raf may be a critical effector of oncogenic *RAS* (Katz and McCormick 1997). Ideally, genetic data in humans would be available to predict the utility of a target. For example, 'driver' kinase mutations in cancers present intriguing target candidates (Greenman et al. 2007). One target that was identified in this way is the B-Raf kinase (Davies et al. 2002); indeed *BRAF* may be the most common protein kinase oncogene (Greenman et al. 2007). PLX4720 and vemurafenib were identified as oncogenic B-Raf^{V600E} kinase inhibitors because of the genetic validation of the *BRAF* oncogene. This will be discussed in more detail below, and focus on the biology is discussed in "Targeting Oncogenic Braf in Human Cancer" and "Beyond Braf in Melanoma" of this volume.

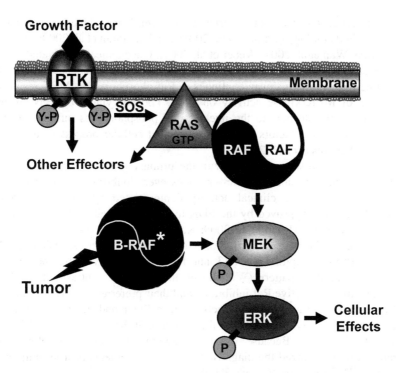

Fig. 1 Diagram of Raf signaling. Normal cellular signals often start with binding of growth factors to their receptors, releasing the receptor tyrosine kinase (RTK) activity to autophosphorylate and phosphorylate downstream substrates (such as SOS) that in turn effect exchange of GDP for GTP on the RAS proteins. Note that alternate effectors are also turned on by the RTK. GTP-bound RAS, which is anchored to the membrane, recruits RAF proteins and activates their ability to phosphorylate MEK on two serine residues. Mounting evidence suggests that growth factor stimulated RAF is dimeric or heterodimeric (comprised of one or more RAF isozymes: A-, B- or C-RAF). Alternatively, tumors bearing the *BRAF* oncogene, predominantly the V600E mutation, unleash constitutive MEK phosphorylation by the B-RAF* (oncogenic) kinase. Phosphorylated MEK in turn phosphorylates ERK, which translocates to the nucleus and phosphorylates a plethora of substrates that include transcription factors. The subsequent reprogramming of transcription results in an assortment of cellular effects that include proliferation, differentiation, survival, motility, or senescence

To illustrate the points made in this chapter, it is helpful to briefly consider some aspects of Raf biology. A diagram depicting the biology and biochemistry of the Ras/Raf pathway is shown in Fig. 1. Normally, the binding of a growth factor to its receptor will activate intrinsic tyrosine kinase activity, resulting in autophosphorylation as well as substrate phosphorylation. Multiple pathways are subsequently activated, including the Ras/Raf pathway. Upon growth factor stimulated exchange of GTP for GDP on the Ras GTPase, Ras-GTP recruits Raf to the membrane. 'Raf' could indicate any of the three Raf isoforms, A-Raf, B-Raf, and/or C-Raf, depending on the cell type, and the figure shows a Raf dimer since recent evidence suggests that dimerization or even hetero-dimerization of Raf is important in its biology (Garnett et al. 2005; Rajakulendran et al. 2009; Rushworth et al. 2006; Wan et al. 2004; Weber et al. 2001). Oncogenically activated B-Raf is independent of upstream signaling, and appears to signal independently of C-Raf. Signaling through the pathway continues as Raf phosphorylates MEK resulting in activation of MEK kinase activity on ERK. Phosphorylated ERK is an active kinase which translocates to the nucleus and phosphorylates nuclear substrates such as transcription factors which in turn effect cellular processes such as proliferation (Schubbert et al. 2007).

While sorafenib was identified with the primary purpose of inhibiting C-Raf kinase activity, it remains unclear—perhaps even doubtful—if C-Raf inhibition bears relevance to the clinical activity demonstrated by sorafenib. To date, sorafenib has been approved by the FDA to treat renal cell carcinoma and hepatocellular carcinoma (Kane et al. 2009; Kane et al. 2006). However, sorafenib is also a potent inhibitor of a selection of tyrosine kinase receptors, including VEGF receptors, PDGF receptors, Kit, Flt3, and Ret; clinical activity may be due to the composite inhibition pattern (Wilhelm et al. 2004). By contrast, PLX4720 and vemurafenib are selective Raf inhibitors, and their preferred affinity for oncogenic B-Raf translates to remarkable selectivity in cellular and in vivo models: antitumor activity is evident only if the tumor cell bears the $BRAF^{V600E}$ gene (Tsai et al. 2008). Because of this requirement, clinical development of vemurafenib has utilized the diagnostic selection of patients bearing tumors with the $BRAF^{V600E}$ mutation (Garber 2009).

Note that Raf is a serine-threonine kinase, while most of the targets of marketed kinase inhibitors (including the other targets of sorafenib) are tyrosine kinases. While it was originally believed that distinct chemo types would be required to inhibit these two different types of phosphorylation events, it is now clear that chemotypes can readily crossover to other branches of the kinase family tree.

Once a target is chosen, a series of assays must be developed, and a screening paradigm must be implemented. The assays include biochemical assays for the kinase target and selected counterscreening (non-target) kinases, cell-based assays for showing target inhibition in vitro and appropriate effects on cellular pharmacology, and in vivo models to measure pharmacodynamics and efficacy. Potency and selectivity metrics for each of the assays should be identified that allow filtering through the screening funnel. After proof-of-concept efficacy has been established, the metrics generally become more stringent and additional parameters monitoring pharmacokinetics and Absorption, Distribution, Metabolism, Excretion (ADME) are measured. Often, the bulk of the drug discovery effort focuses on the optimization of pharmacological properties. In other words, potent and selective compounds may be identified quite early in the project, but oral bioavailability is only achieved many months (or even years) later. These steps are described in detail below.

3 Biochemical Assays for Screening and Counter Screening

Determination of kinase inhibitory activity can be achieved in many ways. Thus, inhibition of substrate phosphorylation, inhibition of ATP hydrolysis, or direct binding of compound to kinase can all be employed in setting up a biochemical assay. Furthermore, each of these different biochemical events can be monitored using different technologies (Charter et al. 2006; Eglen and Reisine 2009; Hastie et al. 2006; Li et al. 2008; Riddle et al. 2006; Warner et al. 2004). There are advantages and disadvantages to each of these assays, and—importantly—it is likely that a different compound would emerge depending on the technology used to screen. Fundamentally, the preferred biochemical assay format would most closely mimic the native kinase as it participates in the oncogenic process. In the case of sorafenib, direct enzymatic activity was measured using radioactive ATP as substrate and readout (Wilhelm et al. 2004). For PLX4720, again the primary assay measured direct enzymatic activity, but in this case the readout used an antibody to phospho-MEK and measured the proximity between the labeled antibody and the epitope tag (in this case biotin) on MEK (Tsai et al. 2008; Warner et al. 2004).

Of great importance is the source of the kinase enzyme. Ideally, the enzyme should reflect the native form that exists within the target cell. Often, expression of kinase protein for enzymatic assays is carried out in baculovirus-infected insect cells. Baculoviruses are natural insect pathogens that readily infect cultured insect cells and can be engineered to express very high levels of recombinant protein (Summers 2006). Because insect cells are eukaryotic and possess many of the same post-translational modification systems as human cells, baculovirus-mediated expression is often preferred. Furthermore, co-expression of multiple enzymes is often desirable, and this can be relatively easily executed by co-infecting insect cells with multiple baculoviruses.

The source of Raf enzymes for both the sorafenib and the B-Raf^{V600E}-selective projects derived from baculovirus-based expression, and this was key to the progress. For the sorafenib project, C-Raf protein was purified from insect cells that had been co-infected with three different baculoviruses: epitope-tagged C-Raf, v-Src, and v-Ras (Macdonald et al. 1993). This triple-infection yielded highly active protein, as Ras-aided Src-dependent tyrosine phosphorylation causes significant stimulation of kinase activity. The target protein for guiding discovery of B-Raf^{V600E}-selective compounds was purified from insect cells that had been co-infected with a truncated form of B-Raf^{V600E} (encoding residues D448 through K723) and the co-chaperone CDC37 (Tsai et al. 2008). CDC37 recruits the insect cell-derived HSP90 protein to stabilize a ternary complex with B-Raf^{V600E}, resulting in optimal activity and stability (Wan et al. 2004).

One additional consideration in devising the biochemical assay involves the constitution of the reaction conditions. Typically, buffers, pH, and salts (including magnesium and/or manganese ions) are adjusted for optimal activity. Furthermore, the source and concentration of substrates—both ATP and phosphate-acceptor—can critically affect the outcome. For example, kinase-inactive MEK protein was used in both screens described above, so that Raf activity would not be complicated by MEK activation. Notably, in the discovery path leading to sorafenib, initial hits from the screens were tested at different ATP concentrations so that compounds with minimal dependence on ATP would be prioritized. This small but significant variation resulted in an initial scaffold that bound outside the adenine binding site of the Raf enzyme, in turn determining that the final lead—sorafenib—itself, would bind to a form of the enzyme that disfavors ATP-binding (Wan et al. 2004).

4 Lead Optimization Using Crystallography and Cellular Assays

The first three-dimensional structure of the kinase domain of B-Raf was published in 2004 (Wan et al. 2004). Interestingly, solution of this X-ray structure was dependent on the presence of sorafenib in the crystallization reaction, and the binding interactions of sorafenib were elegantly revealed. Sorafenib had been discovered without the guidance of co-crystallography, and the solved co-structure nicely rationalized the structure–activity relationships that had been empirically determined (Wilhelm et al. 2006).

By contrast, the discovery effort that led to the identification of PLX4720 and vemurafenib was heavily dependent on the use of X-ray co-crystallography. Indeed, over 100 co-crystal structures of analogs from several different series were solved in the process of optimizing compounds. To aid in this labor-intensive effort, an engineered form of the B-Raf kinase domain was devised by molecular biology and protein informatics techniques. This engineering effort resulted in a B-Raf kinase domain bearing 16 amino acid substitutions, with either valine or glutamate at residue 600 (Tsai et al. 2008).

The solved crystal structure reveals a dimeric architecture. Furthermore, the two protomers generally present in two different conformations, so the structure actually represents a heterodimer. Recent work suggests that this heterodimeric structure may reflect a true physiological entity (Rajakulendran et al. 2009). Indeed, while both subunits in the crystal structure are B-Raf protomers, the relevant form in the tumor may contain Raf homodimers, B-Raf/C-Raf heterodimers, or even other macromolecular complexes of the Rafs with scaffolding proteins or chaperones. Thus, analysis of the binding modes of different compounds in the crystal structure is highly informative. Comparison of the two subunits reveals many key differences, but perhaps most striking is the alternative conformation of a key loop, called the DFG (aspartate-phenylalanine-glycine) loop. When the phenylalanine of this loop points in toward the active site (DFG-in), ATP-binding is favored, and conversely the DFG-out conformation disfavors ATP-binding.

As shown in Fig. 2, sorafenib and PLX4720 each bind to alternate protomers of the heterodimer. In the sorafenib co-structure, electron density for the compound is

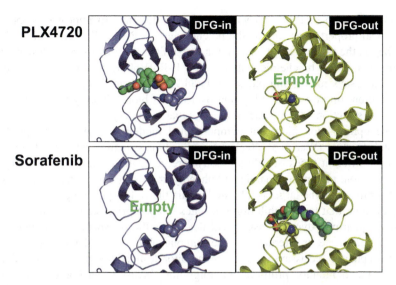

Fig. 2 Three-dimensional co-crystal structures of PLX4720 and sorafenib bound to B-Raf. B-Raf crystallizes to reveal a dimeric X-ray structure. One protomer of the dimer adopts a conformation that could accommodate ATP-binding as reflected by the conformation of the aspartate-phenylalanine-glycine loop (DFG, residues 594-596 of B-Raf). When the phenylalanine of this loop is directed toward the inside of the protein (DFG-in, loop shown using *blue* carbon spheres in the *left* protomers), ATP-binding is feasible. The DFG-out conformation (*right* protomer, loop shown using *yellow* carbon spheres) disallows ATP-binding. Electron density from co-crystals of PLX4720/B-Raf reveals binding exclusively to the DFG-in conformation (*top left*, PLX4720 shown with *green* carbon spheres); by contrast, sorafenib binds solely to the DFG-out conformation (*bottom right*, sorafenib shown with *green* carbon spheres). The DFG-in conformation is stabilized by the V600E mutation, explaining the preferred affinity of PLX4720 for the oncogenically activated form of *BRAF*

found almost exclusively in the DFG-out conformation. By contrast, PLX4720 binds to the DFG-in conformation. Therefore, PLX4720 behaves as a competitive inhibitor of ATP-binding, while sorafenib stabilizes a form of the kinase that disfavors ATP-binding. This property is perhaps fundamental in understanding differences between the two compounds. Since PLX4720 and vemurafenib bind preferably to the more activated form of the kinase—and because the V600E mutation stabilizes this same form—this class of compounds becomes oncogene-selective.

While most of this chapter has focused on sorafenib and PLX4720/vemurafenib to make points about kinase drug development, it should be noted that several additional Raf inhibitors have made it through drug development projects and into the clinic. These include RAF-265, XL281, and GSK2118436. At this time, only the molecular structure of RAF-265 has been disclosed. RAF-265 is derived from a drug discovery effort that used sorafenib as starting point and selected for improved potency on oncogenic B-Raf (Montagut and Settleman 2009; Ramurthy et al. 2008). Like sorafenib, RAF-265 also inhibits growth factor receptors such as VEGFR and PDGFR.

Optimization of RAF-265 was specifically designed to improve the physico-chemical properties as well as the potency against B-Raf (Ramurthy et al. 2008). To begin, the urea was tied back into a benzimidazole ring, then substituents were optimized using biochemical assays for B-RafV600E and C-Raf, as well as cellular assays monitoring phosphorylated ERK and proliferation in tumor cells. In addition, improved solubility and overall oral bioavailability were achieved in the final selection of RAF-265. It appears that X-ray crystallography was not part of the optimization plan, but computational modeling based on the published crystal structure (Wan et al. 2004) rationalized the structure–activity relationships.

Two different types of cellular assays are generally essential for guiding lead optimization: pharmacodynamic and phenotypic. A pharmacodynamic assay seeks to determine that the target is inhibited within the cell. A phenotypic assay seeks to demonstrate that target inhibition translates to appropriate cellular efficacy. Typically, a pharmacodynamic assay will determine the phosphorylation state of the target's substrate or alternatively the autophosphorylation of the target directly. Typical phenotypic assays for a kinase inhibitor destined for an oncology indication would be to monitor proliferation, migration, invasion, anchorage-independent growth, or downstream pathway readouts such as transcription or growth factor production. It is important that both sets of assays be configured in a relatively high-throughput format so that many compounds can be analyzed very quickly.

To measure cellular Raf inhibition it is most common to use antibodies to phosphorylated MEK or phosphorylated ERK. This can be done in a variety of compound-treatment formats: unstimulated cells, growth factor stimulated cells, or cells in which Raf proteins are conditionally or constitutively activated. All of these methods were used in the development of both sorafenib and PLX4720/vemurafenib. Although B-Raf mutations had not yet been discovered, a conditionally activated form of B-Raf was used to select compounds that inhibit B-Raf kinase activity using a high-throughput immunoprecipitation assay for MEK activity (Lyons et al. 2001). Note that B-Raf was used, since the activity of B-Raf is basally elevated by two asparates at residues 447 and 448, equivalent to the tyrosines 340 and 341 of C-Raf that require phosphorylation for full activity (Pritchard et al. 1995). The higher-intrinsic activity of B-Raf is likely also the reason that *BRAF* and not *CRAF* is the predominant oncogene. Sorafenib was also shown to inhibit phosphorylation of MEK and ERK in unstimulated and stimulated tumor cell lines (Lyons et al. 2001; Wilhelm et al. 2004).

After the discovery of the BRAF oncogene (Davies et al. 2002) and the determination that *BRAF* oncogene-dependent tumors are highly dependent on the RAF/MEK/ERK pathway (Solit et al. 2006), it became clear that projects focusing on the discovery of oncogenic B-Raf-selective compounds should rely primarily on cell lines that express oncogenic BRAF. Thus, the discovery program that identified PLX4720 and vemurafenib utilized B-Raf^{V600E} cell lines for both pharmacodynamic and proliferation assays. Indeed, PLX4720 displays remarkable selectivity for inhibition of MEK and ERK phosphorylation as well as proliferation in melanoma and colorectal cell lines harboring B-Raf^{V600E}, with essentially no inhibitory activity in cell lines lacking oncogenic *BRAF* (Tsai et al. 2008).

This contrasts sharply with the data for sorafenib; while MEK and ERK phosphorylation are inhibited in many cell lines, there is no selectivity for oncogenic B-Raf, and cellular proliferation is comparably inhibited in most cell lines tested (Wilhelm et al. 2004).

5 Improving Pharmaceutical Properties

An additional set of hurdles encountered during lead optimization address the pharmaceutical properties necessary to safely achieve appropriate systemic compound levels (Wan and Holmen 2009). Typical assays that are used to monitor 'ADME properties' include measures of solubility, ionization potential, lipophilicity, serum protein binding, permeability, and stability to metabolic enzymes from hepatocytes.

Information about absorption can be derived from dissolution, lipophilicity, and permeability. Solubility in the gut is necessary for proper uptake, and balanced lipophilicity aids uptake into cells. For kinase inhibitors generally, improving solubility by adjusting drug product formulation is often critical. For example, ionization potential at different pH values can suggest salt forms that can increase solubility. Cellular permeability, looking at transit in both directions (apical-to-basal and basal-to-apical), can be measured in surrogate gut cells such as Caco-2 cells. High permeability, similar in both directions is desirable. These same parameters also play into determining distribution. The avidity of the compound to serum proteins can markedly affect distribution through circulation and into target tissues. Furthermore, determining whether the compound of interest is a substrate for active transporters can give insight into mechanisms of excretion. Both sorafenib and PLX4720 are poorly soluble and lipophilic, and have very high-serum protein-binding affinity, but they also have good permeability.

In vitro measurements of metabolism deserve special attention, as metabolic stability is a key variable that can distinguish compounds (Bjornsson et al. 2003). Metabolism primarily involves liver enzymes that are grouped into phase I enzymes involved in enzymatic transformations such as oxidation, and phase II enzymes that include transferases that conjugate compounds or their oxidation products to aid their elimination. Obviously, the body has multiple mechanisms to eliminate xenobiotics, and the medicinal chemist attempts to steer around these obstacles. A first measure of metabolism can be determined by exposing compounds to intact hepatocytes or 'S9 fractions' (subcellular fractions enriched for metabolic enzymes). Typically, it is desirable to retain at least half of the parent compound following 30–60 min incubations.

Key phase I enzymes include the family of cytochrome P450 oxidases (CYPs). Determining inhibition of about seven different family members (e.g. isozymes 1A2, 3A4, 2B6, 2C8, 2C9, 2C19, and 2D6) is often monitored during lead optimization. Furthermore, identifying which CYP isozymes can transform the parent compound is generally followed in the clinic. Since many marketed drugs are

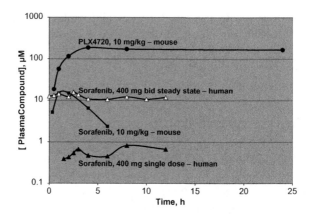

Fig. 3 Pharmacokinetic analysis of PLX4720 and sorafenib. Plasma levels of PLX4720 or sorafenib were measured at the indicated times following compound administration. For PLX4720, compound was administered as a 10 mg/ml suspension in 10% DMSO, and 1% carboxymethylcellulose to mice (Tsai et al. 2008). In mice, sorafenib was administered as a 10 mg/ml suspension in Cremophor EL/95% ethanol/water (12.5/12.5/75, v/v/v) (Sparidans et al. 2009). In humans, sorafenib tosylate was administered as a 200 mg tablet; results are shown for a 400 mg single dose, and for a 400 mg dose taken twice a day (the recommended clinical dose) after reaching steady state (Strumberg et al. 2005)

metabolized by different CYP isozymes, a potent inhibitor has the potential to alter the metabolism of concomitant medications. Sorafenib is a modest inhibitor of CYPs, CYP2B6, and CYP2C8, and is itself transformed by CYP3A4 (Kane et al. 2006, 2009). Nonetheless, clinical studies to evaluate the possibility of drug–drug interactions between sorafenib and concomitant medications have revealed minimal cause for concern (Lathia et al. 2006), perhaps because the high-serum-protein binding serves to shield the compound from the enzymes.

As mentioned above, optimizing for high-oral bioavailability is often the most time-intensive part of a kinase drug development project. Thus, compounds with appropriate potency and selectivity are often poorly active in animal efficacy models. Medicinal and computational chemistry tools help guide this process (Lipinski et al. 2001), but in the end much of the progress relies on empirical iterations.

Examination of the pharmacokinetics of sorafenib and PLX4720 may be instructive to illustrate the challenges of bioavailability. In Fig. 3 compound levels of sorafenib (Sparidans et al. 2009) and PLX4720 (Tsai et al. 2008) in mouse plasma are graphed as a function of time after administration of a 10 mg/kg dose by oral gavage. At this low dose, high-oral bioavailability in a simple formulation is relatively easy to achieve. While bioavailability is high for both compounds, the half-lives are quite different as sorafenib shows a 2–3 h half-life and PLX4720 shows a half-life exceeding 24 h. Note that the relatively modest exposure of sorafenib was nonetheless sufficient for efficacy in multiple models (Wilhelm et al. 2004). While it makes sense that constant high-plasma levels may be required for optimal efficacy, there is increasing interest in the idea that intermittent high exposures could be sufficient or even preferred (Shah et al. 2008). For such an approach, compounds with shorter half-lives would be preferable.

The exposure of sorafenib in human subjects is markedly higher, as also shown in Fig. 3 in large part due to its substantial half-life of 25–48 h (Kane et al. 2006; Strumberg et al. 2005). Note that a single dose of 400 mg leads to very modest plasma levels, while the current recommended human dose of 400 mg twice daily results in considerable accumulation of the drug in plasma (Strumberg et al. 2005). Since kinase inhibitors like sorafenib and PLX4720 are poorly soluble in water, formulation strategies to improve solubility in the gut are critical. In the case of sorafenib, this was aided by the conversion of the free-base to the crystalline tosylate salt, the current clinical dosage form (Kane et al. 2006).

6 Efficacy Studies in Mice

The standard animal model in oncology drug discovery projects remains the tumor xenograft; this is in spite of the substantial limitations of this model (Sharpless and Depinho 2006). Briefly, human tumor cells are implanted, typically subcutaneously, into immunocompromised mice and these cells grow into a mass that is easily measured. This means that human cells are growing in an environment that is quite different from their native micro-environment. Despite its many imperfections, the tumor xenograft model does help to monitor how effectively compounds can be delivered in vivo. Pharmacodynamic measurements similar to those used to monitor activity in cellular assays can be used to determine the effectiveness of target inhibition, and the rate of tumor growth determines the degree of efficacy.

Both sorafenib and PLX4720 show significant efficacy in xenograft studies. Using careful pharmacodynamic studies, it was shown that in certain models sorafenib-dependent tumor growth inhibition correlates with blockade of the RAF/MEK/ERK pathway, while in other models the inhibition correlates with inhibition of tumor angiogenesis (Wilhelm et al. 2004). By contrast, PLX4720 shows efficacy exclusively in xenografts bearing B-Raf^{V600E} tumors, and the corresponding efficacy correlates with inhibition of the target pathway (Tsai et al. 2008).

During the in vivo efficacy studies, important information about tolerability of the compound can be gleaned from monitoring body weight and mortality. Often, precursor studies determine the maximal tolerated dose (MTD), and efficacy is then determined as a function of dose up to the MTD. A therapeutic index can be estimated by comparing the minimal efficacious dose to the MTD. Indeed, during the drug development process sorafenib was selected from among a series of analogs as having the highest-therapeutic index (Wilhelm et al. 2006).

As described in the next chapter, genetically engineered mouse models are being developed that promise to yield much more predictive efficacy data, but those models are not yet in widespread use during early drug discovery efforts.

7 Toxicology and Safety Studies

Once a kinase inhibitor has cleared all the hurdles discussed above, a series of toxicology and safety pharmacology studies are performed to assess the suitability to advance into clinical studies (Baldrick 2008a, b). Since kinase inhibitors are generally designed to be dosed continuously, multiple dose studies are the norm. Typically, these studies include 28-day general toxicology studies in one rodent species (often rat) and one non-rodent species (often dog), along with studies to determine respiratory safety (often in dogs), cardiovascular safety (often in dogs), and central nervous system safety (often in rats). Since small molecules can affect ion channels as an off-target activity, cardiovascular safety studies are often preceded by in vitro electrophysiology tests of the hERG (human ether-a-go-go) potassium channel. Indeed, this test is sometimes conducted during the lead optimization phase of the project, before selecting compounds for the extensive studies required to submit an IND (Investigational New Drug) application to initiate human clinical studies. Genetic toxicology studies including carcinogenicity testing in vitro (often using the Ames test) and in vivo (often using a micronucleus test in mice) are also performed.

Note that key to conducting these studies is the availability of significant quantities of compound, typically on the kilogram scale. Compounds can be synthesized using carefully controlled standard operating procedures that conform to good manufacturing practices (GMP), and this is required by the FDA for the human studies but not necessarily for IND-enabling studies. At a minimum, the compound purity must be quite high, and the synthetic route must be monitored with detailed analyses using validated protocols at each step. Often, this can take 3–6 months, or more depending on the difficulty of compound synthesis.

Once high-quality compound is available, the toxicology and the safety pharmacology studies must be carried out using good laboratory practices (GLP), again using carefully controlled standard operating procedures. Often, preliminary dose range-finding studies are conducted ahead of the GLP-toxicology studies to help select the most informative doses. While the in-life duration of these studies is carefully defined, much of the time to complete these studies involves preparing tissues and carefully analyzing each critical organ from each animal by histopathology. Often, the GLP-toxicology and safety pharmacology studies can take 6–9 months from first dose to produce the final reports.

8 Future Perspectives

Cancer often causes severe dysregulation of intracellular signaling pathways. Indeed, the more advanced a malignancy, the more mutations and pathways become involved. Thus, it makes good sense to target each of these many signaling pathways with small molecule inhibitors. Since kinases play key roles in essentially all of these processes–and since they are druggable—many different kinases have become targets of pharmaceutical drug discovery projects.

However, the central signaling role of kinases is not limited to tumor cells. Indeed, these same kinases are often crucial to the function of many cells in many different tissues. Therefore, the therapeutic index of a kinase inhibitor is reduced to a very complex balance: the kinase activity must be more essential for the tumor than for all the non-diseased organs. Complicating this analysis further, tumor cells and normal cells alike have myriad mechanisms to compensate for the blockade of specific pathways. The therapeutic index would increase if these compensatory pathways would be more robust in non-diseased tissues. However, the inherent plasticity of cancer cells could make them more adept at bypassing the inhibitor. These considerations will differ markedly from one kinase target to another.

Two alternative drug discovery strategies can lead to improved efficacy and safety: inhibiting one key target with exquisite specificity, or targeting a selection of kinases that collaborate to support tumor growth. The inhibitors discussed in this chapter provide examples of both strategies, each with distinct advantages. The future will likely see an increasing number of highly selective kinase inhibitors, which can then be rationally combined to personalize co-targeting to each individual cancer.

It should be mentioned that co-targeting kinases in the context of synergistic inactivation of two or more pathways at once most likely requires the compound(s) to act in the same cell at the same time. This introduces a new complexity when combining two agents with different pharmacokinetics and tissue distribution. Therefore, it can be envisioned that co-targeting these kinases with a single molecule may afford great advantages.

Since tumor cells possess multiple adaptive mechanisms, resistance to a single kinase inhibitor is very likely to occur. Therefore, additional compounds, targeting the same kinase or a compensatory pathway will be highly desired in order to achieve durable control and preferably eradication of tumors.

The tools to discover and develop novel kinase inhibitors are getting ever better. Hence, there is reason for great optimism for the future of kinase-directed therapy for cancer.

References

Baldrick P (2008a) Safety evaluation to support first-in-man investigations I: kinetic and safety pharmacology studies. Regul Toxicol Pharmacol 51:230–236

Baldrick P (2008b) Safety evaluation to support first-in-man investigations II: toxicology studies. Regul Toxicol Pharmacol 51:237–243

Bjornsson TD, Callaghan JT, Einolf HJ, Fischer V, Gan L, Grimm S, Kao J, King SP, Miwa G, Ni L, Kumar G, McLeod J, Obach RS, Roberts S, Roe A, Shah A, Snikeris F, Sullivan JT, Tweedie D, Vega JM, Walsh J, Wrighton SA (2003) The conduct of in vitro and in vivo drug–drug interaction studies: a pharmaceutical research and manufacturers of america (PhRMA) perspective. Drug Metab Dispos 31:815–832

Charter NW, Kauffman L, Singh R, Eglen RM (2006) A generic, homogenous method for measuring kinase and inhibitor activity via adenosine 5'-diphosphate accumulation. J Biomol Screen 11:390–399

Davies H, Bignell GR, Cox C, Stephens P, Edkins S, Clegg S, Teague J, Woffendin H, Garnett MJ, Bottomley W, Davis N, Dicks E, Ewing R, Floyd Y, Gray K, Hall S, Hawes R, Hughes J, Kosmidou V, Menzies A, Mould C, Parker A, Stevens C, Watt S, Hooper S, Wilson R, Jayatilake H, Gusterson BA, Cooper C, Shipley J, Hargrave D, Pritchard-Jones K, Maitland N, Chenevix-Trench G, Riggins GJ, Bigner DD, Palmieri G, Cossu A, Flanagan A, Nicholson A, Ho JW, Leung SY, Yuen ST, Weber BL, Seigler HF, Darrow TL, Paterson H, Marais R, Marshall CJ, Wooster R, Stratton MR, Futreal PA (2002) Mutations of the BRAF gene in human cancer. Nature 417:949–954

Eglen RM, Reisine T (2009) The current status of drug discovery against the human kinome. Assay Drug Dev Technol 7:22–43

Garber K (2009) Trial offers early test case for personalized medicine. J Natl Cancer Inst 101:136–138

Garnett MJ, Rana S, Paterson H, Barford D, Marais R (2005) Wild-type and mutant B-RAF activate C-RAF through distinct mechanisms involving heterodimerization. Mol Cell 20:963–969

Greenman C, Stephens P, Smith R, Dalgliesh GL, Hunter C, Bignell G, Davies H, Teague J, Butler A, Stevens C, Edkins S, O'Meara S, Vastrik I, Schmidt EE, Avis T, Barthorpe S, Bhamra G, Buck G, Choudhury B, Clements J, Cole J, Dicks E, Forbes S, Gray K, Halliday K, Harrison R, Hills K, Hinton J, Jenkinson A, Jones D, Menzies A, Mironenko T, Perry J, Raine K, Richardson D, Shepherd R, Small A, Tofts C, Varian J, Webb T, West S, Widaa S, Yates A, Cahill DP, Louis DN, Goldstraw P, Nicholson AG, Brasseur F, Looijenga L, Weber BL, Chiew YE, DeFazio A, Greaves MF, Green AR, Campbell P, Birney E, Easton DF, Chenevix-Trench G, Tan MH, Khoo SK, Teh BT, Yuen ST, Leung SY, Wooster R, Futreal PA, Stratton MR (2007) Patterns of somatic mutation in human cancer genomes. Nature 446:153–158

Hastie CJ, McLauchlan HJ, Cohen P (2006) Assay of protein kinases using radiolabeled ATP: a protocol. Nat Protoc 1:968–971

Kane RC, Farrell AT, Saber H, Tang S, Williams G, Jee JM, Liang C, Booth B, Chidambaram N, Morse D, Sridhara R, Garvey P, Justice R, Pazdur R (2006) Sorafenib for the treatment of advanced renal cell carcinoma. Clin Cancer Res 12:7271–7278

Kane RC, Farrell AT, Madabushi R, Booth B, Chattopadhyay S, Sridhara R, Justice R, Pazdur R (2009) Sorafenib for the treatment of unresectable hepatocellular carcinoma. Oncologist 14:95–100

Katz ME, McCormick F (1997) Signal transduction from multiple Ras effectors. Curr Opin Genet Dev 7:75–79

Lathia C, Lettieri J, Cihon F, Gallentine M, Radtke M, Sundaresan P (2006) Lack of effect of ketoconazole-mediated CYP3A inhibition on sorafenib clinical pharmacokinetics. Cancer Chemother Pharmacol 57:685–692

Li Y, Xie W, Fang G (2008) Fluorescence detection techniques for protein kinase assay. Anal Bioanal Chem 390:2049–2057

Lipinski CA, Lombardo F, Dominy BW, Feeney PJ (2001) Experimental and computational approaches to estimate solubility and permeability in drug discovery and development settings. Adv Drug Deliv Rev 46:3–26

Lyons JF, Wilhelm S, Hibner B, Bollag G (2001) Discovery of a novel Raf kinase inhibitor. Endocr Relat Cancer 8:219–225

Macdonald SG, Crews CM, Wu L, Driller J, Clark R, Erikson RL, McCormick F (1993) Reconstitution of the Raf-1-MEK-ERK signal transduction pathway in vitro. Mol Cell Biol 13:6615–6620

Montagut C, Settleman J (2009) Targeting the RAF-MEK-ERK pathway in cancer therapy. Cancer Lett 283:125–134

Pritchard CA, Samuels ML, Bosch E, McMahon M (1995) Conditionally oncogenic forms of the A-Raf and B-Raf protein kinases display different biological and biochemical properties in NIH 3T3 cells. Mol Cell Biol 15:6430–6442

Quintas-Cardama A, Kantarjian H, Cortes J (2007) Flying under the radar: the new wave of BCR-ABL inhibitors. Nat Rev Drug Discov 6:834–848

Rajakulendran T, Sahmi M, Lefrancois M, Sicheri F, Therrien M (2009) A dimerization-dependent mechanism drives RAF catalytic activation. Nature 461:542–545

Ramurthy S, Subramanian S, Aikawa M, Amiri P, Costales A, Dove J, Fong S, Jansen JM, Levine B, Ma S, McBride CM, Michaelian J, Pick T, Poon DJ, Girish S, Shafer CM, Stuart D, Sung L, Renhowe PA (2008) Design and synthesis of orally bioavailable benzimidazoles as Raf kinase inhibitors. J Med Chem 51:7049–7052

Riddle SM, Vedvik KL, Hanson GT, Vogel KW (2006) Time-resolved fluorescence resonance energy transfer kinase assays using physiological protein substrates: applications of terbium-fluorescein and terbium-green fluorescent protein fluorescence resonance energy transfer pairs. Anal Biochem 356:108–116

Rushworth LK, Hindley AD, O'Neill E, Kolch W (2006) Regulation and role of Raf-1/B-Raf heterodimerization. Mol Cell Biol 26:2262–2272

Schubbert S, Shannon K, Bollag G (2007) Hyperactive Ras in developmental disorders and cancer. Nat Rev Cancer 7:295–308

Shah NP, Kasap C, Weier C, Balbas M, Nicoll JM, Bleickardt E, Nicaise C, Sawyers CL (2008) Transient potent BCR-ABL inhibition is sufficient to commit chronic myeloid leukemia cells irreversibly to apoptosis. Cancer Cell 14:485–493

Sharpless NE, Depinho RA (2006) The mighty mouse: genetically engineered mouse models in cancer drug development. Nat Rev Drug Discov 5:741–754

Solit DB, Garraway LA, Pratilas CA, Sawai A, Getz G, Basso A, Ye Q, Lobo JM, She Y, Osman I, Golub TR, Sebolt-Leopold J, Sellers WR, Rosen N (2006) BRAF mutation predicts sensitivity to MEK inhibition. Nature 439:358–362

Sparidans RW, Vlaming ML, Lagas JS, Schinkel AH, Schellens JH, Beijnen JH (2009) Liquid chromatography-tandem mass spectrometric assay for sorafenib and sorafenib-glucuronide in mouse plasma and liver homogenate and identification of the glucuronide metabolite. J Chromatogr B Analyt Technol Biomed Life Sci 877:269–276

Strumberg D, Richly H, Hilger RA, Schleucher N, Korfee S, Tewes M, Faghih M, Brendel E, Voliotis D, Haase CG, Schwartz B, Awada A, Voigtmann R, Scheulen ME, Seeber S (2005) Phase I clinical and pharmacokinetic study of the novel Raf kinase and vascular endothelial growth factor receptor inhibitor BAY 43–9006 in patients with advanced refractory solid tumors. J Clin Oncol 23:965–972

Summers MD (2006) Milestones leading to the genetic engineering of baculoviruses as expression vector systems and viral pesticides. Adv Virus Res 68:3–73

Tsai J, Lee JT, Wang W, Zhang J, Cho H, Mamo S, Bremer R, Gillette S, Kong J, Haass NK, Sproesser K, Li L, Smalley KS, Fong D, Zhu YL, Marimuthu A, Nguyen H, Lam B, Liu J, Cheung I, Rice J, Suzuki Y, Luu C, Settachatgul C, Shellooe R, Cantwell J, Kim SH, Schlessinger J, Zhang KY, West BL, Powell B, Habets G, Zhang C, Ibrahim PN, Hirth P, Artis DR, Herlyn M, Bollag G (2008) Discovery of a selective inhibitor of oncogenic B-Raf kinase with potent antimelanoma activity. Proc Natl Acad Sci USA 105:3041–3046

Wan H, Holmen AG (2009) High throughput screening of physicochemical properties and in vitro ADME profiling in drug discovery. Comb Chem High Throughput Screen 12:315–329

Wan PT, Garnett MJ, Roe SM, Lee S, Niculescu-Duvaz D, Good VM, Jones CM, Marshall CJ, Springer CJ, Barford D, Marais R (2004) Mechanism of activation of the RAF-ERK signaling pathway by oncogenic mutations of B-RAF. Cell 116:855–867

Warner G, Illy C, Pedro L, Roby P, Bosse R (2004) AlphaScreen kinase HTS platforms. Curr Med Chem 11:721–730

Weber CK, Slupsky JR, Kalmes HA, Rapp UR (2001) Active Ras induces heterodimerization of cRaf and BRaf. Cancer Res 61:3595–3598

Wilhelm SM, Carter C, Tang L, Wilkie D, McNabola A, Rong H, Chen C, Zhang X, Vincent P, McHugh M, Cao Y, Shujath J, Gawlak S, Eveleigh D, Rowley B, Liu L, Adnane L, Lynch M, Auclair D, Taylor I, Gedrich R, Voznesensky A, Riedl B, Post LE, Bollag G, Trail PA (2004) BAY 43–9006 exhibits broad spectrum oral antitumor activity and targets the RAF/MEK/ ERK pathway and receptor tyrosine kinases involved in tumor progression and angiogenesis. Cancer Res 64:7099–7109

Wilhelm S, Carter C, Lynch M, Lowinger T, Dumas J, Smith RA, Schwartz B, Simantov R, Kelley S (2006) Discovery and development of sorafenib: a multikinase inhibitor for treating cancer. Nat Rev Drug Discov 5:835–844

Drug Efficacy Testing in Mice

William Y. Kim and Norman E. Sharpless

Abstract The traditional path of drug development passes from in vitro screening and response assessment to validation of drug efficacy in cell line xenografts. While xenografts have their merits, historically, more often than not, they have not served as an accurate predictor of drug efficacy in humans. The refinement and increased availability of genetically engineered mouse models (GEMMs) of cancer has made GEMMs an attractive avenue for the preclinical testing of therapeutic agents. The histopathologic and genetic resemblance of GEMMs to human cancer are an important measure to evaluate their suitability for pre-clinical studies and a number of studies using kinase inhibitors have now been performed in GEMMs. We have highlighted several of the salient advantages and challenges associated with GEMM studies. Well-characterized GEM models of human cancer should aide in the prioritization of both established and novel therapeutics.

Keywords Genetically engineered mouse models · Drug development · Oncomouse · Attrition · Preclinical models · Kinase inhibitor

---

W. Y. Kim · N. E. Sharpless (✉)
The Lineberger Comprehensive Cancer Center,
The University of North Carolina,
CB# 7295, Chapel Hill,
NC 27599-7295, USA
e-mail: nes@med.unc.edu

W. Y. Kim
e-mail: wykim@med.unc.edu

Current Topics in Microbiology and Immunology (2012) 355: 19–38
DOI: 10.1007/82_2011_160
© Springer-Verlag Berlin Heidelberg 2011
Published Online: 7 August 2011

Contents

1 Introduction 20
2 Classical Preclinical Testing in Xenograft Models 20
3 Harnessing Genetically Engineered Murine Models for Drug Efficacy Testing 22
4 Comparing the Track Record of Xenograft and GEM Models 24
5 Refining Kinase Inhibitor Therapy in GEMMs 26
6 "Credentialing" GEMMs as Genetically Faithful Models 28
7 Logistic Considerations in Developing a "Mouse Clinic" 31
8 Future Perspectives 32
References 33

1 Introduction

Although a cancer researcher might become optimistic in these heady days of rationally targeted anti-cancer therapies, three trends remain a cause for concern (reviewed in Kola and Landis 2004; Peterson and Houghton 2004; Sharpless and Depinho 2006). First, the number of registered pharmaceutical new chemical entities (NCEs) is not growing rapidly, but instead is leveling off or even declining over the last decade. As registration of an NCE is the first real stage of drug development, this observation suggests that novel anti-cancer drugs are still very difficult and expensive to produce. This fact reflects the second concerning trend: the failure rate of oncologic drugs that enter human testing is still very high, perhaps greater than 95%. This observation in turn reflects the third worrisome trend: by a variety of metrics, most novel anti-cancer therapies fail in human testing because of the lack of efficacy. For example, the attrition rate of compounds at the Phase II stage may be over 70%, and the response rate of phase I trials remains low compared to the incidence of toxicity in such studies (Decoster et al. 1990; Roberts et al. 2004). In aggregate, these trends indicate that oncologic drugs remain very hard to develop, largely because the rare successes have to subsidize the testing of ineffective compounds in humans, and that these problems will be with us for much time. Clearly, one reason for the high attrition rate of anti-cancer compounds is the lack of predictive preclinical models for drug efficacy testing prior to human use. Several approaches have been suggested to prioritize would-be therapeutics, and in this chapter, we will focus on efforts to improve drug efficacy testing in mice using human cancer xenografts and genetically engineered murine models (GEMMs).

2 Classical Preclinical Testing in Xenograft Models

As described in the previous chapter, drug development usually follows a defined course. Potential cancer therapies are discovered through in vitro screens or more recently by targeted drug design. Such compounds are then tested for activity in vitro using a variety of cancer cell lines, and if sufficiently promising, then tested

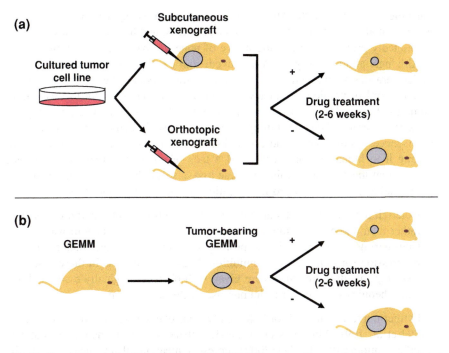

Fig. 1 Generation of mice bearing xenograft or GEMM tumors. **a** Xenograft tumors are generated by bolus injections of human cell lines derived from cell cultures. The cells are amplified to sufficient numbers in vitro and then injected subcutaneously, (or far more rarely orthotopically) and allowed to develop tumors. Drug treatment can be initiated prior to tumor formation or in the setting of a measurable tumor. Subcutaneous xenograft tumor growth is typically assessed by bidimensional tumor measurements using calipers. **b** GEMM tumors occur spontaneously or after conditional oncogene activation or tumor suppressor gene inactivation. Depending on the GEM model and site of tumor development, mice are screened for tumor formation by palpation (e.g. melanoma or breast GEMMs) or radiographically (e.g. MRI or microCT for lung tumors). Drug treatment is usually initiated after tumor formation with the intent of shrinking a measurable tumor

in vivo. In vivo testing typically consists of several parts including an analysis of pharmacology, pharmacodynamics and toxicology. For several decades, in vivo efficacy testing has largely been done in one way: through the use of xenograft models. In these models, cell lines are grown, generally subcutaneously, in immunodeficient (e.g. *SCID*) mice. Typically, 10^6 malignant cells are injected subcutaneously into the flank, a brief wait occurs, and then therapy with the potential anti-neoplastic is begun at the first sign of tumor growth, or even before a tumor appears. An agent is usually considered "active" in these assays if it slows tumor development (i.e. decreases progression) (Fig. 1a).

Xenograft models offer a number of advantages, including their ease of use, public availability, and relatively modest infrastructural needs (e.g. long-term animal housing, imaging, etc). Assuredly, many important studies leading to changes in clinical care have been done using representative samples of human cancers grown as xenografts (see for example Peterson and Houghton 2004;

Sausville and Burger 2006). Moreover, in some instances, e.g. certain rare cancers, no other small animal model for such cancers exists, and their use in these cases is undoubtedly preferable to the alternative of none in vivo efficacy testing.

Although almost every FDA-approved, anti-cancer agent developed in the modern era has shown activity in some xenograft system, these systems have a mixed record of predicting efficacy in humans (Johnson et al. 2001; Voskoglou-Nomikos et al. 2003). It is clear that many ineffective compounds are passing the xenograft filter and then later failing, at great expense, in human phase II trials. Of equal concern, however, is the possibility that potentially active agents are not making it to human testing because of a lack of efficacy in these systems. We contend that the predictive value of these assays would be sharply improved with three relatively straightforward modifications to standard xenograft testing:

1. Determining a compound's activity in several cell lines of a given tumor type rather than one or two examples, usually chosen in a non-random way.
2. Considering tumor regression or prolonged stabilization, rather than mere non-progression (or tumor growth inhibition "TGI"), as success in these assays.
3. Assuring that drug treatments are given with pharmacologically realistic doses and schedules with regard to human use of the same agent.

Furthermore, the use of orthotopically transplanted xenograft tumors (e.g. Kerbel et al. 1991; Mitsiades et al. 2003; Rofstad 1994) or uncultured, patient-specific 'tumorgrafts' (Garber 2009) represent meaningful advances over traditional xenografting of established human cancer cell lines.

Although these changes seem straightforward, the current literature suggests that much academic xenograft testing fails to meet even these modest standards. When carefully done, drug efficacy testing in xenograft models has clear merit and will continue to play an important role for years to come. However, the limited predictive power of these models suggests that drug development decisions should not be based solely on drug performance in these models and instead be complemented by drug efficacy testing in other disease-relevant animal models. In the following section, we will suggest that GEMMs could fill this important void in the current drug development paradigm.

3 Harnessing Genetically Engineered Murine Models for Drug Efficacy Testing

The design and production of GEMMs have been described at length elsewhere (Frese and Tuveson 2007; Jonkers and Berns 2002). In brief, transgenic and knockout alleles are combined to produce strains of mice that are predisposed to autochthonous tumors. Generally, such models rely on the use of transgenic alleles directing the expression of oncogenic "driver" proteins in the tissue of interest. For example, expression of mutant K-Ras can be induced in the adult murine pancreas or lung to cause pancreatic adenocarcinomas (Bardeesy et al. 2006;

Table 1 Comparison of xenograft models and genetically engineered mouse models (GEMMS)

	Xenograft	GEMM
Functional immune system	No	Yes
Intact DNA repair mechanisms	No	Yes
Stochastic genetic events during tumor progression	No	Yes
Faithful tumor stromal interactions	No	Yes
Variability of tumor penetrance	No	Yes
Tumor latency	Short	Long
Ease of tumor response assessment	Easy	Difficult (imaging)
Infrastructure needed	Small	Large
Differences in human and mouse genomes	N/A	Yes

Hingorani et al. 2005) or non-small cell lung cancer (Johnson et al. 2001; Meuwissen et al. 2001) respectively. To shorten tumor latency, such systems often also include deletion of relevant tumor suppressor genes (e.g. $p16^{Ink4a}$, $p53$, $Pten$) in the same tissues (see for example Ji et al. 2007). Importantly, the use of modern CRE-Lox and doxycycline-inducible technologies allows for the somatic and tissue-specific induction of these genetic lesions, thereby providing an opportunity to direct almost any combination of oncogene and tumor suppressor mutations to the presumed cell of origin of the cancer type under investigation.

Compared to their widespread use in the study of human cancer biology, the use of GEMMs for the development of novel anti-cancer therapeutics, such as kinase inhibitors, is far less established. In this latter scenario, genetically predisposed animals are observed for tumor development, and therapy is usually begun after advanced tumors develop. An agent is considered 'active' if it causes significant tumor regression, or at the very least, prolonged stable disease (Fig. 1b). Tumors arising in GEMMs can also be used to derive a large number of genetically related cell lines which can help to better define the activity of agents that have already shown at least some activity in xenograft assays. For example, inhibitors of poly-ADP-Ribosylase (PARP) demonstrated considerable activity in combination with cytotoxics in a variety of xenograft assays (see e.g. Donawho et al. 2007), but GEMM studies from Jonkers and colleagues were instrumental in convincingly defining the potent single-agent activity of these compounds specifically in BRCA1/2-deficient, as opposed to proficient, cancers (Evers et al. 2008; Rottenberg et al. 2008). This specific efficacy of PARP inhibitors in BRCA1/2-deficient tumors, which has been convincingly confirmed in human patients (Fong et al. 2009), was not evident solely from the xenograft testing of these compounds.

GEMMs differ from xenografts in several important aspects that may be very relevant for drug efficacy testing (Table 1). First, GEMM tumors occur in animals with an intact immune system and unperturbed DNA repair mechanisms. Second, as GEMMs rely on the accumulation of stochastic genetic events for tumor progression, these models follow a stepwise progression and recapitulation of the tumor heterogeneity of human solid tumors. Third, as cancers occur autochthonously in these models, GEMMs afford a more faithful recapitulation of tumor–stroma interactions found in human cancer. Which of these differences between

GEMMs and xenografts is most relevant for the evaluation of any particular new agent is currently unclear, but a number of recent observations clearly point toward an important role of the tumor microenvironment in the initiation, progression and maintenance of tumors. Chronic inflammation, for example, is a risk factor for certain cancers, and once tumors have formed, the interaction between neoplastic cells with various components of the surrounding microenvironment including inflammatory cells, vascular and lymphatic networks, and the extracellular matrix can either promote or inhibit tumor growth (reviewed in Mueller and Fusenig 2004). It is not hard to see why xenograft models might not accurately recapitulate this aspect of cancer biology: fully transformed cells—often selected for their propensity to grow as rapidly as possible after transplantation—are injected as a bolus into a stroma that is deranged and disorganized by the ectopic transplant of a large number of foreign cells. In contrast, the neoplastic cells of GEM tumors form in a stepwise manner similar to in situ human tumors in the setting of an appropriately responsive tumor microenvironment. Such differences between tumor development in the xenograft versus autochthonous setting have been suggested to explain the marked differences observed in the role of hypoxia and Id proteins in tumor angiogenesis in the two settings (Ruzinova et al. 2003; Sikder et al. 2003). Likewise, recent work from Pollard and colleagues has suggested differences in the gene expression of tumor-associated macrophages (TAMs) in xenograft versus GEM models (Ojalvo et al. 2009). We expect these differences to be of significance as TAMs have been suggested to augment tumor angiogenesis, invasion and matrix remodeling; modulate drug delivery, and modulate a host anti-tumor immune response. Given these multiple differences in the reaction of diverse stromal elements, the ability to more faithfully model the stroma–tumor interaction appears to be a particular strength of GEMMs compared to xenograft assays.

4 Comparing the Track Record of Xenograft and GEM Models

While many arguments can be made for and against the utility of xenografts versus GEMMs for in vivo drug efficacy testing, the most relevant question ultimately is which model better predicts the clinical efficacy of anti-cancer therapeutics in humans. There currently is not a large body of drug development experience using both xenograft and GEMM approaches to allow a rigorous comparison between both approaches. However, a few examples do exist.

One of the oldest examples involves the use of the peroxisome proliferator-activated receptor γ (PPARγ) agonists for the treatment of colorectal cancer. Previous work had shown that PPARγ agonists could promote the differentiation and cell cycle arrest of primary cells derived from human liposarcomas (Demetri et al. 1999). Because PPARγ was noted to be highly expressed in colonic epithelium as well as the wealth of epidemiologic data connecting dietary fat intake with colorectal cancer risk, two separate groups evaluated the effect of PPARγ

agonists on colorectal cancer, using different systems, publishing starkly contrasting results. PPARγ agonist treatment of subcutaneous xenografts derived from established colorectal cancer cell lines appeared to slow their growth rate and promote their differentiation (Sarraf et al. 1998). In contrast, PPARγ agonist treatment of mice genetically engineered to develop intestinal polyps secondary to germ line deletion of a single copy of the *Apc* gene (Min mice) resulted in tumorigenic acceleration, causing an increased number of colonic polyps (Saez et al. 1998). The xenograft studies led to a single institution, phase II clinical trial evaluating the effectiveness of an FDA-approved PPARγ agonists, troglitazone, in patients with metastatic colorectal cancer. Of the 25 patients enrolled, there were no objective responses noted and the median progression-free survival (PFS) was a mere 1.6 months (Kulke et al. 2002), which compares poorly even to historical PFS noted with best supportive care.

A second example of discrepant results of drug efficacy testing between xenografts and GEMMs comes from the experience of testing anti-angiogenic agents such as endostatin and angiostatin. These agents demonstrated impressive activity in xenograft studies (O'Reilly et al. 1997; O'Reilly et al. 1996; O'Reilly et al. 1994) compared to a much more limited activity in GEMMs (Bergers et al. 1999). These discrepancies may be explained by the described differences in angiogenesis between xenograft and autochthonous tumor models (reviewed in Alani et al. 2004); but in any event, the results in GEMMs were more consistent with the limited anti-tumor activity of these agents in clinical trials in humans.

A more recent example is the comparison of gemcitabine efficacy in autochthonous versus transplanted pancreatic tumors (Olive et al. 2009). Pancreatic cancer GEMMs, like human pancreatic cancers, are generally resistant to gemcitabine chemotherapy (objective response rates of 5–10%). This chemoresistance however, does not appear to be cell-autonomous as transplantation of cell lines derived from pancreatic cancer GEMMs into a syngeneic flank increases the sensitivity of these tumors to gemcitabine to that of cultured human cell line xenografts. Indeed, the relative chemoresistance of autochthonous tumors appears to be a reflection of suboptimal drug delivery into fibrotic and poorly vascularized pancreatic GEM tumors, a characteristic that accurately reflects its human counterpart and speaks to the importance of the interactions between tumor cells and stroma discussed in our previous section. Our group has measured intra tumoral drug levels in GEMM versus xenograft models, and seen large and unanticipated differences in drug exposure between the two types of systems (NES, WYK and William Zamboni, submitted). Ongoing efforts will attempt to further determine the physiologic bases for these differences between GEMMs and xenografts with regard to intra-tumor drug delivery.

To more systematically address the utility of GEMMs for drug development, Johnson and colleagues recently examined this issue in *KRas* mutant lung and pancreatic cancers (Singh et al. 2010), examining the effects of combining cytotoxic chemotherapy with agents inhibiting epidermal growth factor receptor (EGFR) and vascular endothalial growth factor receptor (VEGFR) in highly faithful GEMMs. Comparison of data from large phase III randomized trials in humans with the results seen in lung and pancreatic cancer GEMMs treated similarly suggests many similarities. For example, the combination of EGFR inhibition and chemotherapy worsens survival of both mice and humans with *KRas* mutant NSCLC. Importantly, some discrepancies were noted as well. For example, combined gemcitabine and VEGF inhibition in *KRas* mutant pancreatic cancer prolonged survival in GEM models of pancreatic cancer, while this approach has not been of benefit in human patients with pancreatic cancer. This particular discrepancy appeared to result from heterogeneity among the GEMM tumors, with a subset benefitting from angiogenesis inhibition, and another subset displaying behavior more similar to the human disease. This heterogeneity may provide an opportunity to better understand the efficacy of anti-VEGF agents in human tumors. Such discrepancies were modest, however, and the authors concluded that for these models, GEMMs performed well in predicting human Phase III results.

5 Refining Kinase Inhibitor Therapy in GEMMs

There are several examples demonstrating the utility of GEMMs for the development of kinase inhibitors and related molecules (e.g. rapamycin) for solid tumors. Even when these results only confirm established findings in cancer patients (e.g. the demonstration of efficacy of anti-EGFR agents in EGFR-mutant lung cancer), the tractability of GEM systems compared to human testing is of significant value as these systems can be used to rapidly test novel combinations of therapeutics and model secondary resistance in ways not possible in human clinical trials. A few particularly instructive examples are:

1. *EGFR mutant lung cancer in GEMMs*: As discussed in detail in "EGFR Mutant Lung Cancer", most patients with non-small cell lung cancer do not respond to therapeutic inhibition of the EGFR. However, a subset of patients experience rapid and dramatic responses (Shepherd et al. 2005). This sensitivity has subsequently been shown to correlate with somatic activating mutations in the EGFR kinase domain (Lynch et al. 2004; Paez et al. 2004; Pao et al. 2004). In mice, transgenic expression of tetracycline inducible alleles of either of the two most common EGFR activating mutations (the point mutant, L858R, in exon 21 or deletion of a four amino acid sequence LREA in exon 19) is sufficient for the development of lung adenocarcinoma with brochioloalveolar features (BAC) (Ji et al. 2006a; Politi et al. 2006). Furthermore, confirming the effects seen in humans, treatment of established EGFR-driven tumors with the small molecule EGFR inhibitors, erlotinib and HKI-272, resulted in dramatic radiographic responses. Notably however, foretelling the results to be shown in both human lung and colorectal cancer, mutant K-Ras driven lung tumors appeared to be relatively resistant to EGFR inhibitor therapy.

In addition to the activating mutations in the kinase domain of EGFR, in-frame deletions of the extracellular domain of EGFR, so-called EGFRvIII, have been found in other solid tumors (most notably in glioblastoma) as well as a small subset of lung cancers. In contrast to EGFR kinase domain mutants, however, which showed equivalent tumor response to both reversible (erlotinib) and irreversible (HKI-272) inhibitors of EGFR, EGFRvIII-driven lung tumors were considerably more sensitive to irreversible inhibitors of EGFR than reversible inhibitors such as erlotinib (Ji et al. 2006b). These data suggest that irreversible inhibitors of EGFR may be more effective in the treatment of tumors harboring EGFRvIII mutations such as glioblastomas (GBM).

Lung cancers treated with EGFR inhibitors eventually develop resistance to therapy. The majority of patients who develop drug resistance also acquire a secondary mutation in the kinase domain of EGFR, T790M, which is thought to sterically hinder the binding of reversible inhibitors (Balak et al. 2006; Kosaka et al. 2006; Pao et al. 2005). Generation of a doxycycline inducible GEMM that expressed both the L858R and the T790M alleles demonstrated, as predicted, that these bitransgenic mice were resistant to erlotinib but remained relatively sensitive to HKI-272 (Li et al. 2007). In a separate report, Pao and colleagues show that L858R/T790M tumors were resistant to erlotinib, but could be rendered sensitive by simultaneous treatment with the anti-EGFR monoclonal antibody, cetuximab (Regales et al. 2009). While yet to be tested clinically, these results suggest a possible therapeutic value of irreversible EGFR inhibitors and/or combined EGFR targeting.

2. *Ras-mutant lung cancer in GEMMs*: Ras and related small GTPases have been considered 'undruggable' based on biochemical characteristics as well as the discouraging number of failed anti-RAS efforts. Unlike the successful development of nM binding ATP-competitive inhibitors for blocking the low μM ATP binding activity of protein kinases, it has not been feasible to develop analogous inhibitors to block the 10 pM Kd of GTP-binding to RAS (Bos et al. 2007). Instead, more recent anti-RAS drug discovery efforts have focused on blocking key downstream signaling molecules such as AKT and RAF/MEK/ERK (Cox and Der 2002). As predicted from our knowledge of signaling redundancies, K-Ras driven murine lung adenocarcinomas do not respond substantially to pharmacologic inhibition of MEK, EGFR or the PI3K alone. When MEK inhibitors and PI3K inhibitors were combined, however, marked and unexpected synergy was observed (Engelman et al. 2008). This therapeutic combination appears to be effective in both HER2 and EGFR driven lung cancers as well (Faber et al. 2009). This synergy, first convincingly demonstrated in GEMMs, has led to related human clinical trials in RAS-mutant cancers. Moreover, while inactivation of *LKB1* on a background of *KRas* activation imparts resistance to dual MEK and PI3K inhibition, sensitivity can be restored by the addition of the Src inhibitor, dasatinib (Carretero et al. 2010).

An additional attractive therapeutic target in K-Ras driven lung cancers is c-MET. K-Ras-driven murine lung cancers express high levels of activated c-MET as well as increased levels of its ligand hepatocyte growth factor (HGF) (Yang et al. 2008). Preclinical testing of the c-MET inhibitor, PHA-665752, in K-Ras driven lung cancer GEMM, results in a decreased number of tumors as well as an increase in apoptosis of both tumor and endothelial cells (Yang et al. 2008). While this result has yet to be confirmed in the clinic, trials are in progress using various strategies to inhibit the c-MET pathway.

3. *Prostate Cancer GEMs with PI(3)K Pathway Activation*: Prostate adenocarcinomas are characterized by a high rate of inactivation of the *PTEN* tumor suppressor gene with consequent upregulation of the PI3K/AKT/mTOR pathway. There are now several well-characterized GEMMs of prostate cancer based on *PTEN* inactivation or Akt activation in prostate epithelial cells, which result with variable penetrance and latency in prostate intraepithelial neoplasia (PIN) and prostate adenocarcinoma (Shappell et al. 2004). Of the numerous downstream effector pathways of activated Akt, early studies demonstrated that treatment of Akt-driven PIN with the inhibitor of the mammalian target of rapamycin (mTOR) inhibitor, RAD001 (everolimus), resulted in complete reversal of established PIN, suggesting that the mTOR pathway is a critical mediator of Akt-driven prostate adenocarcinomas (Majumder et al. 2004). Furthermore, in a separate prostate cancer GEM model built on the combined inactivation of the *Nkx*3.1 homeobox gene and *Pten,* while inhibition of either mTOR or the MEK/ERK pathway using rapamycin and PD0325901 appeared to restrain tumor growth, combined mTOR and MEK inhibition had marked synergistic effects (Kinkade et al. 2008). Based in part on this work, there are now ongoing clinical trials evaluating the effectiveness of mTOR inhibitors in prostate cancer (Figlin et al. 2008).

4. *BRAF Mutant Melanoma in GEMMs*: Malignant melanoma is characterized by a frequent incidence of concomitant *B-Raf* activation and *PTEN* loss (Daniotti et al. 2004; Tsao et al. 2004). Correspondingly, melanocyte-specific expression of mutant, activated $BRaf^{V600E}$ with concomitant *Pten* deletion results in the rapid formation of pigmented and highly metastatic melanoma (Dankort et al. 2009). These genetic lesions result in the activation of both the PI3K and mTOR pathways. In keeping with the above results, therapeutic treatment of established *Pten* deficient, *B-Raf* mutant melanomas with either a MEK inhibitor (PD325901) or the mTORC1 inhibitor, rapamycin, modestly inhibited their growth, but did not result in tumor regression. As in the other aforementioned systems, concurrent inhibition of both pathways results in tumor regression that correlates with inhibition of MEK and mTOR signaling, suggesting that dual inhibition of the MEK/ERK and PI3K/AKT/mTOR pathways may be efficacious in *B-Raf/PTEN* mutant cancers.

6 "Credentialing" GEMMs as Genetically Faithful Models

Human and murine genomes differ in important ways, and these differences may affect the nature of cooperating tumorigenic events and suitability of these models for drug efficacy testing. While there have been relatively few comprehensive comparisons between the transcriptional profiles and genetic complexity of cancer GEMMs and their human counterparts, a few analyses in this regard have proven informative and are described below:

Drug Efficacy Testing in Mice

1. *Cooperating Genetic Events in GEMMs*: With regard to genetic lesions in GEM tumors, the published results have suggested that GEMMs may not possess the same degree of genetic complexity in terms of copy-number variants, aneuploidy and point mutations as human tumors (see for example Ellwood-Yen et al. 2003; Kim et al. 2006). A period of telomere dysfunction which may occur at an early stage of most human but not murine tumor progression has been suggested as one cause for this discrepancy, and tumor-bearing mice with 'humanized' telomere length exhibit increased cytogenetic complexity reminiscent of the human disease (Artandi et al. 2000; Maser et al. 2007). Despite these genome-wide differences, a number of secondary genetic events important in the evolution of human tumors appear to be conserved in the progression and metastasis of GEM tumors such as the amplification of *KRas2* and *Myc* in pancreatic ductal adenocarinomas, *Nedd9* in Ras induced melanomas, and loss of *Fbxw7* and *Pten* in *Atm;p53* deficient lymphomas (Bardeesy et al. 2006; Ellwood-Yen et al. 2003; Kim et al. 2006; Maser et al. 2007). In a similar light, murine hepatocellular carcinomas (HCCs) induced by transplanted, genetically defined, liver progenitor cells were found to have focal amplifications of *Myc* and *Yap*, both known oncogenic events in the development of HCC (Zender et al. 2006).

2. *Genome-Wide Expression Profiling*: A recent study by Perou et al. of GEMM transcriptional profiles is particularly informative. The authors performed a microarray-based, comprehensive assessment of gene expression in more than 20 breast cancer GEMMs, and compared these expression profiles with a large number of human tumors using a novel cross-platform method for transcriptome normalization (Herschkowitz et al. 2007). The authors found great heterogeneity among breast cancer GEMMs, and were able to identify a few models with significant transcriptional overlap to human breast cancer subtypes. For example, the C3-Large T Antigen model appeared transcriptionally similar to the basal-like subtype of breast cancer. In retrospect, this similarity likely reflects the fact that RB and p53 inactivation are signature events of most basal-like cancers, and Large T Antigen similarly inactivates these two archetypal tumor suppressor genes. Likewise, the MMTV-Her2/Neu model was transcriptionally similar to human Her2 + breast cancer, again consistent with the molecular genetics of these tumors. Surprisingly, no good murine model was identified for human estrogen receptor expressing (ER + or luminal) breast cancer, at least in terms of transcriptional profiles.

Expression profiling and assessment of copy number alterations by array CGH of *PTEN*, *TP53* and *Rb* deficient mouse gliomas showed remarkable similarity in syntenic regions of gene amplification and loss (Chow et al. 2011). In contrast to the expression profiling of breast cancer GEMMs, which suggested that each GEMM can be classified into a single molecular subtype of human breast cancer, subgroups of these mice resembled the proneural, proliferative and mesenchymal molecular subtypes of glioblastoma previously shown to have prognostic significance suggesting that secondary genetic events are driving the molecular classification of glioblastomas. Similar studies using a Myc gene signature derived from a Myc-driven prostate cancer GEMM indicates that this model faithfully recapitulates the molecular changes seen in a subset of human prostate cancers

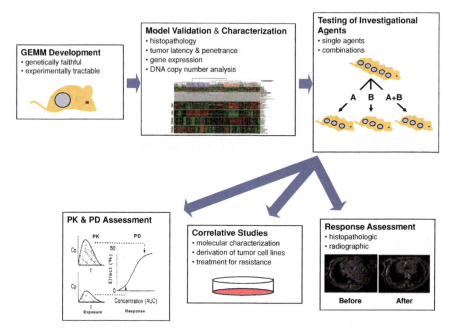

Fig. 2 Workflow and infrastructural needs for GEMM testing. GEM models are first designed and developed based on genetic events faithful to human cancers. The model is then characterized and validated histopathologically and molecularly prior to therapeutic testing. Once a model is characterized, investigational agents are tested as single agents or in combination. Treated and untreated mice are assessed for tumor response (typically radiographically or other imaging modalities using RECIST-like criteria) with pharmacokinetic (PK) and pharmacodymanic (PD) monitoring. Other correlative studies such as the molecular characterization of treated tumors and culture and in vitro evaluation of GEMM tumor cell lines can be performed as indicated

harboring Myc activation (Ellwood-Yen et al. 2003). These observations suggest that faithful GEM models of some, but probably not all, human cancers can be identified, and reiterate the importance of GEMM credentialing.

In summary, the available genomic data suggests that some aspects of human tumor progression are recapitulated in GEMMs, but that relevant inter-species differences also exist. Therefore, characterization and validation (e.g. 'credentialing') of a GEMM is requisite prior to widespread use for pre-clinical testing (Fig. 2). It is worth noting in this context that established human cancer cell lines—the alternative source of cancer cells for in vivo drug efficacy testing—are far from perfect with regard to genetic faithfulness to human cancer. Many tumor lines have been in culture for years or decades, and therefore subject to ex vivo genetic events associated with in vitro progression and drift. Moreover, the ability to be grown in vitro may differ markedly depending on a tumor's attendant genetic lesions. For example, $p16^{INK4a}$ expression is an important barrier to in vitro growth for many cell types, and therefore not unexpectedly, the frequency of $p16^{INK4a}$

inactivation in cell lines often greatly exceeds the in vivo mutation frequency of $p16^{INK4a}$ in the same tumor type. Therefore, in vitro drift and the need for culture strongly influence in vitro and xenograft approaches.

7 Logistic Considerations in Developing a "Mouse Clinic"

An important consideration when one considers the use of GEMMs for drug efficacy testing is the amount of time required to breed a sufficiently large cohort of animals for informative preclinical drug testing. While GEMMs possess one or more index genetic lesions, the neoplastic cells in these models require the acquisition of subsequent genetic alterations to progress into cancer. These secondary genetic events occur stochastically resulting in genetic heterogeneity as well as differences in penetrance, tumor latency and therapeutic responsiveness. Our experience has been that many efficacious therapeutics will cause tumor regression in only a subset of animals within a given GEM model. For example, some classical cytotoxics can induce profound tumor regression in a small fraction of breast GEM models, but such agents are not active in most tumors from animals of this genotype (unpublished data NES, WYK and Charles Perou). As these mice are syngeneic, this heterogeneity of response likely reflects the differences in cooperating genetic events during tumor progression in this model. While this presence of responders and non-responders within a given model is clearly similar to the experience of Phase II/III testing in humans with a given tumor type, such heterogeneity also necessitates the study of larger numbers of mice. For these reasons, we typically analyze 12–16 mice per initial therapeutic cohort, as opposed to cohort sizes of 4–8 mice that we use for xenograft testing.

Additionally, many cancer GEMMs are multiallelic, typically requiring a conditional knock-out, activatable knock-in, or transgenic allele as well as a Cre or tetracycline-inducible allele to control spatial expression of the genes of interest. The need for multiple alleles can decrease breeding efficiency if the employed alleles cannot be homozygosed, and also produces a need for rapid and accurate animal genotyping. Inefficient breeding and mutli-allele genotyping in turn can increase the needed cage space for GEMM testing and also significantly augment the experimental cost. One approach to these problems is to identify GEMMs that are relatively simple to use. For example, for the testing of anti-RAS therapeutics, we have relied extensively on the *Tyr-RASInk4a/Arf-/-* model from Chin and colleagues (Chin et al. 1997). This model is very faithful to the genetics of human melanoma featuring a melanocyte-specific, activated RAS transgene integrated on the Y-chromosome combined with germ line $p16^{INK4a}$ and Arf inactivation (*Ink4a/Arf-/-*), an allele which can be homozygosed. Therefore, by crossing *Tyr-RASInk4a/Arf-/-* males with *Ink4a/Arf-/-* females, a cohort is produced where no genotyping is required (all the males get cancer) and all the progeny mice are useful (the males develop tumors and the females are used for future breeding). While this degree of efficiency is not possible for all models, often more efficient breeding schemes can be developed to allow for low-cost and rapid cohort development.

Drug efficacy testing in GEMMs requires substantial expertise, infrastructure to set up mouse colonies for efficient drug efficacy testing in GEMs (Fig. 2), and a commitment to test multiple agents, including 'boring' older cytotoxic agents in addition to more novel targeted therapies. Without assessment of multiple agents, we believe it is hard to assess the activity of any single compound. Likewise, several challenges must be solved including access to adequate cage space, the development of well-defined processes for animal husbandry and genotyping, meticulous record keeping, and for some models, infrastructure to permit serial animal imaging. Moreover, access to expertise in cancer histopathology is a critical and, in our view, still under appreciated need in GEMM experiments. Lastly, we believe in the modern era, where GEMM experiments require a modest amount of companion pharmacologic (PK) and pharmacodynamic (PD) monitoring to be fully informative. For example, the demonstration that a compound has activity in a given model is only helpful if complementary PK analyses indicate that drug levels associated with efficacy are levels that could be reasonably achieved in humans. Perhaps even more difficult is understanding why compounds that should work based on our understanding of tumor signaling still fail in certain models. In these instances, PD monitoring can be particularly informative; for example sometimes showing that failure of an agent correlates with a lack of in vivo inhibition of the relevant drug target. For these reasons, we have come to believe that GEMM analyses must necessarily be complemented by PK/PD monitoring.

A historical impediment regarding GEMM testing involves a series of legal issues related to the involved technologies. In particular, the topic of 'Oncomouse' patents has been covered extensively elsewhere (Hanahan et al. 2007; Marshall 2002; Sharpless and Depinho 2006). In our view, however, several recent developments have conspired to mitigate this problem including the expiration of some of these patents, the licensing of these patents by many large Pharma entities and decisions in the US and Canadian Supreme Courts that have limited the scope of these patents and bolstered the legal notion of 'safe harbor' which may shelter some GEMM testing. For whichever of these reasons, in the last few years, GEMM testing of novel therapeutics has now become commonplace in many institutions and has begun to be more widely embraced by large Pharma. While these patents may still pose problems for those industry workers in entities that have not taken license for these patents, this issue appears to no longer be a major experimental impediment in most settings.

8 Future Perspectives

Despite the relatively recent introduction of GEMMs for pre-clinical drug development, we believe that there have already been some remarkable successes that

Drug Efficacy Testing in Mice

will speed up the development of active human therapeutics. In particular, there has been significant work with kinase inhibitors and related molecules in several GEM models of lung adenocarcinoma, prostate carcinoma and melanoma; and we expect publication of a raft of additional GEMM therapeutic stories in many other tumor types in the next few years.We believe the published experience suggests that GEMM testing adds immediate value to xenograft testing for pre-clinical efficacy studies.

Some cancer researchers believe that while GEMM testing is clearly of benefit, it is better left to the industry, which has the in-house wherewithal to meet the challenges of GEMM testing. In fact, these researchers are partially correct, as the forward-thinking industry has begun to move into GEMM testing with great enthusiasm, a move we wholeheartedly endorse. Unfortunately, however, we believe that such a desire to compartmentalize academic versus industry science may have contributed to a hesitation among large funding agencies to support laudable and highly translational GEMM efforts As a reflection of this, the most ambitious academic GEMM efforts have relied extensively on private, state and industry funding. Nonetheless, we believe that this line of research is too important to cede solely to the industry, and see an increasing need for such investigation in federally financed academic labs that have no commercial interest in the development of the agents that they are testing.

We have highlighted several of the challenges associated with GEMM studies, most notably the need for requisite infrastructure to support this work. Despite these challenges, we feel GEMM testing can be done cost-effectively with sufficient rapidity to directly shape human clinical trials of novel agents. Lastly, as mentioned, while we are cheered by significant recent industry investments in GEMM testing, it is crucial that widespread and vibrant GEMM testing also proceed in academia conducted by dispassionate scientists interested in improving clinical cancer care.

Acknowledgments We would like to thank N. Bardeesy for useful discussions and K. Wong for MRI images.

References

Alani RM, Silverthorn CF, Orosz K (2004) Tumor angiogenesis in mice and men. Cancer Biol Ther 3:498–500

Artandi SE, Chang S, Lee SL, Alson S, Gottlieb GJ, Chin L, DePinho RA (2000) Telomere dysfunction promotes non-reciprocal translocations and epithelial cancers in mice. Nature 406:641–645

Balak MN, Gong Y, Riely GJ, Somwar R, Li AR, Zakowski MF, Chiang A, Yang G, Ouerfelli O, Kris MG, Ladanyi M, Miller VA, Pao W (2006) Novel D761Y and common secondary T790M mutations in epidermal growth factor receptor-mutant lung adenocarcinomas with acquired resistance to kinase inhibitors. Clin Cancer Res 12:6494–6501. doi:12/21/6494[pii] 10.1158/1078-0432.CCR-06-1570

Bardeesy N, Aguirre AJ, Chu GC, Cheng KH, Lopez LV, Hezel AF, Feng B, Brennan C, Weissleder R, Mahmood U, Hanahan D, Redston MS, Chin L, Depinho RA (2006) Both p16(Ink4a) and the p19(Arf)-p53 pathway constrain progression of pancreatic adenocarcinoma in the mouse. Proc Natl Acad Sci USA 103:5947–5952. doi:0601273103[pii]10.1073/pnas.0601273103

Bergers G, Javaherian K, Lo KM, Folkman J, Hanahan D (1999) Effects of angiogenesis inhibitors on multistage carcinogenesis in mice. Science 284:808–812

Bos JL, Rehmann H, Wittinghofer A (2007) GEFs and GAPs: critical elements in the control of small G proteins. Cell 129:865–877. doi:S0092-8674(07)00655-1[pii]10.1016/j.cell.2007.05.018

Carretero J, Shimamura T, Rikova K, Jackson AL, Wilkerson MD, Borgman CL, Buttarazzi MS, Sanofsky BA, McNamara KL, Brandstetter KA, Walton ZE, Gu TL, Silva JC, Crosby K, Shapiro GI, Maira SM, Ji H, Castrillon DH, Kim CF, Garcia-Echeverria C, Bardeesy N, Sharpless NE, Hayes ND, Kim WY, Engelman JA, Wong KK (2010) Integrative genomic and proteomic analyses identify targets for Lkb1-deficient metastatic lung tumors. Cancer Cell 17:547–559

Chin L, Pomerantz J, Polsky D, Jacobson M, Cohen C, Cordon-Cardo C, Horner JW II, DePinho RA (1997) Cooperative effects of INK4a and ras in melanoma susceptibility in vivo. Genes Dev 11:2822–2834

Chow LM, Endersby R, Zhu X, Rankin S, Qu C, Zhang J, Broniscer A, Ellison DW, Baker SJ (2011) Cooperativity within and among Pten, p53, and Rb pathways induces high-grade astrocytoma in adult brain. Cancer Cell 19:305–316. doi:S1535-6108(11)00051-1[pii]10.1016/j.ccr.2011.01.039

Cox AD, Der CJ (2002) Ras family signaling: therapeutic targeting. Cancer Biol Ther 1:599–606. doi:306[pii]

Daniotti M, Oggionni M, Ranzani T, Vallacchi V, Campi V, Di Stasi D, Torre GD, Perrone F, Luoni C, Suardi S, Frattini M, Pilotti S, Anichini A, Tragni G, Parmiani G, Pierotti MA, Rodolfo M (2004) BRAF alterations are associated with complex mutational profiles in malignant melanoma. Oncogene 23:5968–5977

Dankort D, Curley DP, Cartlidge RA, Nelson B, Karnezis AN, Damsky WE Jr, You MJ, DePinho RA, McMahon M, Bosenberg M (2009) Braf(V600E) cooperates with Pten loss to induce metastatic melanoma. Nat Genet 41:544–552

Decoster G, Stein G, Holdener EE (1990) Responses and toxic deaths in phase I clinical trials. Ann Oncol 1:175–181

Demetri GD, Fletcher CD, Mueller E, Sarraf P, Naujoks R, Campbell N, Spiegelman BM, Singer S (1999) Induction of solid tumor differentiation by the peroxisome proliferator-activated receptor-gamma ligand troglitazone in patients with liposarcoma. Proc Natl Acad Sci USA 96:3951–3956

Donawho CK, Luo Y, Luo Y, Penning TD, Bauch JL, Bouska JJ, Bontcheva-Diaz VD, Cox BF, DeWeese TL, Dillehay LE, Ferguson DC, Ghoreishi-Haack NS, Grimm DR, Guan R, Han EK, Holley-Shanks RR, Hristov B, Idler KB, Jarvis K, Johnson EF, Kleinberg LR, Klinghofer V, Lasko LM, Liu X, Marsh KC, McGonigal TP, Meulbroek JA, Olson AM, Palma JP, Rodriguez LE, Shi Y, Stavropoulos JA, Tsurutani AC, Zhu GD, Rosenberg SH, Giranda VL, Frost DJ (2007) ABT-888, an orally active poly(ADP-ribose) polymerase inhibitor that potentiates DNA-damaging agents in preclinical tumor models. Clin Cancer Res 13:2728–2737

Ellwood-Yen K, Graeber TG, Wongvipat J, Iruela-Arispe ML, Zhang J, Matusik R, Thomas GV, Sawyers CL (2003) Myc-driven murine prostate cancer shares molecular features with human prostate tumors. Cancer Cell 4:223–238. doi:S1535610803001971[pii]

Engelman JA, Chen L, Tan X, Crosby K, Guimaraes AR, Upadhyay R, Maira M, McNamara K, Perera SA, Song Y, Chirieac LR, Kaur R, Lightbown A, Simendinger J, Li T, Padera RF, Garcia-Echeverria C, Weissleder R, Mahmood U, Cantley LC, Wong KK (2008) Effective use of PI3K and MEK inhibitors to treat mutant Kras G12D and PIK3CA H1047R murine lung cancers. Nat Med 14:1351–1356. doi:nm.1890[pii]10.1038/nm.1890

Evers B, Drost R, Schut E, de Bruin M, van der Burg E, Derksen PW, Holstege H, Liu X, van Drunen E, Beverloo HB, Smith GC, Martin NM, Lau A, O'Connor MJ, Jonkers J (2008) Selective inhibition of BRCA2-deficient mammary tumor cell growth by AZD2281 and cisplatin. Clin Cancer Res 14:3916–3925

Faber AC, Li D, Song Y, Liang MC, Yeap BY, Bronson RT, Lifshits E, Chen Z, Maira SM, Garcia-Echeverria C, Wong KK, Engelman JA (2009) Differential induction of apoptosis in HER2 and EGFR addicted cancers following PI3K inhibition. Proc Natl Acad Sci USA 106:19503–19508. doi:0905056106[pii]10.1073/pnas.0905056106

Figlin RA, Brown E, Armstrong AJ, Akerley W, Benson AB III, Burstein HJ, Ettinger DS, Febbo PG, Fury MG, Hudes GR, Kies MS, Kwak EL, Morgan RJ Jr, Mortimer J, Reckamp K, Venook AP, Worden F, Yen Y (2008) NCCN task force report: mTOR inhibition in solid tumors. J Natl Compr Canc Netw 6(Suppl 5):S1–S20 quiz S21-S22

Fong PC, Boss DS, Yap TA, Tutt A, Wu P, Mergui-Roelvink M, Mortimer P, Swaisland H, Lau A, O'Connor MJ, Ashworth A, Carmichael J, Kaye SB, Schellens JH, de Bono JS (2009) Inhibition of poly(ADP-ribose) polymerase in tumors from BRCA mutation carriers. N Engl J Med 361:123–134

Frese KK, Tuveson DA (2007) Maximizing mouse cancer models. Nat Rev Cancer 7:645–658

Garber K (2009) From human to mouse and back: 'tumorgraft' models surge in popularity. J Natl Cancer Inst 101:6–8

Hanahan D, Wagner EF, Palmiter RD (2007) The origins of oncomice: a history of the first transgenic mice genetically engineered to develop cancer. Genes Dev 21:2258–2270

Herschkowitz JI, Simin K, Weigman VJ, Mikaelian I, Usary J, Hu Z, Rasmussen KE, Jones LP, Assefnia S, Chandrasekharan S, Backlund MG, Yin Y, Khramtsov AI, Bastein R, Quackenbush J, Glazer RI, Brown PH, Green JE, Kopelovich L, Furth PA, Palazzo JP, Olopade OI, Bernard PS, Churchill GA, Van Dyke T, Perou CM (2007) Identification of conserved gene expression features between murine mammary carcinoma models and human breast tumors. Genome Biol 8:R76

Hingorani SR, Wang L, Multani AS, Combs C, Deramaudt TB, Hruban RH, Rustgi AK, Chang S, Tuveson DA (2005) Trp53R172H and KrasG12D cooperate to promote chromosomal instability and widely metastatic pancreatic ductal adenocarcinoma in mice. Cancer Cell 7:469–483

Ji H, Li D, Chen L, Shimamura T, Kobayashi S, McNamara K, Mahmood U, Mitchell A, Sun Y, Al-Hashem R, Chirieac LR, Padera R, Bronson RT, Kim W, Janne PA, Shapiro GI, Tenen D, Johnson BE, Weissleder R, Sharpless NE, Wong KK (2006a) The impact of human EGFR kinase domain mutations on lung tumorigenesis and in vivo sensitivity to EGFR-targeted therapies. Cancer Cell 9:485–495

Ji H, Zhao X, Yuza Y, Shimamura T, Li D, Protopopov A, Jung BL, McNamara K, Xia H, Glatt KA, Thomas RK, Sasaki H, Horner JW, Eck M, Mitchell A, Sun Y, Al-Hashem R, Bronson RT, Rabindran SK, Discafani CM, Maher E, Shapiro GI, Meyerson M, Wong KK (2006b) Epidermal growth factor receptor variant III mutations in lung tumorigenesis and sensitivity to tyrosine kinase inhibitors. Proc Natl Acad Sci USA 103:7817–7822. doi:0510284103[pii] 10.1073/pnas.0510284103

Ji H, Ramsey MR, Hayes DN, Fan C, McNamara K, Kozlowski P, Torrice C, Wu MC, Shimamura T, Perera SA, Liang MC, Cai D, Naumov GN, Bao L, Contreras CM, Li D, Chen L, Krishnamurthy J, Koivunen J, Chirieac LR, Padera RF, Bronson RT, Lindeman NI, Christiani DC, Lin X, Shapiro GI, Janne PA, Johnson BE, Meyerson M, Kwiatkowski DJ, Castrillon DH, Bardeesy N, Sharpless NE, Wong KK (2007) LKB1 modulates lung cancer differentiation and metastasis. Nature 448:807–810

Johnson L, Mercer K, Greenbaum D, Bronson RT, Crowley D, Tuveson DA, Jacks T (2001) Somatic activation of the K-ras oncogene causes early onset lung cancer in mice. Nature 410:1111–1116

Jonkers J, Berns A (2002) Conditional mouse models of sporadic cancer. Nat Rev Cancer 2:251–265. doi:10.1038/nrc777

Kerbel RS, Cornil I, Theodorescu D (1991) Importance of orthotopic transplantation procedures in assessing the effects of transfected genes on human tumor growth and metastasis. Cancer Metastasis Rev 10:201–215

Kim M, Gans JD, Nogueira C, Wang A, Paik JH, Feng B, Brennan C, Hahn WC, Cordon-Cardo C, Wagner SN, Flotte TJ, Duncan LM, Granter SR, Chin L (2006) Comparative oncogenomics identifies NEDD9 as a melanoma metastasis gene. Cell 125:1269–1281

Kinkade CW, Castillo-Martin M, Puzio-Kuter A, Yan J, Foster TH, Gao H, Sun Y, Ouyang X, Gerald WL, Cordon-Cardo C, Abate-Shen C (2008) Targeting AKT/mTOR and ERK MAPK signaling inhibits hormone-refractory prostate cancer in a preclinical mouse model. J Clin Invest 118:3051–3064. doi:10.1172/JCI34764

Kola I, Landis J (2004) Can the pharmaceutical industry reduce attrition rates? Nat Rev Drug Discov 3:711–715

Kosaka T, Yatabe Y, Endoh H, Yoshida K, Hida T, Tsuboi M, Tada H, Kuwano H, Mitsudomi T (2006) Analysis of epidermal growth factor receptor gene mutation in patients with non-small cell lung cancer and acquired resistance to gefitinib. Clin Cancer Res 12:5764–5769. doi: 12/19/5764[pii]10.1158/1078-0432.CCR-06-0714

Kulke MH, Demetri GD, Sharpless NE, Ryan DP, Shivdasani R, Clark JS, Spiegelman BM, Kim H, Mayer RJ, Fuchs CS (2002) A phase II study of troglitazone, an activator of the PPARgamma receptor, in patients with chemotherapy-resistant metastatic colorectal cancer. Cancer J 8:395–399

Li D, Shimamura T, Ji H, Chen L, Haringsma HJ, McNamara K, Liang MC, Perera SA, Zaghlul S, Borgman CL, Kubo S, Takahashi M, Sun Y, Chirieac LR, Padera RF, Lindeman NI, Janne PA, Thomas RK, Meyerson ML, Eck MJ, Engelman JA, Shapiro GI, Wong KK (2007) Bronchial and peripheral murine lung carcinomas induced by T790M–L858R mutant EGFR respond to HKI-272 and rapamycin combination therapy. Cancer Cell 12:81–93

Lynch TJ, Bell DW, Sordella R, Gurubhagavatula S, Okimoto RA, Brannigan BW, Harris PL, Haserlat SM, Supko JG, Haluska FG, Louis DN, Christiani DC, Settleman J, Haber DA (2004) Activating mutations in the epidermal growth factor receptor underlying responsiveness of non-small-cell lung cancer to gefitinib. N Engl J Med 350:2129–2139

Majumder PK, Febbo PG, Bikoff R, Berger R, Xue Q, McMahon LM, Manola J, Brugarolas J, McDonnell TJ, Golub TR, Loda M, Lane HA, Sellers WR (2004) mTOR inhibition reverses Akt-dependent prostate intraepithelial neoplasia through regulation of apoptotic and HIF-1-dependent pathways. Nat Med 10:594–601

Marshall E (2002) Intellectual property. DuPont ups ante on use of Harvard's OncoMouse. Science 296:1212

Maser RS, Choudhury B, Campbell PJ, Feng B, Wong KK, Protopopov A, O'Neil J, Gutierrez A, Ivanova E, Perna I, Lin E, Mani V, Jiang S, McNamara K, Zaghlul S, Edkins S, Stevens C, Brennan C, Martin ES, Wiedemeyer R, Kabbarah O, Nogueira C, Histen G, Aster J, Mansour M, Duke V, Foroni L, Fielding AK, Goldstone AH, Rowe JM, Wang YA, Look AT, Stratton MR, Chin L, Futreal PA, DePinho RA (2007) Chromosomally unstable mouse tumours have genomic alterations similar to diverse human cancers. Nature 447:966–971. doi: nature05886[pii]10.1038/nature05886

Meuwissen R, Linn SC, van der Valk M, Mooi WJ, Berns A (2001) Mouse model for lung tumorigenesis through cre/lox controlled sporadic activation of the K-ras oncogene. Oncogene 20:6551–6558

Mitsiades CS, Mitsiades NS, Bronson RT, Chauhan D, Munshi N, Treon SP, Maxwell CA, Pilarski L, Hideshima T, Hoffman RM, Anderson KC (2003) Fluorescence imaging of multiple myeloma cells in a clinically relevant SCID/NOD in vivo model: biologic and clinical implications. Cancer Res 63:6689–6696

Mueller MM, Fusenig NE (2004) Friends or foes: bipolar effects of the tumour stroma in cancer. Nat Rev Cancer 4:839–849. doi:nrc1477[pii]10.1038/nrc1477

Ojalvo LS, King W, Cox D, Pollard JW (2009) High-density gene expression analysis of tumor-associated macrophages from mouse mammary tumors. Am J Pathol 174:1048–1064

Olive KP, Jacobetz MA, Davidson CJ, Gopinathan A, McIntyre D, Honess D, Madhu B, Goldgraben MA, Caldwell ME, Allard D, Frese KK, Denicola G, Feig C, Combs C, Winter SP, Ireland-Zecchini H, Reichelt S, Howat WJ, Chang A, Dhara M, Wang L, Ruckert F, Grutzmann R, Pilarsky C, Izeradjene K, Hingorani SR, Huang P, Davies SE, Plunkett W, Egorin M, Hruban RH, Whitebread N, McGovern K, Adams J, Iacobuzio-Donahue C, Griffiths J, Tuveson DA (2009) Inhibition of Hedgehog signaling enhances delivery of chemotherapy in a mouse model of pancreatic cancer. Science 324:1457–1461

O'Reilly MS, Holmgren L, Shing Y, Chen C, Rosenthal RA, Moses M, Lane WS, Cao Y, Sage EH, Folkman J (1994) Angiostatin: a novel angiogenesis inhibitor that mediates the suppression of metastases by a Lewis lung carcinoma. Cell 79:315–328

O'Reilly MS, Holmgren L, Chen C, Folkman J (1996) Angiostatin induces and sustains dormancy of human primary tumors in mice. Nat Med 2:689–692

O'Reilly MS, Boehm T, Shing Y, Fukai N, Vasios G, Lane WS, Flynn E, Birkhead JR, Olsen BR, Folkman J (1997) Endostatin: an endogenous inhibitor of angiogenesis and tumor growth. Cell 88:277–285

Paez JG, Janne PA, Lee JC, Tracy S, Greulich H, Gabriel S, Herman P, Kaye FJ, Lindeman N, Boggon TJ, Naoki K, Sasaki H, Fujii Y, Eck MJ, Sellers WR, Johnson BE, Meyerson M (2004) EGFR mutations in lung cancer: correlation with clinical response to gefitinib therapy. Science 304:1497–1500

Pao W, Miller V, Zakowski M, Doherty J, Politi K, Sarkaria I, Singh B, Heelan R, Rusch V, Fulton L, Mardis E, Kupfer D, Wilson R, Kris M, Varmus H (2004) EGF receptor gene mutations are common in lung cancers from "never smokers" and are associated with sensitivity of tumors to gefitinib and erlotinib. Proc Natl Acad Sci USA 101:13306–13311

Pao W, Miller VA, Politi KA, Riely GJ, Somwar R, Zakowski MF, Kris MG, Varmus H (2005) Acquired resistance of lung adenocarcinomas to gefitinib or erlotinib is associated with a second mutation in the EGFR kinase domain. PLoS Med 2:e73

Peterson JK, Houghton PJ (2004) Integrating pharmacology and in vivo cancer models in preclinical and clinical drug development. Eur J Cancer 40:837–844

Politi K, Zakowski MF, Fan PD, Schonfeld EA, Pao W, Varmus HE (2006) Lung adenocarcinomas induced in mice by mutant EGF receptors found in human lung cancers respond to a tyrosine kinase inhibitor or to down-regulation of the receptors. Genes Dev 20:1496–1510

Regales L, Gong Y, Shen R, de Stanchina E, Vivanco I, Goel A, Koutcher JA, Spassova M, Ouerfelli O, Mellinghoff IK, Zakowski MF, Politi KA, Pao W (2009) Dual targeting of EGFR can overcome a major drug resistance mutation in mouse models of EGFR mutant lung cancer. J Clin Invest 119:3000–3010. doi:38746[pii]10.1172/JCI38746

Roberts TG Jr, Goulart BH, Squitieri L, Stallings SC, Halpern EF, Chabner BA, Gazelle GS, Finkelstein SN, Clark JW (2004) Trends in the risks and benefits to patients with cancer participating in phase 1 clinical trials. Jama 292:2130–2140

Rofstad EK (1994) Orthotopic human melanoma xenograft model systems for studies of tumour angiogenesis, pathophysiology, treatment sensitivity and metastatic pattern. Br J Cancer 70:804–812

Rottenberg S, Jaspers JE, Kersbergen A, van der Burg E, Nygren AO, Zander SA, Derksen PW, de Bruin M, Zevenhoven J, Lau A, Boulter R, Cranston A, O'Connor MJ, Martin NM, Borst P, Jonkers J (2008) High sensitivity of BRCA1-deficient mammary tumors to the PARP inhibitor AZD2281 alone and in combination with platinum drugs. Proc Natl Acad Sci USA 105:17079–17084

Ruzinova MB, Schoer RA, Gerald W, Egan JE, Pandolfi PP, Rafii S, Manova K, Mittal V, Benezra R (2003) Effect of angiogenesis inhibition by Id loss and the contribution of bone-marrow-derived endothelial cells in spontaneous murine tumors. Cancer Cell 4:277–289

Saez E, Tontonoz P, Nelson MC, Alvarez JG, Ming UT, Baird SM, Thomazy VA, Evans RM (1998) Activators of the nuclear receptor PPARgamma enhance colon polyp formation. Nat Med 4:1058–1061

Sarraf P, Mueller E, Jones D, King FJ, DeAngelo DJ, Partridge JB, Holden SA, Chen LB, Singer S, Fletcher C, Spiegelman BM (1998) Differentiation and reversal of malignant changes in colon cancer through PPARgamma. Nat Med 4:1046–1052

Sausville EA, Burger AM (2006) Contributions of human tumor xenografts to anticancer drug development. Cancer Res 66:3351–3354 discussion 3354

Shappell SB, Thomas GV, Roberts RL, Herbert R, Ittmann MM, Rubin MA, Humphrey PA, Sundberg JP, Rozengurt N, Barrios R, Ward JM, Cardiff RD (2004) Prostate pathology of genetically engineered mice: definitions and classification. The consensus report from the Bar Harbor meeting of the mouse models of human cancer consortium prostate pathology committee. Cancer Res 64:2270–2305

Sharpless NE, Depinho RA (2006) The mighty mouse: genetically engineered mouse models in cancer drug development. Nat Rev Drug Discov 5:741–754

Shepherd FA, Rodrigues Pereira J, Ciuleanu T, Tan EH, Hirsh V, Thongprasert S, Campos D, Maoleekoonpiroj S, Smylie M, Martins R, van Kooten M, Dediu M, Findlay B, Tu D, Johnston D, Bezjak A, Clark G, Santabarbara P, Seymour L (2005) Erlotinib in previously treated non-small-cell lung cancer. N Engl J Med 353:123–132

Sikder HA, Devlin MK, Dunlap S, Ryu B, Alani RM (2003) Id proteins in cell growth and tumorigenesis. Cancer Cell 3:525–530

Singh M, Lima A, Molina R, Hamilton P, Clermont AC, Devasthali V, Thompson JD, Cheng JH, Bou Reslan H, Ho CC, Cao TC, Lee CV, Nannini MA, Fuh G, Carano RA, Koeppen H, Yu RX, Forrest WF, Plowman GD, Johnson L (2010) Assessing therapeutic responses in Kras mutant cancers using genetically engineered mouse models. Nat Biotechnol 28:585–593. doi: nbt.1640[pii]10.1038/nbt.1640

Tsao H, Goel V, Wu H, Yang G, Haluska FG (2004) Genetic interaction between NRAS and BRAF mutations and PTEN/MMAC1 inactivation in melanoma. J Invest Dermatol 122:337–341

Voskoglou-Nomikos T, Pater JL, Seymour L (2003) Clinical predictive value of the in vitro cell line, human xenograft, and mouse allograft preclinical cancer models. Clin Cancer Res 9:4227–4239

Yang Y, Wislez M, Fujimoto N, Prudkin L, Izzo JG, Uno F, Ji L, Hanna AE, Langley RR, Liu D, Johnson FM, Wistuba I, Kurie JM (2008) A selective small molecule inhibitor of c-Met, PHA-665752, reverses lung premalignancy induced by mutant K-ras. Mol Cancer Ther 7:952–960. doi:7/4/952[pii]10.1158/1535-7163.MCT-07-2045

Zender L, Spector MS, Xue W, Flemming P, Cordon-Cardo C, Silke J, Fan ST, Luk JM, Wigler M, Hannon GJ, Mu D, Lucito R, Powers S, Lowe SW (2006) Identification and validation of oncogenes in liver cancer using an integrative oncogenomic approach. Cell 125:1253–1267. doi:S0092-8674(06)00720-3[pii]10.1016/j.cell.2006.05.030

Part II
Kinase Targets and Disease

Gastrointestinal Stromal Tumors

Cristina Antonescu

Abstract Gastrointestinal stromal tumor (GIST) is the most common sarcoma of the intestinal tract. Nearly all tumors have a mutation in the *KIT* or, less often, platelet-derived growth factor receptor (*PDGFRA*) or B-rapidly Accelerated Fibrosarcoma (*BRAF*) gene. The discovery of constitutive KIT activation as the central mechanism of GIST pathogenesis, suggested that inhibiting or blocking KIT signaling might be the milestone in the targeted therapy of GISTs. Indeed, imatinib mesylate inhibits KIT kinase activity and represents the front line drug for the treatment of unresectable and advanced GISTs, achieving a partial response or stable disease in about 80% of patients with metastatic GIST. *KIT* mutation status has a significant impact on treatment response. Patients with the most common exon 11 mutation experience higher rates of tumor shrinkage and prolonged survival, as tumors with an exon 9 mutation or wild-type *KIT* are less likely to respond to imatinib. Although imatinib achieves a partial response or stable disease in the majority of GIST patients, complete and lasting responses are rare. About half of the patients who initially benefit from imatinib treatment eventually develop drug resistance. The most common mechanism of resistance is through polyclonal acquisition of second site mutations in the kinase domain, which highlights the future therapeutic challenges in salvaging these patients after failing kinase inhibitor monotherapies. More recently, sunitinib (Sutent, Pfizer, New York, NY), which inhibits vascular endothelial growth factor receptor (VEGFR) in addition to KIT and PDGFRA, has proven efficacious in patients who are intolerant or refractory to imatinib. This review summarizes the recent knowledge on targeted therapy in GIST, based on the central role of KIT oncogenic activation, as well as discussing mechanisms of resistance.

C. Antonescu (✉)
Memorial Sloan-Kettering Cancer Center,
New York, NY 10021, USA
e-mail: antonesc@mskcc.org

Current Topics in Microbiology and Immunology (2012) 355: 41–57
DOI: 10.1007/82_2011_161
© Springer-Verlag Berlin Heidelberg 2011
Published Online: 21 October 2011

Contents

1 Introduction 42
2 KIT Activation as Dominant Pathogenetic Mechanism 42
3 GIST with Wild-Type KIT 44
4 Treatment of GIST with Imatinib 46
    4.1 Imatinib Monotherapy for Advanced GIST 46
    4.2 Imatinib Plus Surgery for Advanced GIST 47
    4.3 Adjuvant Imatinib Therapy After Resection of a Primary GIST 47
    4.4 Evaluation of Tumor Response to Imatinib 48
5 Acquired Imatinib Resistance 50
6 Overcoming Imatinib Resistance 53
7 Future Perspectives 54
References 54

1 Introduction

Gastrointestinal stromal tumor (GIST) is the most common mesenchymal tumor of the GI tract. Until a few years ago, GIST was an enigmatic pathologic entity, being often misdiagnosed as a smooth muscle neoplasm. The revelation of KIT expression in GIST has not only revolutionized the pathologic criteria in classifying GIST, but also shed light into the histogenesis of these tumors (Hirota et al. 1998). KIT is also expressed and plays a critical role in the intestinal pacemaker, the interstitial cells of Cajal (ICC) (Maeda et al. 1992; Ward et al. 1994). Thus, the similarities in KIT expression and ultrastructural appearance between GISTs and the ICC suggested that GISTs derive from the ICC lineage.

GISTs occur with predilection in the stomach and small bowel, and the median age at diagnosis is about 60 years. The clinical spectrum ranges from benign, solitary tumors to multifocal intra-abdominal and/or liver metastases. The pathologic criteria most commonly used to predict clinical behavior in GIST are tumor size and mitotic activity. Before the development of imatinib mesylate, the treatment included surgery for primary tumors and was relatively ineffective for recurrent GIST (DeMatteo et al. 2000). GIST has been notoriously refractory to conventional chemotherapy with response rates of only 5% (Edmonson et al. 1993).

2 KIT Activation as Dominant Pathogenetic Mechanism

KIT was originally identified as the cellular homologue of the retroviral oncogene v-KIT in the Hardy–Zuckerman-4-feline sarcoma virus (Besmer et al. 1986). In humans, the *KIT* gene maps to 4q12–13, in the vicinity of the genes encoding for *PDGFRA* and *FLK1* receptor tyrosine kinases (RTK), and is composed of 21 exons, spanning 65 kb. The KIT protein belongs to the class III of RTK, together with macrophage colony stimulating factor (M-CSF) and platelet-derived growth factor receptor (PDGFR), based on their sequence homology and similar conformational structure. The KIT autophosphorylation on tyrosines and the association of KIT with substrates transduces the signals for various cellular responses, including cell proliferation, survival, adhesion, chemotaxis, and secretory responses. The downstream signaling cascades known to activate KIT include the Ras/MAP kinase, Rac/Rho-JNK, PI3 K/AKT, and src family kinase/signal transducer and activator of transcription (SFK/STAT) signaling networks.

The KIT receptor plays a critical role in the normal development and function of the ICC, as well as in hematopoiesis, gametogenesis, and melanogenesis during embryonic development and in postnatal organism (Maeda et al. 1992). As a consequence, loss-of-function mutations at either KIT or KIT ligand murine loci generate deficiencies in all these major cell systems. In contrast, the presence of KIT receptor activating mutations have been implicated in the pathogenesis of several human tumors, including seminomas (Tian et al. 1999), mastocytosis (Nagata et al. 1995), acute myelogenous leukemias (Gari et al. 1999), and more recently in melanomas (Willmore-Payne et al. 2005), suggesting a central role for KIT in oncogenesis.

In 1998, Kitamura and colleagues reported that GIST is commonly associated with mutations in the gene encoding the KIT receptor tyrosine kinase (Hirota et al. 1998). These mutations result in constitutive activation of KIT signaling. A few years later, Heinrich et al. identified oncogenic mutations in *PDGFRA*, a gene encoding for a closely related member of class III RTK, in a small subset of GIST (Heinrich et al. 2003b). Subsequently, a large number of studies have found that up to 90% of GIST contain activating mutations in either *KIT* or *PDGFRA* (Antonescu et al. 2003; Rubin et al. 2001). The majority of *KIT* mutations in GIST are somatic, although a few families with germ line mutations have been identified (Nishida et al. 1998). The frequency of *KIT* mutation in GIST ranges between 80 and 85%. Nevertheless, even GISTs without a documented mutation nearly all have phosphorylated KIT protein, implying activation (Rubin et al. 2001).

In more than 75% of the cases, *KIT* mutations identified in GISTs are localized within exon 11, which encodes for the juxtamembrane domain of the receptor. The most common site of *KIT* mutations is in the 5'end of exon 11. The types of mutations occurring in this hot-spot are quite heterogeneous, including in-frame deletions of variable sizes, point mutations, or deletions preceded by substitutions. Although mutations at this site are not associated with a specific clinicopathologic phenotype, the presence of deletions rather than substitutions predicts a more aggressive behavior. Specifically, deletions affecting codons WK557–558 indicate a poor prognosis (Wardelmann et al. 2003). A second, less common, hot spot is located at the 3'end of exon 11, which includes mainly internal tandem duplication mutations (ITDs) (Antonescu et al. 2003). GIST patients harboring ITD-type mutations follow a more indolent clinical course and their tumors are with predilection located in the stomach (Antonescu et al. 2003). The second most common site of *KIT* mutations, accounting for 10% of GIST patients, is located in exon

9, coding for the extracellular domain. Most *KIT* exon 9 mutations represent an insertion of two amino acids, AY 502–503. GISTs harboring *KIT* exon 9 mutations are characterized by small bowel location and aggressive clinical behavior (Antonescu et al. 2003). Infrequently, GISTs have a mutation in the kinase domain.

Mutations in *KIT* result in enhanced KIT activity through distinct molecular mechanisms. The integrity of the KIT juxtamembrane domain is important to maintain the kinase in its physiologic auto inhibited state. Deletion of tyr-567 and val-568 in the normal *KIT* gene have been shown to enhance agonist induced KIT signaling by altering the specificity of docking sites for cytoplasmic signaling molecules in the activated KIT receptor. Recently, the crystal structure of the KIT ectodomain was characterized, showing that KIT dimerization is driven by bivalent binding of KIT ligand and stabilized by lateral D4-D4 and D5-D5 interactions of two neighboring KIT ectodomains (Yuzawa et al. 2007). Activating oncogenic mutations within the ectodomain of KIT map to the D5-D5 interface, which presumably stabilize receptor dimers and thus activate the kinase in the absence of ligand.

A recent report identified that ETV1, an E-twenty-six (ETS) transcription factor, is highly overexpressed in GIST as well as in subtypes of ICC involved in KIT-mediated transformation (Chi et al. 2010). The dual requirement of KIT and ETV1 for the ICC normal development and GIST formation suggests a synergistic role in GIST pathogenesis. ETV1 transcriptional program is regulated by activated KIT, which prolongs ETV1 protein stability and cooperates with ETV1 to promote tumor development. These findings indicate that GIST may arise from ICCs with high levels of ETV1 expression which when coupled with an activating KIT mutation turns on an oncogenic ETS transcriptional program (Chi et al. 2010).

3 GIST with Wild-Type KIT

Further genomic profiling of human GIST samples has identified mutations in other growth factor receptor signaling pathways in GIST (Fig. 1). About one-third of GISTs lacking *KIT* mutations harbor a mutation in *PDGFRA*, within exons 12, 14, or 18 (Heinrich et al. 2003b; Lasota et al. 2004). Most GISTs with mutated *PDGFRA* have a distinct phenotype, including gastric location, epithelioid morphology, variable/absent KIT expression by immunohistochemistry, and an indolent clinical course (Lasota et al. 2004).

In about 10% of GIST patients no mutations in either *KIT* or *PDGFRA* have been identified. Among adult patients, the wild-type GIST subset represents a heterogeneous group with no particular association with anatomic location or clinical outcome. In contrast, GISTs occurring in children or in type 1 neurofibromatosis are nearly always wild-type (Agaram et al. 2008a; Mussi et al. 2008). In fact, pediatric GISTs represent a distinct clinicopathologic and molecular subset, with predilection for females, multifocal gastric tumors, and wild-type genotype (Agaram et al. 2008a).

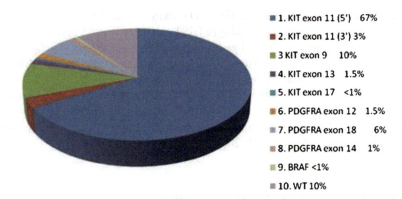

Fig. 1 Pie chart with distribution of *KIT*, *PDGFRA*, and B-rapidly accelerated fibrosarcoma (*BRAF*) mutations in GIST

In a recent study, we have identified a primary *BRAF* exon 15 V600E mutation in 7% of adult GIST patients, lacking *KIT/PDGFRA* mutations (Agaram et al. 2008b). The *BRAF*-mutated GISTs show predilection for small bowel location and high risk of malignancy. This finding delineates a new molecular group of patients who may benefit from selective *BRAF* inhibitors, as an alternative therapeutic option to imatinib.

Another interesting line of evidence is the transcriptional upregulation of IGF1R in pediatric GIST (Agaram et al. 2008a). This finding could indicate drug sensitivity to IGF1R-directed agents, such as the IGF1R antibodies, currently being tested in phase II clinical trials. Furthermore, IGF1R protein overexpression and low levels of IGF1R gene amplification were demonstrated recently in a small number of wild-type GISTs (Tarn et al. 2008). This report also shows that inhibition of IGF1R activity by NVP-AEW541 (a small molecule IGF1R inhibitor, Novartis) in GIST cell lines leads to cytotoxicity and apoptosis via AKT and MAPK signaling.

Although most commonly occurring in sporadic settings, GIST has been described as part of certain syndromes, such as familial GIST, Carney's triad, Carney-Stratakis syndrome (CSS), and neurofibromatosis. The association of multifocal gastric GIST with paragangliomas and pulmonary chondromas affecting mostly females is diagnostic of Carney's triad. More recently, it was recognized that the autosomal dominant inheritance of the dyad "paraganglioma and gastric GIST", or the CSS, represents a separate condition which affects both males and females and lacks the association with pulmonary chondromas. Mutations of genes coding for succinate dehydrogenase (SDH) subunits, typically associated with familial paragangliomas, are also identified in CSS (Pasini et al. 2008). In contrast, the pathogenesis of Carney's triad tumors, including GIST, remains undefined, with a recent comprehensive genetic analysis of 41 tumors from 37 patients failed to identify any activating mutations in the coding region of *KIT*, *PDGFRA*, and *SDH A-D* (Matyakhina et al. 2007). However, more recently, a significant loss in succinate dehydrogenase B (SDHB) protein expression compared to KIT mutant GIST was identified in wild-type/pediatric GIST (Janeway et al. 2011). Genomic DNA sequencing in 34 pediatric and wild-type GIST patients without a personal or family history of paraganglioma showed germline mutations in *SDHB* or *SDHC* in 12% of cases (Janeway et al. 2011). These results suggest that testing for germline *SDH* mutations is recommended in wild-type GIST patients.

GIST occurring in the setting of neurofibromatosis type 1 patients is secondary to a somatic inactivation of the wild-type NF1 allele in the tumor (Maertens et al. 2006). *KIT* or *PDGFRA* mutations have been documented only infrequently in these latter tumors (Mussi et al. 2008).

4 Treatment of GIST with Imatinib

Imatinib mesylate (STI571, Gleevec^{TM}, Novartis Pharmaceuticals, Basel, Switzerland) is a selective tyrosine kinase inhibitor whose targets include Abl, Bcr-Abl, KIT, and PDGFR (see also "JAK-mutant Myeloproliferative Neoplasms"). Imatinib is a 2 phenyl-amino-pyrimidine derivative, which specifically binds to the inactive conformation of the Abl kinase or the inactive form of KIT.

4.1 Imatinib Monotherapy for Advanced GIST

Imatinib mesylate was first applied in 1998 to refractory CML and subsequently to advanced GIST patients in 2000 (Druker et al. 1996; Joensuu et al. 2001). Imatinib achieves partial responses or stable disease in nearly 80% of GIST patients, and remarkably the 2 year survival in advanced GIST is now 75–80% (Demetri et al. 2002). The long-term outcome of imatinib treatment for metastatic GIST has emerged from several large trials. Approximately 45% of patients with metastatic GIST have a measurable response after administration of imatinib, while about 30% will have at least stable disease (Demetri et al. 2002). Only a minority of GIST patients are insensitive to imatinib (so-called "primary resistance").

The response rates of GIST patients to imatinib are influenced by the *KIT* genotype of the tumor (Heinrich et al. 2003a). Patients with KIT exon 11 mutations have a partial response rate of 84% compared with a 0% partial response rate among patients without KIT mutations (Heinrich et al. 2003a). Imatinib therapy in pediatric GIST, predominantly associated with a wild-type genotype for *KIT/PDGFRA/BRAF* has been disappointing (Agaram et al. 2008a). Furthermore, tumors with activation loop mutations particularly show the least response to imatinib inhibition. Patients with a GIST harboring an extracellular domain mutation (*KIT* exon 9) have an intermediate response, with about 45% partial response rate (Heinrich et al. 2003a). Significantly higher progression-free survival in *KIT* exon 9 mutant patients may be achievable with a high-dose imatinib regimen (800 mg daily) (Debiec-Rychter et al. 2006).

Imatinib interruption in patients with advanced GIST controlled with imatinib is often associated with a high risk of disease progression within 1 year. In most patients, however, the disease is controlled with imatinib re-challenge, with no statistically significant differences in imatinib-refractory progression-free survival between interruption and continuation (Lee et al. 2006).

4.2 Imatinib Plus Surgery for Advanced GIST

There are several reasons to consider surgical resection in patients with metastatic GIST who are being treated with molecular therapy. While tyrosine kinase inhibitors (TKI) induce marked tumor regression in the majority of patients, complete responses are rarely achieved. One possible hypothesis is that the chance of resistance is proportional to the amount of residual viable GIST following therapy with TKI. While it has been shown that tumor load can continue to decrease even after a year of imatinib therapy, the median time to best response is approximately 3.5 months and there is little incremental shrinkage after 9 months (Verweij et al. 2004). Thus patients with advanced GIST who have stable or responsive disease on imatinib seem to benefit from elective surgical resection.

The optimal timing of surgery in relation to imatinib therapy for patients with advanced GIST is still debatable, but our experience in responsive disease suggests that surgical resection after 3–6 months with tyrosine kinase inhibition is beneficial if their disease appears completely resectable (DeMatteo et al. 2007). It is critical to continue tyrosine kinase inhibition postoperatively to delay, or possibly even prevent, subsequent progression. Patients with metastatic GIST who were randomized to stop imatinib after 1 year of therapy subsequently developed progressive disease (Blay 2004). The optimal duration of tyrosine kinase inhibitor therapy after resection of metastatic GIST is unknown at this time. Once resistance to imatinib develops, there is currently only a small chance of rescuing the patient and surgical debulking has not shown benefit in patients who develop imatinib resistance (DeMatteo et al. 2007).

There have been initial concerns that targeted therapy might increase postoperative complications. However, long-term cessation of imatinib has been associated with a flare phenomenon, accompanied by marked clinical deterioration. Subsequently, several studies have suggested that continuing imatinib treatment until 1 day before surgery does not increase postoperative complications and that imatinib can be safely restarted within 2 weeks after surgery (Barnes et al. 2005).

4.3 Adjuvant Imatinib Therapy After Resection of a Primary GIST

In a recent randomized phase III, double-blind, placebo-controlled, multicenter trial, following the resection of a primary GIST, adjuvant therapy with imatinib was safe and significantly prolonged recurrence-free survival compared to placebo treatment (Dematteo et al. 2009). Eligible patients had complete gross resection of a primary GIST at least 3 cm in size and positive for the KIT protein by immunohistochemistry. Patients were randomly assigned to imatinib 400 mg or to placebo daily for 1 year after surgical resection. Patients assigned to placebo were eligible to crossover to imatinib treatment in the event of tumor recurrence. The primary endpoint was recurrence-free survival. Accrual was stopped early because the trial results crossed the interim analysis efficacy boundary for recurrence-free survival. However, there was no difference observed in the overall survival in the short-term follow-up available. These findings impacted the management of patients with primary GIST and prompted the FDA approval of imatinib in the adjuvant setting.

4.4 Evaluation of Tumor Response to Imatinib

Clinical response to targeted therapy has been assessed based on imaging methods using conventional Southwest Oncology Group (SWOG)/Response Evaluation Criteria in Solid Tumors (RECIST) criteria on contrast-enhanced CT or MRI images. In addition to size, the attenuation of a lesion, the presence of new lesions and/or sites of involvement, and nodules within any pre-existing lesions are used to determine resistance (Choi 2005) (Figs. 2, 3). Because of the 95% correlation between the information from regular contrast-enhanced CT and PET-CT scans, administration of FDG involves exposure to extra radiation, and intravenous contrast CT has a definition superior to non-contrast PET scans; CT scans with intravenous contrast are the preferred routine imaging modality for GIST patients undergoing TKI therapy.

It is still debatable how accurately these imaging tools correlate with the biology of stable or responsive GIST lesions, and whether they have the sensitivity to detect a subset of tumors or the small region of a tumor undergoing sub-clinical progression. A further unresolved question relates to the heterogeneity of imatinib stable lesions from a pathologic or molecular standpoint. Scaife et al. (2003) compared the radiologic and pathologic responses in imatinib-treated GIST followed by surgical resection and found that CT scans inaccurately predicted the histologic response in 30% of patients, while PET scans failed to predict a pathologic response in 64% of patients.

A recent comprehensive pathologic analysis showed that histologic response of GIST to imatinib therapy is variable and heterogeneous (Agaram et al. 2007). The histologic response varies from nodule to nodule within the same resection, as well as within the same lesion. Some tumors may show only gross tumor necrosis, with large, central areas of cystification and hemorrhage, whereas the remaining solid areas are viable microscopically. Dense hyalinization with complete loss of tumor cells is rare. Even in tumors with a very good histologic response, microscopic foci of viable and mitotically active cells are often present (Fig. 4). The assessment of

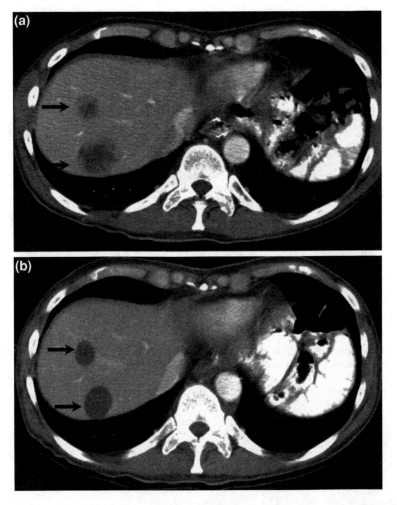

Fig. 2 Effects of imatinib response on CT. **a** Pre-treatment GIST patient with multiple liver metastases. **b** Two months post-treatment showing hepatic metastasis has become homogeneous and hypodense but with minimal change in tumor size

tumor proliferation (Ki67 index) in these viable areas may serve as an indicator of the aggressive nature of the residual viable tumor. A subset of responsive GIST tumors may show weak or even negative KIT immunostaining, compared to the pre-imatinib tumor sample. Furthermore, a small group of imatinib responsive tumors can show well-differentiated smooth muscle features, suggesting that imatinib may induce a trans-differentiation towards a smooth muscle phenotype, through chronic inactivation of KIT signaling (Agaram et al. 2007).

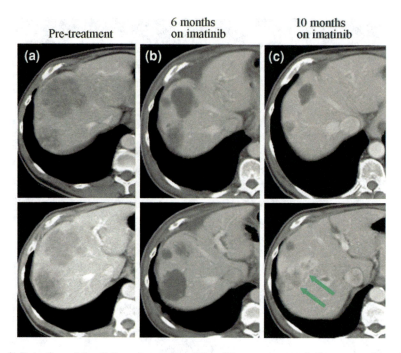

Fig. 3 Detection of imatinib resistance by CT. **a** Liver metastases before start of imatinib therapy. **b** Radiologic evidence of response after 6 months of imatinib treatment showing decrease in tumor density. **c** Development of focal imatinib-resistance after 10 months on therapy, with increase of tumor density and hypervascularization

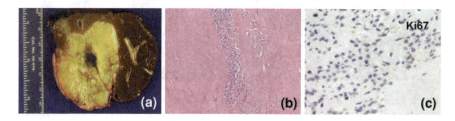

Fig. 4 Pathologic response in a clinically responsive patient to imatinib therapy. **a** Gross appearance of a liver metastasis showing large tumor with myxoid and gelatinous degeneration. **b** Histologic appearance reveals few microscopic foci of viable GIST in a background of extensive-treatment induced changes (*fibrosis*). **c** The viable foci show no proliferative activity by Ki67 proliferation index

5 Acquired Imatinib Resistance

Most GIST patients who initially respond to imatinib therapy eventually experience tumor progression despite continued imatinib therapy. Although the 2 year survival of patients with metastatic GIST treated with imatinib approximates 72%, half of the patients develop disease progression by 2 years (Antonescu et al. 2005). Once resistance to imatinib develops, there is currently only a small chance of rescuing the patient. Dose escalation of imatinib in 133 patients who progressed at 400 mg per day resulted in a median time to progression of only 81 days, and only 18% were progression-free at 1 year (Zalcberg et al. 2005).

The majority of tumors with acquired imatinib resistance show reactivation of KIT and remain KIT dependent (Antonescu et al. 2005). The predominant mechanism of acquired resistance to imatinib is via additional mutations in the *KIT* kinase domain found in 46–67% of patients (Antonescu et al. 2005; Debiec-Rychter et al. 2005). These secondary mutations tend to be single amino acid substitutions in the catalytic domain (exon 17) or in the ATP-binding domain (exons 13 and 14) (Antonescu et al. 2005). The first and the second mutations are consistently located on the same allele of the *KIT* gene (*cis*-location). Second site mutations stabilize the active conformation of the KIT kinase which prevents imatinib binding or interferes with imatinib binding without affecting KIT kinase conformation (Antonescu et al. 2005). Second-site *KIT* mutations are rare in GISTs responsive to imatinib compared with imatinib-resistant tumors (Agaram et al. 2007).

At what point during the disease course these secondary *KIT* mutations occur is currently unclear. Resistant patients with secondary mutations have been treated with imatinib longer than resistant patients lacking secondary mutations (median 27 vs 14.5 months) (Antonescu et al. 2005), suggesting that clonal selection of existing mutations prior to imatinib therapy is unlikely to explain acquired resistance. Furthermore, secondary mutations are typically not seen in the pre-imatinib or primary resistant tumors. The frequency of secondary mutations is also determined by the location of the primary *KIT* mutations, with GISTs harboring *KIT* exon 11 mutations more commonly becoming imatinib-resistant due to acquisition of secondary mutations, as compared to *KIT* exon 9 mutated GIST (Antonescu et al. 2005). This observation further supports that the probability of developing a secondary mutation increases with the duration of imatinib treatment, which is often longer in GISTs harboring exon 11 mutation than in those with exon 9 mutation or wild-type GISTs.

Another level of complexity relies on the fact that long-term imatinib therapy leads to clonal selection of distinct resistant tumor sub clones, the so-called *polyclonal acquired resistance* (Heinrich et al. 2006; Wardelmann et al. 2006). Thus, each tumor nodule under progression may undergo individual clonal evolution, resulting in multiple secondary mutations developed at different metastatic sites within the same patient. As such, designing salvage strategies in these imatinib-resistant settings should address inhibition of all the known genomic activating mutations in the oncoprotein. The complexity of secondary mutations in imatinib-resistant patients argues that single next-generation kinase inhibitors will not be beneficial in all mutant clones.

One third of imatinib-resistant GISTs lack secondary mutations, suggesting that additional mechanisms of resistance might be responsible, such as *KIT* genomic amplification and activation of an alternative receptor tyrosine kinase protein in

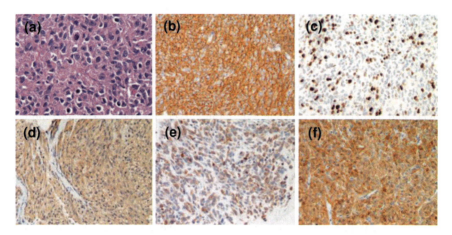

Fig. 5 Pathologic features of imatinib-resistance in a patient with a GIST harboring a primary *KIT exon* 11 *V560D* mutation and a second site mutation in *KIT exon* 17 *N822K*. Morphologic appearance showing increased cellularity (H&E) (**a**), Strong immunoreactivity for KIT (**b**), as well as a high Ki67 proliferation index (**c**), activation of P-AKT (Ser473) (**d**), P-S6(Ser235/236) (**e**), and P-4E-BP1(Thr37/46) (**f**)

the absence of KIT expression. In a recent study we have identified the presence of a *V600E BRAF* exon 15 mutation in one of 28 imatinib resistant GISTs, lacking a defined mechanism of drug resistance. The imatinib resistant tumor, resected after 20 months of imatinib therapy, showed a trans-differentiation into a rhabdomyosarcoma phenotype, with loss of KIT and PDGFRA protein expression. Thus secondary *V600E BRAF* mutations could represent an alternative mechanism of imatinib resistance (Agaram et al. 2008b).

Microscopically, the clinically resistant tumors show marked increased cellularity, and a significantly higher mitotic activity compared to pre-imatinib biopsies (Fig. 5). Both primary and secondary imatinib resistant tumors show strong and diffuse KIT immunopositivity (Antonescu et al. 2005). The degree of KIT phosphorylation appears significantly higher than in non-treated, imatinib-naive GISTs, however, within the resistant subset, the degree of KIT activation is consistently high, regardless of the type of primary *KIT* mutation, the status of secondary *KIT* mutations, or the type of clinical resistance (primary versus secondary) (Antonescu et al. 2005). Rarely is loss of KIT expression noted in imatinib-resistant tumors, suggesting activation of KIT-independent oncogenic pathways. One such example is *dedifferentiated GIST*, defined as tumor progression from a conventional KIT positive GIST to an anaplastic/pleomorphic KIT negative tumor. Changing phenotype after chronic exposure to imatinib includes not only the complete loss of KIT reactivity, but also the aberrant expression of epithelial and muscle markers (Pauwels et al. 2005). More recently, Liegl et al. reported five cases of progressing metastatic GIST with heterologous rhabdomyoblastic differentiation after imatinib treatment. Primary KIT mutations were detected in both the conventional GIST and rhabdomyoblastic components, but no secondary mutations of the type associated with TKI resistance were identified in the dedifferentiated or rhabdomyoblastic areas (Liegl et al. 2009).

6 Overcoming Imatinib Resistance

It is now apparent that during the chronic course of imatinib treatment a significant subset of GIST patients develop resistance, and as a result considerable effort is focused on the development of novel TKI. Sunitinib malate (Pfizer, New York, NY), a multi-targeted TKI with potent anti-angiogenic and direct anti-tumor activities, is the only FDA approved second line therapy for patients with imatinib-resistant or intolerant GIST (February 2006). Sunitinib potently inhibits FLT3, PDGFRA, PDGFRB, vascular endothelial growth factor receptor (VEGFR1, VEGFR2) and KIT. The clinical benefit of sunitinib is genotype-dependent on both the primary and secondary mutations in KIT. It has been shown to give at least short-term clinical benefits in about 65% of GIST patients who are refractory to imatinib. Particularly, it shows superior efficacy in GIST patients hosting *KIT* exon 9 mutations (Demetri et al. 2009). However, only about one-quarter of patients who are switched to sunitinib will continue to have responsive disease a year later (Demetri et al. 2009).

Other KIT inhibitors presently tested in clinical trials of imatinib/sunitinib-resistant GIST include a number of second-generation small molecule inhibitors, such as nilotinib, dasatinib, and sorafenib. According to in vitro data these inhibitors appear to have higher efficacy and potency in the imatinib-resistant mutations (Guo et al. 2007). Nilotinib (Novartis) showed potent inhibition of mutant and wild-type KIT phosphorylation and is now investigated in phase II clinical trials. In our cell-based assays (Guo et al. 2007), dasatinib (Bristol Myers Squibb) inhibited the kinase activity of activation loop mutant KIT isoforms. Furthermore, it also induced cell apoptosis and inhibited cell proliferation in a KIT phosphorylation inhibition-dependent manner.

Given the consistent overexpression of PKCθ in most GISTs, protein kinase C (PKC) inhibitors may inhibit both KIT and PKCθ, and thus may exert higher potency than imatinib in imatinib-sensitive GISTs, as well as in imatinib-resistant GISTs. PKC412 is a novel staurosporine-derived tyrosine kinase inhibitor that targets PKC, kinase insert domain-containing receptor (KDR), Fms-like tyrosine kinase 3 (FLT3), PDGFRA, and KIT. It has been shown in systemic mast cell disease that PKC412 potently inhibits KIT exon 17 mutants D816V and D816Y, which are quite refractory to several kinase inhibitors (Growney et al. 2005). PKC412 was also tested in imatinib-resistant GIST cell lines and showed to reduce KIT autophosphorylation at a level between 500 and 1,000 nm (Debiec-Rychter et al. 2005).

Alternative salvage options other than inhibiting KIT signaling pathway are presently being explored. These strategies promise a therapeutic solution to the challenge of heterogeneous imatinib resistance. Bauer et al. (2006) investigated the activity of heat shock protein 90 (HSP90) inhibitor 17-allylamino-18-demethoxy-geldanamycin (17-AAG) in enhancing cellular degradation of constitutively activated KIT oncoprotein. Thus, 17-AAG was effective in inhibiting KIT-dependent imatinib sensitive and imatinib-resistant GIST cell lines, but not KIT-independent GIST cells, suggesting that its effects result mainly from inactivation of KIT oncoprotein. Taking a different approach, (Sambol et al. 2006) showed the efficacy of flavopiridol, a cyclin-dependent kinase inhibitor, on a primary GIST cell line carrying an imatinib-sensitive KIT K642E exon 13 mutation, by induction of apoptosis and transcriptional down-regulation of KIT. A possible combination of targeted kinase inhibitors with drugs such as flavopiridol or 17-AAG may be more effective in the setting of polyclonal acquired resistance. Other broad therapeutic strategies include targeting KIT downstream targets, such as PI3-K or MAPK/MEK inhibitors.

7 Future Perspectives

The biological complexity encountered in the various molecular subsets of GISTs described in this review, as well as the concomitant increase in patients' life expectancy has enhanced the need for new therapeutic options to overcome the development of primary and secondary resistance to TKI. Furthermore, the clonal evolution exhibited by TKI-resistant GIST, with distinct second site *KIT* mutations in different nodules or different areas of the progressing tumor, underscores the limited effectiveness of a single, next generation TKI, expected to inhibit all permutations. Novel kinase inhibitors such as the allosteric or switch-pocket inhibitors of KIT, which stabilize the auto inhibited conformation of the respective kinase, suggest promising results, but have so far lagged in their development and applicability for clinical use. Future clinical trials should focus more on combination strategies, including both kinase inhibitors and downstream inhibitors. In contrast, the future perspectives in the pediatric and wild-type GIST include targeting the IGF1R and/or the SDH pathways, as two leading directions of drug development and further pre-clinical investigation.

References

Agaram NP, Besmer P, Wong GC, Guo T, Socci ND, Maki RG, DeSantis D, Brennan MF, Singer S, DeMatteo RP, Antonescu CR (2007) Pathologic and molecular heterogeneity in imatinib-stable or imatinib-responsive gastrointestinal stromal tumors. Clin Cancer Res 13:170–181

Agaram NP, Laquaglia MP, Ustun B, Guo T, Wong GC, Socci ND, Maki RG, DeMatteo RP, Besmer P, Antonescu CR (2008a) Molecular characterization of pediatric gastrointestinal stromal tumors. Clin Cancer Res 14:3204–3215

Agaram NP, Wong GC, Guo T, Maki RG, Singer S, Dematteo RP, Besmer P, Antonescu CR (2008b) Novel V600E BRAF mutations in imatinib-naive and imatinib-resistant gastrointestinal stromal tumors. Genes Chromosomes Cancer 47:853–859

Antonescu CR, Sommer G, Sarran L, Tschernyavsky SJ, Riedel E, Woodruff JM, Robson M, Maki R, Brennan MF, Ladanyi M, DeMatteo RP, Besmer P (2003) Association of KIT exon 9 mutations with nongastric primary site and aggressive behavior: KIT mutation analysis and clinical correlates of 120 gastrointestinal stromal tumors. Clin Cancer Res 9:3329–3337

Antonescu CR, Besmer P, Guo T, Arkun K, Hom G, Koryotowski B, Leversha MA, Jeffrey PD, Desantis D, Singer S, Brennan MF, Maki RG, DeMatteo RP (2005) Acquired resistance to imatinib in gastrointestinal stromal tumor occurs through secondary gene mutation. Clin Cancer Res 11:4182–4190

Barnes G, Bulusu VR, Hardwick RH, Carroll N, Hatcher H, Earl HM, Save VE, Balan K, Jamieson NV (2005) A review of the surgical management of metastatic gastrointestinal stromal tumours (GISTs) on imatinib mesylate (Glivec). Int J Surg 3:206–212

Bauer S, Yu LK, Demetri GD, Fletcher JA (2006) Heat shock protein 90 inhibition in imatinib-resistant gastrointestinal stromal tumor. Cancer Res 66:9153–9161

Besmer P, Murphy JE, George PC, Qiu FH, Bergold PJ, Lederman L, Snyder HW Jr, Brodeur D, Zuckerman EE, Hardy WD (1986) A new acute transforming feline retrovirus and relationship of its oncogene v-KIT with the protein kinase gene family. Nature 320:415–421

Blay J, Berthaud P, Perol D et al. (2004) Continuous vs intermittent imatinib treatment in advanced GIST after one year: A prospective randomized phase III trial of the french sarcoma group. ASCO annual meeting

Chi P, Chen Y, Zhang L, Guo X, Wongvipat J, Shamu T, Fletcher JA, Dewell S, Maki RG, Zheng D, Antonescu CR, Allis CD, Sawyers CL (2010) ETV1 is a lineage survival factor that cooperates with KIT in gastrointestinal stromal tumours. Nature 467:849–853

Choi H (2005) Critical issues in response evaluation on computed tomography: lessons from the gastrointestinal stromal tumor model. Curr Oncol Rep 7:307–311

Debiec-Rychter M, Cools J, Dumez H, Sciot R, Stul M, Mentens N, Vranckx H, Wasag B, Prenen H, Roesel J, Hagemeijer A, Van Oosterom A, Marynen P (2005) Mechanisms of resistance to imatinib mesylate in gastrointestinal stromal tumors and activity of the PKC412 inhibitor against imatinib-resistant mutants. Gastroenterology 128:270–279

Debiec-Rychter M, Sciot R, Le Cesne A, Schlemmer M, Hohenberger P, van Oosterom AT, Blay JY, Leyvraz S, Stul M, Casali PG, Zalcberg J, Verweij J, Van Glabbeke M, Hagemeijer A, Judson I (2006) KIT mutations and dose selection for imatinib in patients with advanced gastrointestinal stromal tumours. Eur J Cancer 42:1093–1103

DeMatteo RP, Lewis JJ, Leung D et al (2000) Two hundred gastrointestinal stromal tumors: recurrence patterns and prognostic factors for survival. Ann Surg 231:51–58

DeMatteo RP, Maki RG, Singer S, Gonen M, Brennan MF, Antonescu CR (2007) Results of tyrosine kinase inhibitor therapy followed by surgical resection for metastatic gastrointestinal stromal tumor. Ann Surg 245:347–352

Dematteo RP, Ballman KV, Antonescu CR, Maki RG, Pisters PW, Demetri GD, Blackstein ME, Blanke CD, von Mehren M, Brennan MF, Patel S, McCarter MD, Polikoff JA, Tan BR, Owzar K (2009) Adjuvant imatinib mesylate after resection of localised, primary gastrointestinal stromal tumour: a randomised, double-blind, placebo-controlled trial. Lancet 373:1097–1104

Demetri GD, von Mehren M, Blanke CD et al (2002) Efficacy and safety of imatinib mesylate in advanced gastrointestinal stromal tumors. N Engl J Med 347:472–480

Demetri GD, Heinrich MC, Fletcher JA, Fletcher CD, Van den Abbeele AD, Corless CL, Antonescu CR, George S, Morgan JA, Chen MH, Bello CL, Huang X, Cohen DP, Baum CM, Maki RG (2009) Molecular target modulation, imaging, and clinical evaluation of gastrointestinal stromal tumor patients treated with sunitinib malate after imatinib failure. Clin Cancer Res 15:5902–5909

Druker BJ, Tamura S, Buchdunger E et al (1996) Effects of a selective inhibitor of the Abl tyrosine kinase on the growth of Bcr-Abl positive cells. Nat Med 2:561–566

Edmonson JH, Ryan LM, Blum RH, Brooks JS, Shiraki M, Frytak S, Parkinson DR (1993) Randomized comparison of doxorubicin alone versus ifosfamide plus doxorubicin or mitomycin, doxorubicin, and cisplatin against advanced soft tissue sarcomas. J Clin Oncol 11:1269–1275

Gari M, Goodeve A, Wilson G, Winship P, Langabeer S, Linch D, Vandenberghe E, Peake I, Reilly J (1999) c-KIT proto-oncogene exon 8 in-frame deletion plus insertion mutations in acute myeloid leukaemia. Br J Haematol 105:894–900

Growney JD, Clark JJ, Adelsperger J, Stone R, Fabbro D, Griffin JD, Gilliland DG (2005) Activation mutations of human c-KIT resistant to imatinib mesylate are sensitive to the tyrosine kinase inhibitor PKC412. Blood 106:721–724

Guo T, Agaram NP, Wong GC, Hom G, D'Adamo D, Maki RG, Schwartz GK, Veach D, Clarkson BD, Singer S, DeMatteo RP, Besmer P, Antonescu CR (2007) Sorafenib inhibits the imatinib-resistant KITT670I gatekeeper mutation in gastrointestinal stromal tumor. Clin Cancer Res 13:4874–4881

Heinrich MC, Corless CL, Demetri GD et al (2003a) Kinase mutations and imatinib response in patients with metastatic gastrointestinal stromal tumor. J Clin Oncol 21:4342–4349

Heinrich MC, Corless CL, Duensing A, McGreevey L, Chen CJ, Joseph N, Singer S, Griffith DJ, Haley A, Town A, Demetri GD, Fletcher CD, Fletcher JA (2003b) PDGFRA activating mutations in gastrointestinal stromal tumors. Science 299:708–710

Heinrich MC, Corless CL, Blanke CD, Demetri GD, Joensuu H, Roberts PJ, Eisenberg BL, von Mehren M, Fletcher CD, Sandau K, McDougall K, Ou WB, Chen CJ, Fletcher JA (2006) Molecular correlates of imatinib resistance in gastrointestinal stromal tumors. J Clin Oncol 24:4764–4774

Hirota S, Isozaki K, Moriyama Y, Hashimoto K, Nishida T, Ishiguro S, Kawano K, Hanada M, Kurata A, Takeda M, Muhammad Tunio G, Matsuzawa Y, Kanakura Y, Shinomura Y, Kitamura Y (1998) Gain-of-function mutations of c-KIT in human gastrointestinal stromal tumors. Science 279:577–580

Janeway KA, Kim SY, Lodish M, Nose V, Rustin P, Gaal J, Dahia PL, Liegl B, Ball ER, Raygada M, Lai AH, Kelly L, Hornick JL, O'Sullivan M, de Krijger RR, Dinjens WN, Demetri GD, Antonescu CR, Fletcher JA, Helman L, Stratakis CA (2011) Defects in succinate dehydrogenase in gastrointestinal stromal tumors lacking KIT and PDGFRA mutations. Proc Nat Acad Sci U S A 108:314–318

Joensuu H, Roberts PJ, Sarlomo-Rikala M et al (2001) Effect of the tyrosine kinase inhibitor STI571 in a patient with a metastatic gastrointestinal stromal tumor. N Engl J Med 344:1052–1056

Lasota J, Dansonka-Mieszkowska A, Sobin LH et al (2004) A great majority of GISTs with PDGFRA mutations represent gastric tumors of low or no malignant potential. Lab Invest 84:874–883

Lee JL, Ryu MH, Chang HM, Kim TW, Kang HJ, Sohn HJ, Lee JS, Kang YK (2006) Clinical outcome in gastrointestinal stromal tumor patients who interrupted imatinib after achieving stable disease or better response. Jpn J Clin Oncol 36:704–711

Liegl B, Hornick JL, Antonescu C, Corless C, Fletcher CD (2009) Rhabdomyosarcomatous differentiation in gastrointestinal stromal tumors after tyrosine kinase inhibitor therapy: a novel form of tumor progression. Am J Surg Pathol 33(2):218–226

Maeda H, Yamagata A, Nishikawa S, Yoshinaga K, Kobayashi S, Nishi K (1992) Requirement of c-KIT for development of intestinal pacemaker system. Development 116:369–375

Maertens O, Prenen H, Debiec-Rychter M, Wozniak A, Sciot R, Pauwels P, De Wever I, Vermeesch JR, de Raedt T, De Paepe A, Speleman F, van Oosterom A, Messiaen L, Legius E (2006) Molecular pathogenesis of multiple gastrointestinal stromal tumors in NF1 patients. Hum Mol Genet 15:1015–1023

Matyakhina L, Bei TA, McWhinney SR, Pasini B, Cameron S, Gunawan B, Stergiopoulos SG, Boikos S, Muchow M, Dutra A, Pak E, Campo E, Cid MC, Gomez F, Gaillard RC, Assie G, Fuzesi L, Baysal BE, Eng C, Carney JA, Stratakis CA (2007) Genetics of carney triad: recurrent losses at chromosome 1 but lack of germline mutations in genes associated with paragangliomas and gastrointestinal stromal tumors. J Clin Endocrinol Metab 92:2938–2943

Mussi C, Schildhaus HU, Gronchi A, Wardelmann E, Hohenberger P (2008) Therapeutic consequences from molecular biology for gastrointestinal stromal tumor patients affected by neurofibromatosis type 1. Clin Cancer Res 14:4550–4555

Nagata H, Worobec AS, Oh CK, Chowdhury BA, Tannenbaum S, Suzuki Y, Metcalfe DD (1995) Identification of a point mutation in the catalytic domain of the protooncogene c-KIT in peripheral blood mononuclear cells of patients who have mastocytosis with an associated hematologic disorder. Proc Natl Acad Sci U S A 92:10560–10564

Nishida T, Hirota S, Taniguchi M, Hashimoto K, Isozaki K, Nakamura H, Kanakura Y, Tanaka T, Takabayashi A, Matsuda H, Kitamura Y (1998) Familial gastrointestinal stromal tumours with germline mutation of the KIT gene. Nat Genet 19:323–324

Pasini B, McWhinney SR, Bei T, Matyakhina L, Stergiopoulos S, Muchow M, Boikos SA, Ferrando B, Pacak K, Assie G, Baudin E, Chompret A, Ellison JW, Briere JJ, Rustin P, Gimenez-Roqueplo AP, Eng C, Carney JA, Stratakis CA (2008) Clinical and molecular genetics of patients with the Carney-Stratakis syndrome and germline mutations of the genes coding for the succinate dehydrogenase subunits SDHB, SDHC, and SDHD. Eur J Hum Genet 16:79–88

Pauwels P, Debiec-Rychter M, Stul M, De Wever I, Van Oosterom AT, Sciot R (2005) Changing phenotype of gastrointestinal stromal tumours under imatinib mesylate treatment: a potential diagnostic pitfall. Histopathology 47:41–47

Rubin BP, Singer S, Tsao C, Duensing A, Lux ML, Ruiz R, Hibbard MK, Chen CJ, Xiao S, Tuveson DA, Demetri GD, Fletcher CD, Fletcher JA (2001) KIT activation is a ubiquitous feature of gastrointestinal stromal tumors. Cancer Res 61:8118–8121

Sambol EB, Ambrosini G, Geha RC, Kennealey PT, Decarolis P, O'Connor R, Wu YV, Motwani M, Chen JH, Schwartz GK, Singer S (2006) Flavopiridol targets c-KIT transcription and induces apoptosis in gastrointestinal stromal tumor cells. Cancer Res 66:5858–5866

Scaife CL, Hunt KK, Patel SR, Benjamin RS, Burgess MA, Chen LL, Trent J, Raymond AK, Cormier JN, Pisters PW, Pollock RE, Feig BW (2003) Is there a role for surgery in patients with "unresectable" c-KIT + gastrointestinal stromal tumors treated with imatinib mesylate? Am J Surg 186:665–669

Tarn C, Rink L, Merkel E, Flieder D, Pathak H, Koumbi D, Testa JR, Eisenberg B, von Mehren M, Godwin AK (2008) Insulin-like growth factor 1 receptor is a potential therapeutic target for gastrointestinal stromal tumors. Proc Natl Acad Sci U S A 105:8387–8392

Tian Q, Frierson HF Jr, Krystal GW, Moskaluk CA (1999) Activating c-KIT gene mutations in human germ cell tumors. Am J Pathol 154:1643–1647

Verweij J, Casali PG, Zalcberg J et al (2004) Progression-free survival in gastrointestinal stromal tumours with high-dose imatinib: randomised trial. Lancet 364:1127–1134

Ward SM, Burns AJ, Torihashi S, Sanders KM (1994) Mutation of the proto-oncogene c-KIT blocks development of interstitial cells and electrical rhythmicity in murine intestine. J Physiol 480(Pt 1):91–97

Wardelmann E, Losen I, Hans V, Neidt I, Speidel N, Bierhoff E, Heinicke T, Pietsch T, Buttner R, Merkelbach-Bruse S (2003) Deletion of Trp-557 and Lys-558 in the juxtamembrane domain of the c-KIT protooncogene is associated with metastatic behavior of gastrointestinal stromal tumors. Int J Cancer 106:887–895

Wardelmann E, Merkelbach-Bruse S, Pauls K, Thomas N, Schildhaus HU, Heinicke T, Speidel N, Pietsch T, Buettner R, Pink D, Reichardt P, Hohenberger P (2006) Polyclonal evolution of multiple secondary KIT mutations in gastrointestinal stromal tumors under treatment with imatinib mesylate. Clin Cancer Res 12:1743–1749

Willmore-Payne C, Holden JA, Tripp S, Layfield LJ (2005) Human malignant melanoma: detection of BRAF- and c-KIT-activating mutations by high-resolution amplicon melting analysis. Hum Pathol 36:486–493

Yuzawa S, Opatowsky Y, Zhang Z, Mandiyan V, Lax I, Schlessinger J (2007) Structural basis for activation of the receptor tyrosine kinase KIT by stem cell factor. Cell 130:323–334

Zalcberg JR, Verweij J, Casali PG, Le Cesne A, Reichardt P, Blay JY, Schlemmer M, Van Glabbeke M, Brown M, Judson IR (2005) Outcome of patients with advanced gastro-intestinal stromal tumours crossing over to a daily imatinib dose of 800 mg after progression on 400 mg. Eur J Cancer 41:1751–1757

EGFR Mutant Lung Cancer

Yixuan Gong and William Pao

Abstract Thoracic oncologists traditionally have made treatment decisions based upon tumor histology, distinguishing non-small cell lung cancer (NSCLC) from small cell lung cancer (SCLC). However, recent data has revealed that at least one histological subtype of NSCLC, lung adenocarcinoma comprises multiple molecularly distinct diseases. Lung adenocarcinoma subsets now can be defined by specific 'driver' mutations in genes encoding components of the EGFR signaling pathway. Importantly, these mutations have implications regarding targeted therapy. Here, we focus on *EGFR* mutant NSCLC—a prime example of a clinically relevant molecular subset of lung cancer, with defined mechanisms of drug sensitivity, primary drug resistance, and acquired resistance to EGFR tyrosine kinase inhibitors. Efforts are now being made to overcome mechanisms of acquired resistance. These findings illustrate how knowledge about the genetic drivers of tumors can lead to rational targeted therapy for individual patients.

Contents

1 Introduction.. 60
2 First Generation EGFR Kinase Inhibitors 60
3 EGFR Kinase Domain Mutations 61
4 Primary or "Upfront" Resistance to EGFR TKIs 63
5 Acquired Resistance to EGFR TKIs.. 65
6 New Approaches to Target EGFR Mutant Lung Cancer 67

Y. Gong
Memorial Sloan-Kettering Cancer Center, New York, NY 10065, USA

W. Pao (✉)
Vanderbilt University Medical Center, Nashville, TN 37232, USA
e-mail: william.pao@Vanderbilt.Edu

Current Topics in Microbiology and Immunology (2012) 355: 59–81
DOI: 10.1007/82_2011_171
© Springer-Verlag Berlin Heidelberg 2011
Published Online: 25 August 2011

6.1 Irreversible EGFR Inhibitors	68
6.2 Reversible EGFR Inhibitors with Additional Kinase Targets	70
6.3 Combinations of Targeted Therapy	70
6.4 HSP90 Inhibitors	71
7 A Uniform Clinical Definition of "Acquired Resistance" in NSCLC	72
8 Future Perspectives	72
References	72

1 Introduction

Lung cancer is the leading cause of cancer-related death in men and women in the US and worldwide (Jemal et al. 2009). The median 5-year survival rate is only 15%. Based on histological features, lung cancer is classified into two major categories: small cell lung cancer (SCLC) and non-small cell lung cancer (NSCLC). These comprise ~ 15 and $\sim 85\%$ of cases, respectively. NSCLC is further classified into multiple histological subtypes including adenocarcinoma, squamous cell carcinoma, and large cell carcinoma (Brambilla et al. 2001). Most NSCLC patients are diagnosed with advanced, unresectable disease (stage IIIB or stage IV). Left untreated, these patients have a median survival of <6 months.

Initial treatment of advanced NSCLC involves chemotherapy. The current standard regimen involves a chemotherapy 'doublet': a platinum agent (cisplatin or carboplatin) in combination with a second cytotoxic agent (paclitaxel, gemcitabine, vinorelbine, docetaxel, pemetrexed). In a landmark study of 1,207 patients with advanced NSCLC, treatment with any of four chemotherapy doublets resulted in similar rates of radiographic response (19%) and overall survival (7.9 months) (Schiller et al. 2002). Thus, the efficacy of chemotherapy appears to have reached a plateau in NSCLC. Addition to doublet chemotherapy of a new targeted agent, bevacizumab, increases the median survival of patients by only 2 months (Sandler et al. 2006). Bevacizumab is a recombinant humanized monoclonal antibody that binds and neutralizes the biologic activity of human vascular endothelial growth factor (VEGF). Novel approaches are clearly needed for the treatment of lung cancer. One promising strategy involves targeting the epidermal growth factor receptor (EGFR).

2 First Generation EGFR Kinase Inhibitors

The EGFR is a receptor tyrosine kinase (RTK) of the ERBB family which also includes ERBB2 (HER2), ERBB3 (HER3) and ERBB4 (HER4). Ligands such as epidermal growth factor, transforming growth factor-α, heparin-binding EGF-like growth factor, amphiregulin, and epiregulin, bind to the extracellular domains of these receptors. Ligand binding induces receptor homo- or hetero-dimerization, autophosphorylation of the receptors, and activation of downstream signaling molecules (Hynes and Lane 2005). In normal cells, activation of the EGFR signaling pathway is under tight physiological control. Aberrant activation of EGFR can lead to cancer.

Gefitinib (ZD1839, Iressa®; AstraZeneca, Macclesfield, UK) and erlotinib (OSI-774, Tarceva®, CP-358,774; OSI Pharmaceuticals, Melville, NY) are two small molecule EGFR inhibitors that act by reversibly and competitively binding to the ATP-binding domain of the receptor (Moyer et al. 1997; Wakeling et al. 2002). Gefitinib received accelerated approval from the FDA as second line treatment of NSCLC in 2003 (Cohen et al. 2003), after two phase II trials (IDEAL-1 and -2) in chemotherapy refractory patients demonstrated response rates of 10% in Caucasian cases, 28% in Japanese cases, and an overall survival of 6–8 months (Fukuoka et al. 2003; Kris et al. 2003). Erlotinib was approved in 2004, after a phase III study (BR.21) showed that erlotinib monotherapy conferred a 2 month survival benefit over best supportive care (BSC) in patients with chemo-refractory NSCLC (Shepherd et al. 2005). The response rates were 9% in the erlotinib arm and <1% in the placebo arm.

In a subsequent phase III study (ISEL), gefitinib failed to show a similar survival benefit. This result led to the withdrawal of gefitinib from the US and European (but not Asian) markets. However, gefitinib is still considered an active agent in NSCLC. For example, the INTEREST trial demonstrated in previously treated NSCLC patients that gefitinib and docetaxel treatment were comparable in terms of overall survival, with a lower rate of treatment-related toxicity and a higher quality of life for those receiving gefitinib (Kim et al. 2008). Moreover, gefitinib is active in highly selected populations of patients (see below). Discrepant results between BR.21 and ISEL may be due to differences in patient selection criteria in the two phase III studies (Sharma et al. 2007). The different outcomes may also result from the fact that erlotinib at 150 mg per day is administered closer to its maximum tolerated dose than is gefitinib (at 250 mg per day). Addition of either gefitinib or erlotinib to concurrent chemotherapy in unselected chemo-naïve patients confers no survival benefit over chemotherapy alone (Herbst et al. 2004; Giaccone et al. 2004; Herbst et al. 2005; Gatzemeier et al. 2007).

3 EGFR Kinase Domain Mutations

Because gefitinib and erlotinib induced dramatic clinical and radiographic responses in some NSCLCs, identification of predictive tumor markers prior to treatment became an intense area of interest. Retrospective clinical studies showed that responding patients were more likely to be never smokers (patients who smoked less than 100 cigarettes in a lifetime), female, East Asian, and have tumors with adenocarcinoma histology (Fukuoka et al. 2003; Kris et al. 2003; Shepherd et al. 2005). The molecular basis for these clinical characteristics was not understood until 2004, when gain-of-function somatic mutations of *EGFR* were

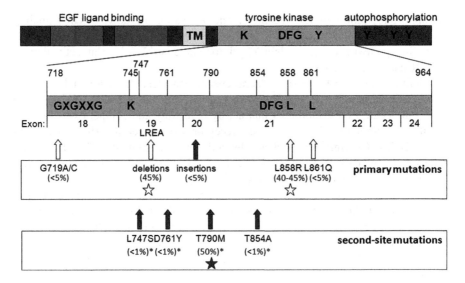

Fig. 1 EGFR mutations associated with EGFR TKI sensitivity and resistance. (*white arrow*: sensitizing mutations; *gray arrow*: resistance mutations; *star*: most common mutations; *asterisk*: percentage of only acquired resistance cases)

found to be associated with increased sensitivity to gefitinib and erlotinib (Fig. 1) (Lynch et al. 2004; Paez et al. 2004; Pao et al. 2004). The frequency of these mutations highly overlaps with the subsets of patients likely to respond to therapy. For example, in unselected cases, drug sensitizing mutations are found in ~ 10 and ~ 30% of Caucasian and East Asian patients, respectively, but in much higher percentages in never smokers with adenocarcinoma histology (Rosell et al. 2009a).

Drug-sensitizing mutations occur in exons 18–21 of *EGFR*, which encode a portion of the tyrosine kinase domain of the receptor (Fig. 1). The most common alterations are a T → G mutation at nucleotide 2,573 in exon 21, leading to substitution of arginine for leucine at position 858 (L858R), and deletions of four amino acids (LREA) encoded by exon 19. These two classes together represent 85–90% of *EGFR* mutations in lung cancer. Two rarer mutants are G719A/C (exon 18) and L861Q (exon 21). Biochemically, *EGFR* kinase domain mutations lead to constitutive activation of the receptor and an increased duration of receptor activation by ligands compared to wild-type EGFR (Lynch et al. 2004). Kinetic analysis of the purified intracellular domains of EGFR L858R and a representative deletion mutant revealed that both mutants display a higher Km for ATP and a lower Ki for erlotinib relative to wild-type receptor, which results in a 100-fold difference in sensitivity to EGFR TKIs (Carey et al. 2006).

Ectopic expression of *EGFR* mutants transforms fibroblast and lung epithelial cells, leading to anchorage-independent growth, focus formation and tumor formation in nude mice (Greulich et al. 2005). Mice with tetracycline-regulated transgenes carrying the exon 19 or 21 mutations develop tumors after *EGFR* expression is induced in lung epithelia. These tumors are highly dependent on expression of the mutant *EGFR* transgenes, as switching off ectopic mutant EGFR expression or treating mice with erlotinib can rapidly eliminate tumors by inducing proliferative arrest and massive cell death (Politi et al. 2006; Ji et al. 2006). Apoptosis is mediated through induction of BIM, a pro-apoptotic protein in the intrinsic pathway of cell death (Gong et al. 2007; Cragg et al. 2007; Costa et al. 2007; Mellinghoff 2007).

It is now clear that *EGFR* mutant tumors represent a distinct clinical subset of NSCLC. First, patients whose tumors harbor *EGFR* mutations have a better prognosis compared to those without such mutations (Marks et al. 2008; Mok et al. 2009). Second, *EGFR* mutant tumors predict for benefit from both gefitinib and erlotinib. In multiple single-arm studies in which patients were treated with either EGFR TKI according to tumor mutation status, response rates of 55–75% were observed in *EGFR* mutant tumors (Sequist et al. 2008; Inoue et al. 2006; Sunaga et al. 2007; Rosell et al. 2009b). Overall survival in many of these studies easily exceeded more than year. Most recently, in a phase III, open label study, previously untreated East Asian patients with lung adenocarcinoma were randomly assigned to receive either gefitinib or carboplatin plus paclitaxel. Patients were never or former light smokers. Patients with *EGFR* mutant tumors displayed a higher response rate and progression-free survival with gefitinib, while mutation-negative patients benefited most from chemotherapy (Mok et al. 2009). Multiple randomized prospective studies comparing an EGFR TKI versus chemotherapy for patients specifically with untreated metastatic *EGFR* mutant tumors have further confirmed the benefit of the TKI over chemotherapy in this patient population (Maemondo et al. 2010; Mitsudomi et al. 2010). Overall survival in these studies has exceeded 2 years.

4 Primary or "Upfront" Resistance to EGFR TKIs

Tumors that do not undergo significant tumor shrinkage to gefitinib or erlotinib display primary resistance. One mechanism involves primary EGFR exon 20 insertions, which occur in <5% of NSCLCs. Preclinical studies (Greulich et al. 2005) and retrospective clinical data (Wu et al. 2008) have demonstrated that tumors with such mutations are generally insensitive to treatment with EGFR TKIs.

Resistance is also mediated by mutant KRAS signaling proteins (Pao et al. 2005b), which are found in about 20% of NSCLCs. KRAS is an enzyme that binds and hydrolyzes guanosine triphosphate (GTP). This GTPase lies downstream of EGFR signaling. When mutated, it is capable of activating cellular signaling independent of *EGFR* (Fig. 2). EGFR and *KRAS* mutations are mutually exclusive. While EGFR mutations are more common in never smokers, *KRAS* mutations are more prevalent in former or current smokers. A recent systematic review and meta-analysis demonstrated that *KRAS* mutations are highly specific negative

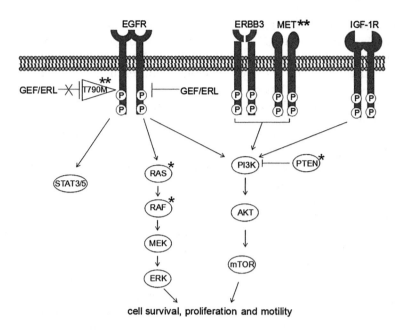

Fig. 2 Schematic of key molecules in the EGFR signaling pathway. *Molecules involved in mediating primary resistance. **Molecules involved in mediating acquired resistance. *GEF/ERL* gefitinib/erlotinib

predictors of response to single-agent EGFR TKIs in advanced NSCLC (Linardou et al. 2008). Whether a poor response to therapy correlates with shorter survival remains to be established.

Mutations found in genes encoding other receptors or components of the EGFR signaling pathway also mediate primary resistance of lung tumors to EGFR TKIs: (i) PTEN (phosphatase and tensin homolog) is a negative regulator of the PI3K/AKT pathway, involved in cell survival. In NSCLC cell lines, homozygous loss of PTEN uncouples EGFR from downstream signaling and activates EGFR, leading to primary resistance (Sos et al. 2009). *PTEN* mutations are rare in NSCLC, but loss of PTEN protein expression occurs in ~24% of tumors. Loss of expression may be due to promoter hypermethylation (Soria et al. 2002); (ii) BRAF is a serine-threonine kinase in the MAPK pathway, downstream of EGFR. *BRAF* mutations (~1–5% of NSCLCs; non-overlapping with *EGFR* mutations) (Fig. 3) confer resistance to EGFR inhibition by activating extracellular signal-regulated kinase (ERK) signaling, independent of EGFR (Pratilas et al. 2008); (iii) ALK fusions are also associated with resistance to EGFR TKIs (Shaw et al. 2009). EML4-ALK alterations arise from fusion of echinoderm microtubule-associated protein-like 4 (EML4) with the anaplastic lymphoma kinase (ALK) (Soda et al. 2007). Found in about 5% of NSCLC patients, ALK fusions are mutually exclusive with *EGFR* mutations and are associated with sensitivity of tumors to ALK inhibitors (Horn and Pao 2009); (iv) through a pooled RNA interference screen, FAS and NF-κB signaling were shown

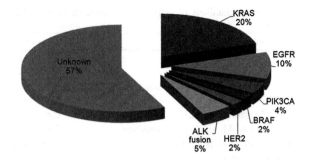

Fig. 3 'Driver' mutations in lung adenocarcinoma

to enhance cell death induced by erlotinib in EGFR-mutant lung cancer cells (Bivona et al. 2011); (v) IGF-1R signaling has also been shown to contribute to disease persistence in EGFR mutant cells (Gong et al. 2009).

Cellular characteristics, such as epithelial to mesenchymal transition (EMT), may be another determinant of sensitivity of NSCLC cells to EGFR inhibition. EMT is a process in which epithelial cells lose polarity, cell–cell contact and epithelial markers and become fibroblastic mesenchymal–like cells. EMT is thought to be a transcriptional reprogramming process that allows tumor cells to become invasive and metastatic. Loss of epithelial markers (e.g., E-cadherin, γ-catenin) and gain of mesenchymal markers (e.g., vimentin and fibronectin) have been associated with resistance to erlotinib (Thomson et al. 2005).

5 Acquired Resistance to EGFR TKIs

Despite deriving substantial clinical benefit from gefitinib or erlotinib, all patients with metastatic EGFR mutant tumors eventually develop acquired resistance. Disease progression usually occurs after about 1 year on therapy (Riely et al. 2006; Jackman et al. 2009).

In about half of cases, growing tumors contain a second-site mutation in the EGFR kinase domain (Table 1) (Kobayashi et al. 2005; Pao et al. 2005a). The most common (>90%) mutation involves a C → T change at nucleotide 2,369 in exon 20, which results in substitution of methionine for threonine at position 790 (T790M) (Balak et al. 2006; Bean et al. 2008). This substitution occurs in the analogous position in other kinases targeted by other kinase inhibitors in different cancers that develop acquired resistance, i.e. T315I in BCR-ABL in patients with imatinib (Gleevec)-resistant chronic myelogenous leukemias (CML), T674I in PDGFRα in imatinib-resistant patients with hypereosinophilic syndrome (HES), and T670I in KIT in imatinib-resistant gastrointestinal stromal tumors (GIST) (Shah et al. 2002; Cools et al. 2003; Tamborini et al. 2004) (Table 2) (see also "Gastrointestinal Stromal Tumors" and "JAK-Mutant Myeloproliferative Neoplasms").

The T790M residue lies within the drug binding cleft of EGFR. Based upon crystal structure analyses of EGFR and the effects of the T315I change on the binding

Table 1 Mechanisms of acquired resistance to EGFR TKIS found in human EGFR mutant tumors

Mechanism	References
Second-site EGFR mutations	Pao et al. (2005b); Kobayashi et al. (2005); Balak et al. (2006); Costa et al. (2007); Bean et al. (2008)
MET amplification	Bean et al. (2007); Engelman et al. (2007b)
Transformation to SCLC	Zakowski et al. (2006)
Epithelial to Mesenchymal Transition	Uramoto et al. (2010); Chung et al. (2010)
Hepatocyte Growth Factor	Yano et al. (2008)
PIK3CA Mutation	Sequist et al. (2011)

of ABL to imatinib, EGFR T790M is predicted to impair binding of either gefitinib or erlotinib to the ATP-binding pocket (Stamos et al. 2002). Alternatively, the amino acid change could alter the relative affinity of ATP versus drug (Yun et al. 2008). The T790M alteration does not diminish the oncogenic activity of EGFR; rather, the amino acid change may, at least in vitro, potentiate the oncogenic activity of drug-sensitive mutations in the EGFR kinase domain already known to have gain-of-function (Godin-Heymann et al. 2008). Expression of the *EGFR T790M* alone in mouse lung epithelia induces lung tumor formation (Regales et al. 2007).

Paradoxically, in an analysis of post-progression survival and characteristics of disease progression in patients with and without T790M, presence of the T790M mutation was found to define a clinical subset with a relatively favorable prognosis and indolent progression (Oxnard et al. 2011). Consistent with this, studies of isogenic TKI-sensitive and resistant pairs of cell lines that mimic the behavior of human tumors showed that T790M-harboring clones can actually grow slower than their parental counterparts (Chmielecki 2011). These data may explain why some patients exhibit disease flares after stopping an EGFR TKI (Riely et al. 2007) and re-responses to therapy when re-starting TKI treatment (Sequist et al. 2011).

A rare germline *T790M* mutation has been linked to inherited susceptibility to lung cancer (Bell et al. 2005). Occasionally, *T790M* mutations can be found in tumors with primary drug resistance (Inukai et al. 2006; Toyooka et al. 2005), but, in EGFR TKI-naïve disease, the mutations are rarely detected by conventional mutation detection methods. Using more sensitive techniques, *T790M* variants have been found to pre-exist treatment at very low levels (Maheswaran et al. 2008). The presence of resistance mutations at such levels does not confer significant primary resistance to EGFR TKIs in tumor cells containing drug sensitizing mutations. However, their presence is associated with a striking difference in progression-free survival, with a median of 7.7 months in patients with a detectable *T790M* allele versus 16.5 months in those without a detectable allele.

Other rare second-site mutations in *EGFR* lead to D761Y, L747S, and T854A substitutions (Fig. 1) (Balak et al. 2006; Costa et al. 2007; Bean et al. 2008). These mutations altogether represent less than 5% of acquired resistance mutations. In surrogate kinase experiments and in growth inhibition assays using cell transfectants (Ba/F3 cells), these mutants confer less resistance to EGFR TKIs

EGFR Mutant Lung Cancer

Table 2 Kinase inhibitor resistance due to "gatekeeper" mutations

Protein	Mutation	Disease	Drug	Reference
BCR-ABL	T315I	CML	Imatinib	Gorre et al. (2001)
BCR-ABL	T315I	CML	Dasatinib	O'Hare et al. (2005)
PDGFRa	T674I	HES	Imatinib	Cools et al. (2003)
KIT	T670I	GIST	Imatinib	Tamborini et al. (2004)
EGFR	T790M	NSCLC	Gefitinib/ Erlotinib	Pao et al. (2005a) Kobayashi et al. (2005)

For BCR-ABL, T315I leads to steric clash, but for mutant EGFR, T790M may restore affinity of kinase for ATP versus drug (Yun et al. 2008)

compared to T790M. Disease progression due to at least the L747S mutant may be overcome clinically by drug dose escalation or switching from gefitinib to the more potent erlotinib (Costa et al. 2008).

Amplification of *MET*, the gene encoding a different membrane bound receptor tyrosine kinase, is a separate mechanism of acquired resistance to EGFR TKIs (Table 1) (Bean et al. 2007; Engelman et al. 2007b). Analysis of tumor samples from multiple independent patient cohorts revealed that *MET* was amplified in about 20% of patients with acquired resistance, although follow-up studies suggest that the frequency may be closer to 10% (Arcila et al. 2011). *MET* amplification occurs regardless of T790M status.

MET amplification in cells originally dependent upon mutant EGFR illustrates the concept of a 'kinase switch'. In 'oncogene addicted' cells, cancer cells depend on signaling from a single mutant kinase for survival. Upon prolonged exposure to EGFR kinase inhibition, some surviving cells become more dependent upon another kinase, such as MET. Currently, it is unclear how many 'kinase switches' can occur in the lifetime of a cancer cell. Activation of the insulin-like growth factor receptor, type 1 (IGF-1R) pathway can lead to gefitinib resistance in vitro in cells with amplified wildtype *EGFR*, and to resistance to CL-387,785 (an experimental irreversible EGFR inhibitor) in H1975 cells (which harbor both *EGFR L858R* and *T790M* alleles) (Shimamura et al. 2008; Guix et al. 2008). However, clinical data supporting these in vitro findings remains to be established.

Other rarer forms of acquired resistance have also been found (Table 3). These include transformation to small cell lung cancer (Zakowski et al. 2006); hepatocyte growth factor (Yano et al. 2008), *PIK3CA* mutation (Sequist et al. 2011), and EMT (Chung et al. 2010; Uramoto et al. 2010). The exact frequencies of these mechanisms remains to be established.

6 New Approaches to Target EGFR Mutant Lung Cancer

As stated above, about 50% of patients with acquired resistance to gefitinib or erlotinib harbor tumors with second-site *EGFR* mutations. Importantly, in the absence of alternative kinase activation, such tumor cells remain dependent upon EGFR signaling for survival. This suggests that new strategies that target the gene products of *EGFR* resistant alleles can overcome acquired resistance. Agents that attack signaling pathways induced by EGFR T790M may also be effective. Currently, at least four approaches are being undertaken: (1) single-agent irreversible EGFR inhibitors (Table 3), (2) single-agent reversible inhibitors with additional kinase targets (Table 3), (3) combinations of EGFR inhibitors with other targeted agents, and (4) HSP90 inhibitors.

6.1 Irreversible EGFR Inhibitors

HKI-272 (neratinib; Wyeth) is an irreversible pan-ERBB family TKI that covalently binds to cysteine 797 of the EGFR kinase domain (Rabindran et al. 2004). In vitro, the ATP-competitive small molecule is more potent than either gefitinib or erlotinib; it inhibits the growth of H1975 cells with an IC_{50} of 223 nM (Kwak et al. 2005). In mouse lung cancer models, the drug induces clear regression of tumors harboring a drug-sensitive L858R mutation (Ji et al. 2006) but leads to mixed results in tumors harboring a drug-resistant *L858R* plus *T790M* allele (Li et al. 2007). In a phase I trial, among 12 evaluable NSCLC patients, no responses were observed, but 5 patients who had progressed on erlotinib or gefitinib achieved stable disease (SD) for over 24 weeks (Wong 2007). In a subsequent three arm phase II study, neratinib showed disappointing results in patients with acquired resistance as well as in patients with untreated EGFR mutant tumors (Sequist et al. 2010a). Because the drug also demonstrated poor activity in untreated EGFR mutant lung cancers, further development of this drug in *EGFR* mutant NSCLC is unclear. Although HKI-272 is more potent than gefitinib/erlotinib, chronic exposure of a NSCLC cell line (PC-9 cells) to HKI-272 in vitro leads to enrichment of EGFR T790M-harboring cells (Godin-Heymann et al. 2008). The same in vitro model using gefitinib has also led to recovery of *EGFR T790M* mutations (Ogino et al. 2007). Collectively, these data suggest that HKI-272 can overcome T790M-mediated resistance, but only at high doses. Such high doses may not be achievable in humans without significant toxicity.

BIBW2992 (afatinib; Boerhinger-Ingelheim) is another irreversible inhibitor with specificity against EGFR and HER2. It potently inhibits the growth of *EGFR* mutant cell lines including H1975 cells at nanomolar concentrations (Bean et al. 2008). In vivo, BIBW2992 induces growth delay of H1975 xenograft tumors and some tumor shrinkage in EGFR L858R plus T790M transgenic mice (Li et al. 2008). Multiple trials are being conducted to evaluate the efficacy of BIBW2992 in various settings against stage IIIB/IV *EGFR* mutant lung adenocarcinoma. Thus far, BIBW2992 appears active in untreated NSCLC patients harboring EGFR activating mutations (Yang et al. 2008; Shih et al. 2009). However, in a study of afatinib versus placebo in patients with EGFR mutant tumors who progressed on gefitinib or erlotinib, afatinib induced only a 7% response rate (Miller et al. 2010). Consistent with these data, similar to HKI-272, BIBW2992 selects for T790M-mediated resistance in vitro (Chmielecki 2011).

Table 3 Second generation EGFR TKIS in clinical trials in NSCLC

Compound name	Target	IC_{50} for EGFR[a]	IC_{50} for H1975 cells	Company	Clinical study	References
HKI-272 (Neratinib)	Irreversible inhibitor of pan-ERBB family	92 nM	222 nM	Wyeth	Phase II	Rabindran et al. (2004) Kwak et al. (2005) Wong (2007)
XL647	Reversible inhibitor of EGFR, ERBB2, VEGFR2, FLT4, and EPHB4	0.3 nM	920 nM	Exelixis	Phase II	Gendreau et al. (2007) Miller et al. (2008) Rizvi et al. (2008)
PF00299804	Irreversible inhibitor of pan-ERBB family	5.8 nM	440 nM	Pfizer	Phase II	Engelman et al. (2007a) Janne et al. (2009)
BIBW2992	Irreversible inhibitor of EGFR and ERBB2	0.5 nM	<100 nM	Boehringer-Ingelheim	Phase III	Li et al. (2008) Yang et al. (2008) Shih et al. (2009)
BMS-690514	reversible inhibitor of EGFR, HER2, and VEGFR1-3	5 nM	1 μM	Bristol-Myers Squibb	Phase II	de La Motte Rouge et al. (2007) Bahleda et al. (2008) Bahleda et al. (2009)

[a] IC50 for wild-type EGFR based upon in vitro kinase assay

PF-00299804 (Pfizer) is a third irreversible small molecule in development. The pan-ERBB inhibitor suppresses the growth of H1975 cells with an IC_{50} less than 500 nM in vitro and inhibits H1975 xenograft tumor growth (Engelman et al. 2007a; Gonzales et al. 2008). It, too, appears active in TKI-naïve patients. Final results from a trial for patients with acquired resistance have not yet been reported (Janne et al. 2009).

6.2 Reversible EGFR Inhibitors with Additional Kinase Targets

XL647 (EXEL-7647; Exelixis) is an orally available reversible small molecular inhibitor of multiple tyrosine kinases including EGFR, HER2, VEGFR, and EPHB4. In H1975 cells, XL647 ($IC_{50} = 920$ nM) is 11 and 17 times more effective than gefitinib and erlotinib, respectively, at inhibiting cell proliferation in vitro, and it delays the growth of H1975 cell xenografts (Gendreau et al. 2007). The drug is active in untreated EGFR mutant NSCLC (Rizvi et al. 2008) but in patients with acquired resistance, only 1 out of 23 patients had a PR, and seven patients had stable disease (SD) at their first assessment (Miller et al. 2008). Final results of this study are pending.

BMS-690514 (Bristol-Myers Squibb) is a reversible inhibitor that targets VEGFR1-3 in addition to EGFR and HER2 (Wong et al. 2007). In preclinical models, BMS-690514 has activity against cultured *T790M*-harboring cells and has demonstrated potent activity in relevant xenograft models (de La Motte Rouge et al. 2007). In early trials, BMS-690514 was reported to induce PRs and SD in both erlotinib-naïve and -resistant patients (Bahleda et al. 2008, 2009). A randomized phase 2 trial of BMS-690514 versus erlotinib in patients with pretreated (EGFR-TKI-naïve) NSCLC has been completed.

6.3 Combinations of Targeted Therapy

a. *EGFR TKI plus a PI3K/AKT/mTOR inhibitor*: EGFR mutants appear to signal predominantly through the phosphatidylinositol 3-kinase (*PI3K*) pathway, associated with cell proliferation and survival (Engelman et al. 2005). A number of agents that target gene products in this pathway are in development. In preclinical models, combinations of HKI-272 or BIBW2992 with an mTOR (mammalian target of rapamycin) inhibitor, rapamycin, resulted in greater tumor reduction in mice harboring T790M-driven lung tumors compared to HKI-272 or BIBW2992 alone (Li et al. 2007, 2008). mTOR is a serine/threonine kinase downstream of PI3K. Alternative mTOR inhibitors include CCI-779 and RAD-001. Other agents in development target PI3K directly (e.g., BEZ235, BGT226, XL765, XL147, GDC0941), or the serine/threonine kinase downstream of PI3K, AKT (e.g., perifosine,

MK2206, VQD-002, XL418) (Liu et al. 2009). Whether these agents will be effective in patients with acquired resistance to EGFR TKIs is an active area of investigation.

b. *EGFR TKI plus EGFR antibodies*: In transgenic mouse lung tumor models, the irreversible EGFR TKI, BIBW2992, induces radiographic complete responses in mice with a drug-sensitive *EGFR L858R* allele, but only stable disease in animals harboring an *EGFR T790M* mutation (Regales et al. 2009; Li et al. 2008). Similar results are obtained with an anti-EGFR antibody, cetuximab, which binds to the extracellular portion of the receptor. However, co-treatment of tumor-bearing animals with both BIBW2992 and cetuximab appears highly effective at overcoming T790M-mediated resistance, at least in preclinical models (Regales et al. 2009). Combination treatment leads to enhanced targeting of mutant EGFR. Based upon these data, a human trial was performed with afatinib plus cetuximab. This combination was not only tolerable in patients but also induced an unprecedented 40% response rate in patients with acquired resistance (Janjigian et al. 2011).

c. *EGFR TKI plus MET/IGF-1R inhibitors*: As stated above, MET and IGF-1R RTKs can mediate acquired resistance to EGFR TKIs. Multiple MET and IGF-1R inhibitors are in development. Agents that target the MET axis include anti-HGF antibodies (e.g., L2G7, AMG102), anti-MET antibodies (e.g., OA-5D5, DN30) and small molecule MET TKIs (e.g., K252a, SU11274, PHA665752, ARQ197, XL880, SGX523, and JNJ38877605) (Comoglio et al. 2008; Karamouzis et al. 2009). For IGF-1R, drugs include anti-IGF-1R antibodies (e.g., CP-751,871, A12, R1507, h7C10, AVE-1642) and small molecule IGF-1R TKIs (e.g., OSI-906) (Hartog et al. 2007; Dziadziuszko et al. 2008). Efficacy data is eagerly awaited.

6.4 HSP90 Inhibitors

Drugs that indirectly target mutant EGFR are also under development. One class of drugs involves HSP90 inhibitors. HSP90 is a heat shock protein which is required for the stability and function of multiple signaling proteins that promote the growth and/or survival of cancer cells. *EGFR* mutant proteins are more dependent than their wild-type counterparts upon HSP90 to fold properly. Consequently, the mutants are more sensitive to degradation following HSP90 inhibition with geldanamycins (Shimamura et al. 2005). In vitro and in vivo, HSP90 inhibitors induce stabilization or regression of T790M EGFR tumors by causing degradation of mutant receptor. HSP90 inhibitors also sensitize *EGFR* mutant tumors to paclitaxel (Shimamura et al. 2008; Sawai et al. 2008; Regales et al. 2007). Unfortunately, clinical data thus far have been disappointing, at least with the HSP90 inhibitor, IPI-504 (Sequist et al. 2010b).

7 A Uniform Clinical Definition of "Acquired Resistance" in NSCLC

One confounding factor thus far in all trials for patients with acquired resistance is that the clinical definition of "acquired resistance" has not been clear. Genotyping of patients' tumors upon study entry has not been mandated. Moreover, the various studies have employed different inclusion/exclusion criteria, especially with respect to the duration of time patients must be treated with an EGFR TKI prior to enrollment and/or the duration of time patients should be off the EGFR TKI prior to starting therapy. Recently, a multi-institutional group of investigators proposed a clear and consistent definition of secondary resistance to help create standard entry criteria for the studies of such patients (Jackman et al. 2009). This definition should help to facilitate a clearer interpretation of trial results and accelerate the development of therapies that are truly effective at overcoming acquired resistance.

8 Future Perspectives

In the past decade, the development of gefitinib and erlotinib has led to a new treatment paradigm in NSCLC. Instead of basing treatment decisions primarily on the histological features of lung tumors, clinicians are now considering tumor mutation status to prioritize therapy. This notion is best exemplified by the association of *EGFR* mutations with increased sensitivity to first-generation EGFR TKIs. Gefitinib and erlotinib can be considered as first-line therapy for those with *EGFR* mutant tumors, and these patients should be considered as a separate disease entity within NSCLC. Hopefully, EGFR mutant NSCLC represents just one of many molecular subsets of lung cancers that will be treated with specific targeted agents in the near future (Fig. 3).

Acknowledgments This work was supported by the NIH National Cancer Institute (NCI) grants R01-CA121210, P01CA129243, P50-CA90949, and P30-CA68485, and Joan's legacy: the Joan Scarangello Foundation to conquer lung cancer.

References

Arcila ME, Oxnard GR, Nafa K, Riely GJ, Solomon SB, Zakowski MF, Kris MG, Pao W, Miller VA, Ladanyi M (2011) Rebiopsy of lung cancer patients with acquired resistance to EGFR inhibitors and enhanced detection of the T790M mutation using a locked nucleic acid-based assay. Clin Cancer Res 17:1169–1180. doi:1078-0432.CCR-10-2277[pii]10.1158/1078-0432.CCR-10-2277

Bahleda R, Felip E, Herbst RS, Hanna NH, Laurie SA, Shepherd FA, Armand JP, Sweeney CJ, Calvo-Aller E, Soria JC (2008) Phase I multicenter trial of BMS-690514: safety, pharmacokinetic profile, biological effects, and early clinical evaluation in patients with advanced solid tumors and non-small cell lung cancer. J Clin Oncol Meeting Abstracts

Bahleda R, Soria J, Harbison C, Park J, Felip E, Hanna N, Laurie SA, Armand J, Shepherd FA, Herbst R (2009) Tumor regression and pharmacodynamic (PD) biomarker validation in non-small cell lung cancer (NSCLC) patients treated with the ErbB/VEGFR inhibitor BMS-690514. J Clin Oncol Meeting Abstracts

Balak MN, Gong Y, Riely GJ, Somwar R, Li AR, Zakowski MF, Chiang A, Yang G, Ouerfelli O, Kris MG, Ladanyi M, Miller VA, Pao W (2006) Novel D761Y and common secondary T790M mutations in epidermal growth factor receptor-mutant lung adenocarcinomas with acquired resistance to kinase inhibitors. Clin Cancer Res 12:6494–6501

Bean J, Brennan C, Shih JY, Riely G, Viale A, Wang L, Chitale D, Motoi N, Szoke J, Broderick S, Balak M, Chang WC, Yu CJ, Gazdar A, Pass H, Rusch V, Gerald W, Huang SF, Yang PC, Miller V, Ladanyi M, Yang CH, Pao W (2007) MET amplification occurs with or without T790M mutations in EGFR mutant lung tumors with acquired resistance to gefitinib or erlotinib. Proc Natl Acad Sci USA 104:20932–20937. doi:0710370104[pii]10.1073/pnas. 0710370104

Bean J, Riely GJ, Balak M, Marks JL, Ladanyi M, Miller VA, Pao W (2008) Acquired resistance to epidermal growth factor receptor kinase inhibitors associated with a novel T854A mutation in a patient with EGFR-mutant lung adenocarcinoma. Clin Cancer Res 14: 7519–7525. doi:14/22/7519[pii]10.1158/1078-0432.CCR-08-0151

Bell DW, Gore I, Okimoto RA, Godin-Heymann N, Sordella R, Mulloy R, Sharma SV, Brannigan BW, Mohapatra G, Settleman J, Haber DA (2005) Inherited susceptibility to lung cancer may be associated with the T790M drug resistance mutation in EGFR. Nat Genet 37:1315–1316

Bivona TG, Hieronymus H, Parker J, Chang K, Taron M, Rosell R, Moonsamy P, Dahlman K, Miller VA, Costa C, Hannon G, Sawyers CL (2011) FAS and NF-kappaB signalling modulate dependence of lung cancers on mutant EGFR. Nature 471:523–526. doi:nature09870 [pii]10.1038/nature09870

Brambilla E, Travis WD, Colby TV, Corrin B, Shimosato Y (2001) The new world health organization classification of lung tumours. Eur Respir J 18:1059–1068

Carey KD, Garton AJ, Romero MS, Kahler J, Thomson S, Ross S, Park F, Haley JD, Gibson N, Sliwkowski MX (2006) Kinetic analysis of epidermal growth factor receptor somatic mutant proteins shows increased sensitivity to the epidermal growth factor receptor tyrosine kinase inhibitor, erlotinib. Cancer Res 66:8163–8171. doi:66/16/8163[pii]10.1158/0008-5472. CAN-06-0453

Chmielecki J, Foo J, Oxnard GR, Hutchinson K, Ohashi K, Somwar R, Wang L, Amato KR, Arcila M, Sos ML, Socci ND, Viale A, de Stanchina E, Ginsberg MS, Thomas RK, Kris MG, Inoue A, Ladanyi M, Miller VA, Michor F, Pao W (2011) Optimization of dosing for EGFR mutant non-small cell lung cancer with evolutionary cancer modeling. Sci Transl Med 3(90):90ra59

Chung JH, Rho JK, Xu X, Lee JS, Yoon HI, Lee CT, Choi YJ, Kim HR, Kim CH, Lee JC (2010) Clinical and molecular evidences of epithelial to mesenchymal transition in acquired resistance to EGFR-TKIs. Lung Cancer. doi:S0169-5002(10)00546-5[pii]10.1016/j.lungcan. 2010.11.011

Cohen MH, Williams GA, Sridhara R, Chen G, Pazdur R (2003) FDA drug approval summary: gefitinib (ZD1839) (Iressa) tablets. Oncologist 8:303–306

Comoglio PM, Giordano S, Trusolino L (2008) Drug development of MET inhibitors: targeting oncogene addiction and expedience. Nat Rev Drug Discov 7:504–516. doi:nrd2530[pii] 10.1038/nrd2530

Cools J, Stover EH, Boulton CL, Gotlib J, Legare RD, Amaral SM, Curley DP, Duclos N, Rowan R, Kutok JL, Lee BH, Williams IR, Coutre SE, Stone RM, DeAngelo DJ, Marynen P, Manley PW, Meyer T, Fabbro D, Neuberg D, Weisberg E, Griffin JD, Gilliland DG (2003) PKC412 overcomes resistance to imatinib in a murine model of FIP1L1-PDGFRalpha-induced myeloproliferative disease. Cancer Cell 3:459–469

Costa DB, Halmos B, Kumar A, Schumer ST, Huberman MS, Boggon TJ, Tenen DG, Kobayashi S (2007) BIM mediates EGFR tyrosine kinase inhibitor-induced apoptosis in lung cancers with oncogenic EGFR mutations. PLoS Med 4:1669–1679. doi:07-PLME-RA-0425[pii]10.1371/journal.pmed.0040315 discussion 1680

Costa DB, Schumer ST, Tenen DG, Kobayashi S (2008) Differential responses to erlotinib in epidermal growth factor receptor (EGFR)-mutated lung cancers with acquired resistance to gefitinib carrying the L747S or T790M secondary mutations. J Clin Oncol 26:1182–1184. doi:26/7/1182[pii]10.1200/JCO.2007.14.9039 author reply 1184-6

Cragg MS, Kuroda J, Puthalakath H, Huang DC, Strasser A (2007) Gefitinib-induced killing of NSCLC cell lines expressing mutant EGFR requires BIM and can be enhanced by BH3 mimetics. PLoS Med 4:1681–1689. doi:07-PLME-RA-0458[pii]10.1371/journal.pmed.0040316 discussion 1690

de La Motte Rouge T, Galluzzi L, Olaussen KA, Zermati Y, Tasdemir E, Robert T, Ripoche H, Lazar V, Dessen P, Harper F, Pierron G, Pinna G, Araujo N, Harel-Belan A, Armand JP, Wong TW, Soria JC, Kroemer G (2007) A novel epidermal growth factor receptor inhibitor promotes apoptosis in non-small cell lung cancer cells resistant to erlotinib. Cancer Res 67:6253–6262. doi:67/13/6253[pii]10.1158/0008-5472.CAN-07-0538

Dziadziuszko R, Camidge DR, Hirsch FR (2008) The insulin-like growth factor pathway in lung cancer. J Thorac Oncol 3:815–818. doi:10.1097/JTO.0b013e31818180f501243894-200808000-00003[pii]

Engelman JA, Janne PA, Mermel C, Pearlberg J, Mukohara T, Fleet C, Cichowski K, Johnson BE, Cantley LC (2005) ErbB-3 mediates phosphoinositide 3-kinase activity in gefitinib-sensitive non-small cell lung cancer cell lines. Proc Natl Acad Sci USA 102:3788–3793

Engelman JA, Zejnullahu K, Gale CM, Lifshits E, Gonzales AJ, Shimamura T, Zhao F, Vincent PW, Naumov GN, Bradner JE, Althaus IW, Gandhi L, Shapiro GI, Nelson JM, Heymach JV, Meyerson M, Wong KK, Janne PA (2007a) PF00299804, an irreversible pan-ERBB inhibitor, is effective in lung cancer models with EGFR and ERBB2 mutations that are resistant to gefitinib. Cancer Res 67:11924–11932. doi:67/24/11924[pii]10.1158/0008-5472.CAN-07-1885

Engelman JA, Zejnullahu K, Mitsudomi T, Song Y, Hyland C, Park JO, Lindeman N, Gale CM, Zhao X, Christensen J, Kosaka T, Holmes AJ, Rogers AM, Cappuzzo F, Mok T, Lee C, Johnson BE, Cantley LC, Janne PA (2007b) MET amplification leads to gefitinib resistance in lung cancer by activating ERBB3 signaling. Science 316:1039–1043. doi:1141478[pii]10.1126/science.1141478

Fukuoka M, Yano S, Giaccone G, Tamura T, Nakagawa K, Douillard JY, Nishiwaki Y, Vansteenkiste J, Kudoh S, Rischin D, Eek R, Horai T, Noda K, Takata I, Smit E, Averbuch S, Macleod A, Feyereislova A, Dong RP, Baselga J (2003) Multi-institutional randomized phase II trial of gefitinib for previously treated patients with advanced non-small cell lung cancer (The IDEAL 1 trial) [corrected]. J Clin Oncol 21:2237–2246

Gatzemeier U, Pluzanska A, Szczesna A, Kaukel E, Roubec J, De Rosa F, Milanowski J, Karnicka-Mlodkowski H, Pesek M, Serwatowski P, Ramlau R, Janaskova T, Vansteenkiste J, Strausz J, Manikhas GM, Von Pawel J (2007) Phase III study of erlotinib in combination with cisplatin and gemcitabine in advanced non-small-cell lung cancer: the Tarceva lung cancer investigation trial. J Clin Oncol 25:1545–1552. doi:25/12/1545[pii]10.1200/JCO.2005.05.1474

Gendreau SB, Ventura R, Keast P, Laird AD, Yakes FM, Zhang W, Bentzien F, Cancilla B, Lutman J, Chu F, Jackman L, Shi Y, Yu P, Wang J, Aftab DT, Jaeger CT, Meyer SM, De Costa A, Engell K, Chen J, Martini JF, Joly AH (2007) Inhibition of the T790M gatekeeper mutant of the epidermal growth factor receptor by EXEL-7647. Clin Cancer Res 13:3713–3723. doi:13/12/3713[pii]10.1158/1078-0432.CCR-06-2590

Giaccone G, Herbst RS, Manegold C, Scagliotti G, Rosell R, Miller V, Natale RB, Schiller JH, Von Pawel J, Pluzanska A, Gatzemeier U, Grous J, Ochs JS, Averbuch SD, Wolf MK, Rennie P, Fandi A, Johnson DH (2004) Gefitinib in combination with gemcitabine and cisplatin in advanced non-small-cell lung cancer: a phase III trial–INTACT 1. J Clin Oncol 22:777–784. doi:10.1200/JCO.2004.08.001JCO.2004.08.001[pii]

Godin-Heymann N, Ulkus L, Brannigan BW, McDermott U, Lamb J, Maheswaran S, Settleman J, Haber DA (2008) The T790M "gatekeeper" mutation in EGFR mediates resistance to low concentrations of an irreversible EGFR inhibitor. Mol Cancer Ther 7:874–879. doi:7/4/874[pii]10.1158/1535-7163.MCT-07-2387

Gong Y, Somwar R, Politi K, Balak M, Chmielecki J, Jiang X, Pao W (2007) Induction of BIM is essential for apoptosis triggered by EGFR kinase inhibitors in mutant EGFR-dependent lung adenocarcinomas. PLoS Med 4:e294. doi:07-PLME-RA-0231[pii]10.1371/journal.pmed. 0040294

Gong Y, Yao E, Shen R, Goel A, Arcila M, Teruya-Feldstein J, Zakowski MF, Frankel S, Peifer M, Thomas RK, Ladanyi M, Pao W (2009) High expression levels of total IGF-1R and sensitivity of NSCLC cells in vitro to an anti-IGF-1R antibody (R1507). PLoS One 4:e7273. doi:10.1371/journal.pone.0007273

Gonzales AJ, Hook KE, Althaus IW, Ellis PA, Trachet E, Delaney AM, Harvey PJ, Ellis TA, Amato DM, Nelson JM, Fry DW, Zhu T, Loi CM, Fakhoury SA, Schlosser KM, Sexton KE, Winters RT, Reed JE, Bridges AJ, Lettiere DJ, Baker DA, Yang J, Lee HT, Tecle H, Vincent PW (2008) Antitumor activity and pharmacokinetic properties of PF-00299804, a second-generation irreversible pan-erbB receptor tyrosine kinase inhibitor. Mol Cancer Ther 7:1880–1889. doi:1535-7163.MCT-07-2232[pii]10.1158/1535-7163.MCT-07-2232

Gorre ME, Mohammed M, Ellwood K, Hsu N, Paquette R, Rao PN, Sawyers CL (2001) Clinical resistance to STI-571 cancer therapy caused by BCR-ABL gene mutation or amplification. Science 293(5531):876–880

Greulich H, Chen TH, Feng W, Janne PA, Alvarez JV, Zapparterra M, Bulmer SE, Frank DA, Hahn WC, Sellers WR, Meyerson M (2005) Oncogenic transformation by inhibitor-sensitive and resistant EGFR mutants. PLoS Med 2:e313

Guix M, Faber AC, Wang SE, Olivares MG, Song Y, Qu S, Rinehart C, Seidel B, Yee D, Arteaga CL, Engelman JA (2008) Acquired resistance to EGFR tyrosine kinase inhibitors in cancer cells is mediated by loss of IGF-binding proteins. J Clin Invest 118:2609–2619. doi:10.1172/JCI34588

Hartog H, Wesseling J, Boezen HM, van der Graaf WT (2007) The insulin-like growth factor 1 receptor in cancer: old focus, new future. Eur J Cancer 43:1895–1904. doi:S0959-8049 (07)00434-0[pii]10.1016/j.ejca.2007.05.021

Herbst RS, Giaccone G, Schiller JH, Natale RB, Miller V, Manegold C, Scagliotti G, Rosell R, Oliff I, Reeves JA, Wolf MK, Krebs AD, Averbuch SD, Ochs JS, Grous J, Fandi A, Johnson DH (2004) Gefitinib in combination with paclitaxel and carboplatin in advanced non-small-cell lung cancer: a phase III trial–INTACT 2. J Clin Oncol 22:785–794. doi:10.1200/JCO.2004.07.215JCO.2004.07.215[pii]

Herbst RS, Prager D, Hermann R, Fehrenbacher L, Johnson BE, Sandler A, Kris MG, Tran HT, Klein P, Li X, Ramies D, Johnson DH, Miller VA (2005) TRIBUTE: a phase III trial of erlotinib hydrochloride (OSI-774) combined with carboplatin and paclitaxel chemotherapy in advanced non-small-cell lung cancer. J Clin Oncol 23:5892–5899. doi:JCO.2005.02.840 [pii]10.1200/JCO.2005.02.840

Horn L, Pao W (2009) EML4-ALK: honing in on a new target in non-small-cell lung cancer. J Clin Oncol 27:4232–4235. doi:JCO.2009.23.6661[pii]10.1200/JCO.2009.23.6661

Hynes NE, Lane HA (2005) ERBB receptors and cancer: the complexity of targeted inhibitors. Nat Rev Cancer 5:341–354

Inoue A, Suzuki T, Fukuhara T, Maemondo M, Kimura Y, Morikawa N, Watanabe H, Saijo Y, Nukiwa T (2006) Prospective phase II study of gefitinib for chemotherapy-naive patients with advanced non-small-cell lung cancer with epidermal growth factor receptor gene mutations. J Clin Oncol 24:3340–3346. doi:JCO.2005.05.4692[pii]10.1200/JCO.2005.05.4692

Inukai M, Toyooka S, Ito S, Asano H, Ichihara S, Soh J, Suehisa H, Ouchida M, Aoe K, Aoe M, Kiura K, Shimizu N, Date H (2006) Presence of epidermal growth factor receptor gene T790M mutation as a minor clone in non-small cell lung cancer. Cancer Res 66:7854–7858. doi:66/16/7854[pii]10.1158/0008-5472.CAN-06-1951

Jackman DM, Miller VA, Cioffredi LA, Yeap BY, Janne PA, Riely GJ, Ruiz MG, Giaccone G, Sequist LV, Johnson BE (2009) Impact of epidermal growth factor receptor and KRAS mutations on clinical outcomes in previously untreated non-small cell lung cancer patients:

results of an online tumor registry of clinical trials. Clin Cancer Res 15:5267–5273. doi:1078-0432.CCR-09-0888[pii]10.1158/1078-0432.CCR-09-0888

Janjigian Y, Groen HJM, Horn L, Smit EF, Fu Y, Wang F, Shahidi M, Denis L, Pao W, Miller VA (2011) Activity and tolerability of afatinib (BIBW2992) and cetuximab in NSCLC patients with acquired resistance to erlotinib or gefitnib. PASCO

Janne P, Reckamp K, Koczywas M, Engelman JA, Camidge DR, Rajan A, Khuri F, Liang JQ, O'Connell J, Giaccone G (2009) Efficacy and safety of PF-00299804 (PF299) in patients (pt) with advanced NSCLC after failure of at least one prior chemotherapy regimen and prior treatment with erlotinib (E): a two-arm, phase II trial. J Clin Oncol Meeting Abstracts

Jemal A, Siegel R, Ward E, Hao Y, Xu J, Thun MJ (2009) Cancer statistics, 2009. CA Cancer J Clin 59:225–249. doi:caac.20006[pii]10.3322/caac.20006

Ji H, Zhao X, Yuza Y, Shimamura T, Li D, Protopopov A, Jung BL, McNamara K, Xia H, Glatt KA, Thomas RK, Sasaki H, Horner JW, Eck M, Mitchell A, Sun Y, Al-Hashem R, Bronson RT, Rabindran SK, Discafani CM, Maher E, Shapiro GI, Meyerson M, Wong KK (2006) Epidermal growth factor receptor variant III mutations in lung tumorigenesis and sensitivity to tyrosine kinase inhibitors. Proc Natl Acad Sci USA 103:7817–7822

Karamouzis MV, Konstantinopoulos PA, Papavassiliou AG (2009) Targeting MET as a strategy to overcome crosstalk-related resistance to EGFR inhibitors. Lancet Oncol 10:709–717. doi:S1470-2045(09)70137-8[pii]10.1016/S1470-2045(09)70137-8

Kim ES, Hirsh V, Mok T, Socinski MA, Gervais R, Wu YL, Li LY, Watkins CL, Sellers MV, Lowe ES, Sun Y, Liao ML, Osterlind K, Reck M, Armour AA, Shepherd FA, Lippman SM, Douillard JY (2008) Gefitinib versus docetaxel in previously treated non-small-cell lung cancer (INTEREST): a randomised phase III trial. Lancet 372:1809–1818. doi:S0140-6736 (08)61758-4[pii]10.1016/S0140-6736(08)61758-4

Kobayashi S, Boggon TJ, Dayaram T, Janne PA, Kocher O, Meyerson M, Johnson BE, Eck MJ, Tenen DG, Halmos B (2005) EGFR mutation and resistance of non-small-cell lung cancer to gefitinib. N Engl J Med 352:786–792

Kris MG, Natale RB, Herbst RS, Lynch TJ Jr, Prager D, Belani CP, Schiller JH, Kelly K, Spiridonidis H, Sandler A, Albain KS, Cella D, Wolf MK, Averbuch SD, Ochs JJ, Kay AC (2003) Efficacy of gefitinib, an inhibitor of the epidermal growth factor receptor tyrosine kinase, in symptomatic patients with non-small cell lung cancer: a randomized trial. JAMA 290:2149–2158

Kwak EL, Sordella R, Bell DW, Godin-Heymann N, Okimoto RA, Brannigan BW, Harris PL, Driscoll DR, Fidias P, Lynch TJ, Rabindran SK, McGinnis JP, Wissner A, Sharma SV, Isselbacher KJ, Settleman J, Haber DA (2005) Irreversible inhibitors of the EGF receptor may circumvent acquired resistance to gefitinib. Proc Natl Acad Sci USA 102:7665–7670

Li D, Shimamura T, Ji H, Chen L, Haringsma HJ, McNamara K, Liang MC, Perera SA, Zaghlul S, Borgman CL, Kubo S, Takahashi M, Sun Y, Chirieac LR, Padera RF, Lindeman NI, Janne PA, Thomas RK, Meyerson ML, Eck MJ, Engelman JA, Shapiro GI, Wong KK (2007) Bronchial and peripheral murine lung carcinomas induced by T790M–L858R mutant EGFR respond to HKI-272 and rapamycin combination therapy. Cancer Cell 12:81–93. doi:S1535-6108(07)00174-2[pii]10.1016/j.ccr.2007.06.005

Li D, Ambrogio L, Shimamura T, Kubo S, Takahashi M, Chirieac LR, Padera RF, Shapiro GI, Baum A, Himmelsbach F, Rettig WJ, Meyerson M, Solca F, Greulich H, Wong KK (2008) BIBW2992, an irreversible EGFR/HER2 inhibitor highly effective in preclinical lung cancer models. Oncogene 27:4702–4711. doi:onc2008109[pii]10.1038/onc.2008.109

Linardou H, Dahabreh IJ, Kanaloupiti D, Siannis F, Bafaloukos D, Kosmidis P, Papadimitriou CA, Murray S (2008) Assessment of somatic k-RAS mutations as a mechanism associated with resistance to EGFR-targeted agents: a systematic review and meta-analysis of studies in advanced non-small-cell lung cancer and metastatic colorectal cancer. Lancet Oncol 9:962–972. doi:S1470-2045(08)70206-7[pii]10.1016/S1470-2045(08)70206-7

Liu P, Cheng H, Roberts TM, Zhao JJ (2009) Targeting the phosphoinositide 3-kinase pathway in cancer. Nat Rev Drug Discov 8:627–644. doi:nrd2926[pii]10.1038/nrd2926

Lynch TJ, Bell DW, Sordella R, Gurubhagavatula S, Okimoto RA, Brannigan BW, Harris PL, Haserlat SM, Supko JG, Haluska FG, Louis DN, Christiani DC, Settleman J, Haber DA (2004) Activating mutations in the epidermal growth factor receptor underlying responsiveness of non-small-cell lung cancer to gefitinib. N Engl J Med 350:2129–2139

Maemondo M, Inoue A, Kobayashi K, Sugawara S, Oizumi S, Isobe H, Gemma A, Harada M, Yoshizawa H, Kinoshita I, Fujita Y, Okinaga S, Hirano H, Yoshimori K, Harada T, Ogura T, Ando M, Miyazawa H, Tanaka T, Saijo Y, Hagiwara K, Morita S, Nukiwa T (2010) Gefitinib or chemotherapy for non-small-cell lung cancer with mutated EGFR. N Engl J Med 362:2380–2388. doi:362/25/2380[pii]10.1056/NEJMoa0909530

Maheswaran S, Sequist LV, Nagrath S, Ulkus L, Brannigan B, Collura CV, Inserra E, Diederichs S, Iafrate AJ, Bell DW, Digumarthy S, Muzikansky A, Irimia D, Settleman J, Tompkins RG, Lynch TJ, Toner M, Haber DA (2008) Detection of mutations in EGFR in circulating lung-cancer cells. N Engl J Med 359:366–377. doi:NEJMoa0800668[pii]10.1056/NEJMoa0800668

Marks JL, Broderick S, Zhou Q, Chitale D, Li AR, Zakowski MF, Kris MG, Rusch VW, Azzoli CG, Seshan VE, Ladanyi M, Pao W (2008) Prognostic and therapeutic implications of EGFR and KRAS mutations in resected lung adenocarcinoma. J Thorac Oncol 3:111–116. doi:10.1097/JTO.0b013e318160c60701243894-200802000-00004[pii]

Mellinghoff I (2007) Why do cancer cells become "addicted" to oncogenic epidermal growth factor receptor? PLoS Med 4:1620–1622. doi:07-PLME-P-1608[pii]10.1371/journal.pmed.0040321

Miller V, Wakelee HA, Lara PN, Cho J, Chowhan NM, Costa D, Vrindavanam N, Yanagihara R, Pennell N, Lynch TJ (2008) Activity and tolerance of XL647 in NSCLC patients with acquired resistance to EGFR-TKIs: preliminary results of a phase II trial. J Clin Oncol Meeting Abstracts

Miller VA, Hirsh V, Cadranel J, Chen Y-M, Park K, Kim S-W, Caicun Z, Oberdick M, Shahidi M, Yang C-H (2010) Phase IIB/III double-blind randomized trial of afatinib (BIBW 2992, an irreversible inhibitor of EGFR/HER1 and HER2) + best supportive care (BSC) versus placebo + BSC in patients with NSCLC failing 1–2 lines of chemotherapy and erlotinib or gefitinib (LUX-Lung 1). Annals of Oncol 21:LBA1

Mitsudomi T, Morita S, Yatabe Y, Negoro S, Okamoto I, Tsurutani J, Seto T, Satouchi M, Tada H, Hirashima T, Asami K, Katakami N, Takada M, Yoshioka H, Shibata K, Kudoh S, Shimizu E, Saito H, Toyooka S, Nakagawa K, Fukuoka M (2010) Gefitinib versus cisplatin plus docetaxel in patients with non-small-cell lung cancer harbouring mutations of the epidermal growth factor receptor (WJTOG3405): an open label, randomised phase 3 trial. Lancet Oncol 11:121–128. doi:S1470-2045(09)70364-X[pii]10.1016/S1470-2045(09)70364-X

Mok TS, Wu YL, Thongprasert S, Yang CH, Chu DT, Saijo N, Sunpaweravong P, Han B, Margono B, Ichinose Y, Nishiwaki Y, Ohe Y, Yang JJ, Chewaskulyong B, Jiang H, Duffield EL, Watkins CL, Armour AA, Fukuoka M (2009) Gefitinib or carboplatin-paclitaxel in pulmonary adenocarcinoma. N Engl J Med 361:947–957. doi:NEJMoa0810699[pii] 10.1056/NEJMoa0810699

Moyer JD, Barbacci EG, Iwata KK, Arnold L, Boman B, Cunningham A, DiOrio C, Doty J, Morin MJ, Moyer MP, Neveu M, Pollack VA, Pustilnik LR, Reynolds MM, Sloan D, Theleman A, Miller P (1997) Induction of apoptosis and cell cycle arrest by CP-358, 774, an inhibitor of epidermal growth factor receptor tyrosine kinase. Cancer Res 57:4838–4848

Ogino A, Kitao H, Hirano S, Uchida A, Ishiai M, Kozuki T, Takigawa N, Takata M, Kiura K, Tanimoto M (2007) Emergence of epidermal growth factor receptor T790M mutation during chronic exposure to gefitinib in a non small cell lung cancer cell line. Cancer Res 67:7807–7814. doi:67/16/7807[pii]10.1158/0008-5472.CAN-07-0681

O'Hare T, Walters DK, Stoffregen EP, Sherbenou DW, Heinrich MC, Deininger MW, Druker BJ (2005) Combined Abl inhibitor therapy for minimizing drug resistance in chronic myeloid leukemia: Src/Abl inhibitors are compatible with imatinib. Clin Cancer Res 11(19 Pt 1): 6987–6993

Oxnard G, Arcila ME, Sima C, Riely GJ, Chmielecki J, Kris MG, Pao W, Ladanyi M, Miller VA (2011) Acquired resistance to EGFR tyrosine kinase inhibitors in EGFR mutant lung cancer:

distinct natural history of patients with tumors harboring the T790M mutation. Clin Cancer Res 17(6):1616–1622. doi:1078-0432.CCR-10-2692[pii]10.1158/1078-0432.CCR-10-2692

Paez JG, Janne PA, Lee JC, Tracy S, Greulich H, Gabriel S, Herman P, Kaye FJ, Lindeman N, Boggon TJ, Naoki K, Sasaki H, Fujii Y, Eck MJ, Sellers WR, Johnson BE, Meyerson M (2004) EGFR mutations in lung cancer: correlation with clinical response to gefitinib therapy. Science 304:1497–1500

Pao W, Miller V, Zakowski M, Doherty J, Politi K, Sarkaria I, Singh B, Heelan R, Rusch V, Fulton L, Mardis E, Kupfer D, Wilson R, Kris M, Varmus H (2004) EGF receptor gene mutations are common in lung cancers from "never smokers" and are associated with sensitivity of tumors to gefitinib and erlotinib. Proc Natl Acad Sci USA 101:13306–13311

Pao W, Miller VA, Politi KA, Riely GJ, Somwar R, Zakowski MF, Kris MG, Varmus H (2005a) Acquired resistance of lung adenocarcinomas to gefitinib or erlotinib is associated with a second mutation in the EGFR kinase domain. PLoS Med 2:e73

Pao W, Wang TY, Riely GJ, Miller VA, Pan Q, Ladanyi M, Zakowski MF, Heelan RT, Kris MG, Varmus HE (2005b) KRAS mutations and primary resistance of lung adenocarcinomas to gefitinib or erlotinib. PLoS Med 2:e17. doi:04-PLME-RA-0242R1[pii]10.1371/journal.pmed. 0020017

Politi K, Zakowski MF, Fan PD, Schonfeld EA, Pao W, Varmus HE (2006) Lung adenocarcinomas induced in mice by mutant EGF receptors found in human lung cancers respond to a tyrosine kinase inhibitor or to down-regulation of the receptors. Genes Dev 20:1496–1510

Pratilas CA, Hanrahan AJ, Halilovic E, Persaud Y, Soh J, Chitale D, Shigematsu H, Yamamoto H, Sawai A, Janakiraman M, Taylor BS, Pao W, Toyooka S, Ladanyi M, Gazdar A, Rosen N, Solit DB (2008) Genetic predictors of MEK dependence in non-small cell lung cancer. Cancer Res 68:9375–9383. doi:68/22/9375[pii]10.1158/0008-5472.CAN-08-2223

Rabindran SK, Discafani CM, Rosfjord EC, Baxter M, Floyd MB, Golas J, Hallett WA, Johnson BD, Nilakantan R, Overbeek E, Reich MF, Shen R, Shi X, Tsou HR, Wang YF, Wissner A (2004) Antitumor activity of HKI-272, an orally active, irreversible inhibitor of the HER-2 tyrosine kinase. Cancer Res 64:3958–3965. doi:10.1158/0008-5472.CAN-03-286864/11/3958[pii]

Regales L, Balak MN, Gong Y, Politi K, Sawai A, Le C, Koutcher JA, Solit DB, Rosen N, Zakowski MF, Pao W (2007) Development of new mouse lung tumor models expressing EGFR T790M mutants associated with clinical resistance to kinase inhibitors. PLoS One 2:e810. doi:10.1371/journal.pone.0000810

Regales L, Gong Y, Shen R, de Stanchina E, Vivanco I, Goel A, Koutcher JA, Spassova M, Ouerfelli O, Mellinghoff IK, Zakowski MF, Politi KA, Pao W (2009) Dual targeting of EGFR can overcome a major drug resistance mutation in mouse models of EGFR mutant lung cancer. J Clin Invest 119:3000–3010. doi:38746[pii]10.1172/JCI38746

Riely GJ, Pao W, Pham D, Li AR, Rizvi N, Venkatraman ES, Zakowski MF, Kris MG, Ladanyi M, Miller VA (2006) Clinical course of patients with non-small cell lung cancer and epidermal growth factor receptor exon 19 and exon 21 mutations treated with gefitinib or erlotinib. Clin Cancer Res 12:839–844. doi:12/3/839[pii]10.1158/1078-0432.CCR-05-1846

Riely GJ, Kris MG, Zhao B, Akhurst T, Milton DT, Moore E, Tyson L, Pao W, Rizvi NA, Schwartz LH, Miller VA (2007) Prospective assessment of discontinuation and reinitiation of erlotinib or gefitinib in patients with acquired resistance to erlotinib or gefitinib followed by the addition of everolimus. Clin Cancer Res 13:5150–5155. doi:13/17/5150[pii]10.1158/1078-0432.CCR-07-0560

Rizvi N, Kris MG, Miller VA, Krug LM, Bekele S, Dowlati A, Rowland KM, Salgia R, Aggarwal N, Gadgeel SM (2008) Activity of XL647 in clinically selected NSCLC patients (pts) enriched for the presence of EGFR mutations: results from phase 2. J Clin Oncol Meeting Abstracts

Rosell R, Moran T, Queralt C, Porta R, Cardenal F, Camps C, Majem M, Lopez-Vivanco G, Isla D, Provencio M, Insa A, Massuti B, Gonzalez-Larriba JL, Paz-Ares L, Bover I, Garcia-Campelo R, Moreno MA, Catot S, Rolfo C, Reguart N, Palmero R, Sanchez JM,

Bastus R, Mayo C, Bertran-Alamillo J, Molina MA, Sanchez JJ, Taron M (2009a) Screening for epidermal growth factor receptor mutations in lung cancer. N Engl J Med 361:958–967. doi:NEJMoa0904554[pii]10.1056/NEJMoa0904554

Rosell R, Perez-Roca L, Sanchez JJ, Cobo M, Moran T, Chaib I, Provencio M, Domine M, Sala MA, Jimenez U, Diz P, Barneto I, Macias JA, de Las Penas R, Catot S, Isla D, Sanchez JM, Ibeas R, Lopez-Vivanco G, Oramas J, Mendez P, Reguart N, Blanco R, Taron M (2009b) Customized treatment in non-small-cell lung cancer based on EGFR mutations and BRCA1 mRNA expression. PLoS One 4:e5133. doi:10.1371/journal.pone.0005133

Sandler A, Gray R, Perry MC, Brahmer J, Schiller JH, Dowlati A, Lilenbaum R, Johnson DH (2006) Paclitaxel-carboplatin alone or with bevacizumab for non-small-cell lung cancer. N Engl J Med 355:2542–2550. doi:355/24/2542[pii]10.1056/NEJMoa061884

Sawai A, Chandarlapaty S, Greulich H, Gonen M, Ye Q, Arteaga CL, Sellers W, Rosen N, Solit DB (2008) Inhibition of Hsp90 down-regulates mutant epidermal growth factor receptor (EGFR) expression and sensitizes EGFR mutant tumors to paclitaxel. Cancer Res 68:589–596. doi:68/2/589[pii]10.1158/0008-5472.CAN-07-1570

Schiller JH, Harrington D, Belani CP, Langer C, Sandler A, Krook J, Zhu J, Johnson DH TECOG (2002) Comparison of four chemotherapy regimens for advanced non-small-cell lung cancer. N Engl J Med 346:92–98. doi:10.1056/NEJMoa011954346/2/92[pii]

Sequist L, Waltman BA, Dias-Santagata D, Digumarthy S, Turke AB, Fidias P, Bergethon K, Shaw AT, Gettinger S, Cosper AK, Akhavanfard S, Heist RS, Temel J, Christensen J, Wain J, Lynch TJ, Vernovsky K, Mark EJ, Lanuti M, Iafrate AJ, Mino-Kenudson M, Engelman JA (2011) Genotypic and histological evolution of EGFR mutant NSCLCs upon development of resistance to EGFR kinase inhibitors. Science Transl Med

Sequist LV, Martins RG, Spigel D, Grunberg SM, Spira A, Janne PA, Joshi VA, McCollum D, Evans TL, Muzikansky A, Kuhlmann GL, Han M, Goldberg JS, Settleman J, Iafrate AJ, Engelman JA, Haber DA, Johnson BE, Lynch TJ (2008) First-line gefitinib in patients with advanced non-small-cell lung cancer harboring somatic EGFR mutations. J Clin Oncol 26:2442–2449. doi:JCO.2007.14.8494[pii]10.1200/JCO.2007.14.8494

Sequist LV, Besse B, Lynch TJ, Miller VA, Wong KK, Gitlitz B, Eaton K, Zacharchuk C, Freyman A, Powell C, Ananthakrishnan R, Quinn S, Soria JC (2010a) Neratinib, an irreversible pan-ErbB receptor tyrosine kinase inhibitor: results of a phase II trial in patients with advanced non-small-cell lung cancer. J Clin Oncol 28:3076–3083. doi:JCO.2009.27.9414[pii]10.1200/JCO.2009.27.9414

Sequist LV, Gettinger S, Senzer NN, Martins RG, Janne PA, Lilenbaum R, Gray JE, Iafrate AJ, Katayama R, Hafeez N, Sweeney J, Walker JR, Fritz C, Ross RW, Grayzel D, Engelman JA, Borger DR, Paez G, Natale R (2010b) Activity of IPI-504, a novel heat-shock protein 90 inhibitor, in patients with molecularly defined non-small-cell lung cancer. J Clin Oncol 28:4953–4960. doi:JCO.2010.30.8338[pii]10.1200/JCO.2010.30.8338

Shah NP, Nicoll JM, Nagar B, Gorre ME, Paquette RL, Kuriyan J, Sawyers CL (2002) Multiple BCR-ABL kinase domain mutations confer polyclonal resistance to the tyrosine kinase inhibitor imatinib (STI571) in chronic phase and blast crisis chronic myeloid leukemia. Cancer Cell 2:117–125

Sharma SV, Bell DW, Settleman J, Haber DA (2007) Epidermal growth factor receptor mutations in lung cancer. Nat Rev Cancer 7:169–181. doi:nrc2088[pii]10.1038/nrc2088

Shaw AT, Yeap BY, Mino-Kenudson M, Digumarthy SR, Costa DB, Heist RS, Solomon B, Stubbs H, Admane S, McDermott U, Settleman J, Kobayashi S, Mark EJ, Rodig SJ, Chirieac LR, Kwak EL, Lynch TJ, Iafrate AJ (2009) Clinical features and outcome of patients with non-small-cell lung cancer who harbor EML4-ALK. J Clin Oncol 27:4247–4253. doi:JCO.2009.22.6993[pii]10.1200/JCO.2009.22.6993

Shepherd FA, Rodrigues Pereira J, Ciuleanu T, Tan EH, Hirsh V, Thongprasert S, Campos D, Maoleekoonpiroj S, Smylie M, Martins R, van Kooten M, Dediu M, Findlay B, Tu D, Johnston D, Bezjak A, Clark G, Santabarbara P, Seymour L (2005) Erlotinib in previously treated non-small-cell lung cancer. N Engl J Med 353:123–132

Shih J, Yang C, Su W, Hsia T, Tsai C, Chen Y, Chang H, Terlizzi E, Shahidi M, Miller VA (2009) A phase II study of BIBW 2992, a novel irreversible dual EGFR and HER2 tyrosine kinase inhibitor (TKI), in patients with adenocarcinoma of the lung and activating EGFR mutations after failure of one line of chemotherapy (LUX-Lung 2). J Clin Oncol Meeting Abstracts

Shimamura T, Lowell AM, Engelman JA, Shapiro GI (2005) Epidermal growth factor receptors harboring kinase domain mutations associate with the heat shock protein 90 chaperone and are destabilized following exposure to geldanamycins. Cancer Res 65:6401–6408. doi:65/14/6401[pii]10.1158/0008-5472.CAN-05-0933

Shimamura T, Li D, Ji H, Haringsma HJ, Liniker E, Borgman CL, Lowell AM, Minami Y, McNamara K, Perera SA, Zaghlul S, Thomas RK, Greulich H, Kobayashi S, Chirieac LR, Padera RF, Kubo S, Takahashi M, Tenen DG, Meyerson M, Wong KK, Shapiro GI (2008) Hsp90 inhibition suppresses mutant EGFR-T790M signaling and overcomes kinase inhibitor resistance. Cancer Res 68:5827–5838. doi:68/14/5827[pii]10.1158/0008-5472.CAN-07-5428

Soda M, Choi YL, Enomoto M, Takada S, Yamashita Y, Ishikawa S, Fujiwara S, Watanabe H, Kurashina K, Hatanaka H, Bando M, Ohno S, Ishikawa Y, Aburatani H, Niki T, Sohara Y, Sugiyama Y, Mano H (2007) Identification of the transforming EML4-ALK fusion gene in non-small-cell lung cancer. Nature 448:561–566. doi:nature05945[pii]10.1038/nature05945

Soria JC, Lee HY, Lee JI, Wang L, Issa JP, Kemp BL, Liu DD, Kurie JM, Mao L, Khuri FR (2002) Lack of PTEN expression in non-small cell lung cancer could be related to promoter methylation. Clin Cancer Res 8:1178–1184

Sos ML, Koker M, Weir BA, Heynck S, Rabinovsky R, Zander T, Seeger JM, Weiss J, Fischer F, Frommolt P, Michel K, Peifer M, Mermel C, Girard L, Peyton M, Gazdar AF, Minna JD, Garraway LA, Kashkar H, Pao W, Meyerson M, Thomas RK (2009) PTEN loss contributes to erlotinib resistance in EGFR-mutant lung cancer by activation of Akt and EGFR. Cancer Res 69:3256–3261. doi:0008-5472.CAN-08-4055[pii]10.1158/0008-5472.CAN-08-4055

Stamos J, Sliwkowski MX, Eigenbrot C (2002) Structure of the epidermal growth factor receptor kinase domain alone and in complex with a 4-anilinoquinazoline inhibitor. J Biol Chem 277:46265–46272

Sunaga N, Tomizawa Y, Yanagitani N, Iijima H, Kaira K, Shimizu K, Tanaka S, Suga T, Hisada T, Ishizuka T, Saito R, Dobashi K, Mori M (2007) Phase II prospective study of the efficacy of gefitinib for the treatment of stage III/IV non-small cell lung cancer with EGFR mutations, irrespective of previous chemotherapy. Lung Cancer 56:383–389. doi:S0169-5002(07)00078-5[pii]10.1016/j.lungcan.2007.01.025

Tamborini E, Bonadiman L, Greco A, Albertini V, Negri T, Gronchi A, Bertulli R, Colecchia M, Casali PG, Pierotti MA, Pilotti S (2004) A new mutation in the KIT ATP pocket causes acquired resistance to imatinib in a gastrointestinal stromal tumor patient. Gastroenterology 127:294–299. doi:S0016508504002203[pii]

Thomson S, Buck E, Petti F, Griffin G, Brown E, Ramnarine N, Iwata KK, Gibson N, Haley JD (2005) Epithelial to mesenchymal transition is a determinant of sensitivity of non-small-cell lung carcinoma cell lines and xenografts to epidermal growth factor receptor inhibition. Cancer Res 65:9455–9462. doi:65/20/9455[pii]10.1158/0008-5472.CAN-05-1058

Toyooka S, Kiura K, Mitsudomi T (2005) EGFR mutation and response of lung cancer to gefitinib. N Engl J Med 352:2136. doi:352/20/2136[pii]10.1056/NEJM200505193522019 author reply 2136

Uramoto H, Iwata T, Onitsuka T, Shimokawa H, Hanagiri T, Oyama T (2010) Epithelial-mesenchymal transition in EGFR-TKI acquired resistant lung adenocarcinoma. Anticancer Res 30:2513–2517. doi:30/7/2513[pii]

Wakeling AE, Guy SP, Woodburn JR, Ashton SE, Curry BJ, Barker AJ, Gibson KH (2002) ZD1839 (Iressa): an orally active inhibitor of epidermal growth factor signaling with potential for cancer therapy. Cancer Res 62:5749–5754

Wong KK (2007) HKI-272 in non small cell lung cancer. Clin Cancer Res 13:s4593–s4596. doi:13/15/4593s[pii]10.1158/1078-0432.CCR-07-0369

Wong T, Ayers M, Emanuel S, Fargnoli J, Harbison C, Lee F, Oppenheimer S, Yu C, Krishnan B, Zhang H, Chen P, Fink B, Norris D, Vite G, Gavai A (2007) Inhibition of EGFR/HER2 signaling in tumor cells and VEGFR2 activity in tumor endothelium contribute to the preclinical anti-tumor activity of BMS-690514. AACR Meeting Abstracts

Wu JY, Wu SG, Yang CH, Gow CH, Chang YL, Yu CJ, Shih JY, Yang PC (2008) Lung cancer with epidermal growth factor receptor exon 20 mutations is associated with poor gefitinib treatment response. Clin Cancer Res 14:4877–4882. doi:14/15/4877[pii]10.1158/1078-0432.CCR-07-5123

Yang C, Shih J, Chao T, Tsai C, Yu C, Yang P, Streit M, Shahidi M, Miller VA (2008) Use of BIBW 2992, a novel irreversible EGFR/HER2 TKI, to induce regression in patients with adenocarcinoma of the lung and activating EGFR mutations: preliminary results of a single-arm phase II clinical trial. J Clin Oncol Meeting Abstracts

Yano S, Wang W, Li Q, Matsumoto K, Sakurama H, Nakamura T, Ogino H, Kakiuchi S, Hanibuchi M, Nishioka Y, Uehara H, Mitsudomi T, Yatabe Y, Sone S (2008) Hepatocyte growth factor induces gefitinib resistance of lung adenocarcinoma with epidermal growth factor receptor-activating mutations. Cancer Res 68:9479–9487. doi:68/22/9479[pii]10.1158/0008-5472.CAN-08-1643

Yun CH, Mengwasser KE, Toms AV, Woo MS, Greulich H, Wong KK, Meyerson M, Eck MJ (2008) The T790M mutation in EGFR kinase causes drug resistance by increasing the affinity for ATP. Proc Natl Acad Sci USA 105:2070–2075. doi:0709662105[pii]10.1073/pnas.0709662105

Zakowski MF, Ladanyi M, Kris MG (2006) EGFR mutations in small-cell lung cancers in patients who have never smoked. N Engl J Med 355:213–215. doi:355/2/213[pii]10.1056/NEJMc053610

Targeting Oncogenic BRAF in Human Cancer

Christine A. Pratilas, Feng Xing and David B. Solit

Abstract Mitogen Activated Protein Kinase (MAPK) pathway activation is a frequent event in human cancer and is often the result of activating mutations in the BRAF and RAS oncogenes. BRAF missense mutations, the vast majority of which are V600E, occur in approximately 8% of human tumors. These kinase domain mutations, which are non-overlapping in distribution with RAS mutations, are observed most frequently in melanoma but are also common in tumors arising in the colon, thyroid, lung, and other sites. Supporting its classification as an oncogene, ^{V600E}BRAF stimulates ERK signaling, induces proliferation, and is capable of promoting transformation. Given the frequent occurrence of BRAF mutations in human cancer and the continued requirement for BRAF activity in the tumors in which it is mutated, efforts are underway to develop targeted inhibitors of BRAF and its downstream effectors. These agents offer the possibility of greater efficacy and less toxicity than the systemic therapies currently available for tumors driven by activating mutations of MAPK pathway components. Early clinical results with the BRAF-selective inhibitors PLX4032 and GSK2118436 suggest that this strategy will prove successful in a select group of patients whose tumors are driven by oncogenic BRAF.

Contents

1	Introduction	84
2	Somatic BRAF Mutations in Human Tumors	84
3	Disabling Physiologic Feedback as a Requirement for RAS-MAPK Activation	86
4	MEK Kinase Inhibitors	88

C. A. Pratilas · F. Xing · D. B. Solit (✉)
Memorial Sloan-Kettering Cancer Center, New York, NY 10065, USA
e-mail: solitd@mskcc.org

Current Topics in Microbiology and Immunology (2012) 355: 83–98
DOI: 10.1007/82_2011_162
© Springer-Verlag Berlin Heidelberg 2011
Published Online: 5 August 2011

5	RAF Kinase Inhibitors	91
6	Future Perspective	93
References		93

1 Introduction

Thirty years have passed since oncogenic RAS was first identified as the transforming factor in the Harvey and Kirsten strains of the Mouse Sarcoma Virus (Chang et al. 1982; Der et al. 1982; Malumbres and Barbacid 2003; Shimizu et al. 1983). Homologous mutations were later identified in a broad range of human cancers including tumors of the pancreas, colon, and lung. RAS mutations, single amino acid missense mutations most commonly at residues G12, G13, or Q61, impair GTP hydrolysis and thus promote formation of constitutively activated GTP-bound RAS. RAS can also be activated in human tumors as a result of upstream activation of receptor tyrosine kinases (RTKs) or by loss of function of the NF-1 tumor suppressor.

Activated RAS promotes transformation through its downstream effectors, the best studied of which include RAF proteins, PI3'-kinases, and RalGEFs. These downstream effectors contain a RAS binding domain, which interacts with the core-effector domain of GTP-bound RAS. RAS binding induces effector activation through alterations in effector localization, intrinsic catalytic activity, or by facilitating complex formation with other signaling components (Repasky et al. 2004).

Oncogenic RAS through activation of RAF proteins induces constitutive activation of the classical mitogen activated protein kinase (MAPK) cascade. The RAF proteins (B-RAF, C-RAF (RAF1), and A-RAF) are serine/threonine protein kinases that phosphorylate and thus activate MAPK/ERK kinase 1 and 2 (MEK1/MEK2), which in turn phosphorylate and activate extracellular signal-regulated kinases 1 and 2 (ERK1/ERK2) (Catling et al. 1995; Moodie et al. 1993). ERK regulates gene expression by phosphorylating several nuclear transcription factors (including Ets, Elk, and Myc) or indirectly by targeting other intracellular signaling molecules (p90-RSK and others).

2 Somatic BRAF Mutations in Human Tumors

Somatic mutations in BRAF were first reported in 2002, and occur in approximately 8% of human tumors, most frequently in melanoma, colorectal, and thyroid cancers (Davies et al. 2002; Gorden et al. 2003) (Table 1). BRAF mutations are found, with rare exceptions, in a mutually exclusive pattern with RAS mutations, suggesting that these alterations activate common downstream effectors of transformation. In tumors, BRAF mutations are found clustered within the P-loop

Table 1 Frequency of BRAF mutations in human cancer

Melanoma	27–67%
Papillary thyroid	36–69%
Colon cancer	5–17%
Head and neck	3–5%
Pancreatic cancer	4–7%
Glioblastoma	3–6%
Lung cancer	1–3%
Ovarian Cancer	0–27%
Gastric	0–11%
Cholangiocarcinoma	0–22%
Prostate	0–10%
Endometrial	0–21%

(exon 11) and activation segment (exon 15) of the kinase domain. A single point mutation within the activation segment of the kinase domain, a glutamic acid for valine substitution at codon 600 (V600E, initially designated V599E), accounts for approximately 90% of BRAF mutants found in human tumors (Brose et al. 2002; Davies et al. 2002). Structural analysis of the V600E mutation suggests that it disrupts an interaction between the P-loop and the activation segment, which normally locks the kinase in the inactive conformation (Wan et al. 2004). In functional studies, the majority of BRAF mutations exhibit elevated kinase activity compared to the wild-type protein (Wan et al. 2004). Several BRAF mutations, however, demonstrate reduced kinase activity in vitro (designated as low-activity mutants). These low-activity mutants activate ERK indirectly through the formation of BRAF/CRAF heterodimers (Wan et al. 2004).

The high frequency of BRAF mutations in human cancer suggests that BRAF functions as an oncogene in the tumors in which it is mutated. In cell culture studies, mutant forms of BRAF are capable of inducing transformation of NIH-3T3 cells (Davies et al. 2002). Expression of [V600E]BRAF in non-transformed melanocytes also promotes the ability of these cells to form tumors in nude mice (Wellbrock et al. 2004). Conversely, BRAF suppression by RNAi in [V600E]BRAF mutant models induces growth arrest and apoptosis and slows tumor growth in xenograft models (Hingorani et al. 2003; Hoeflich et al. 2006). Activating BRAF mutations are, however, present in the majority of melanocytic nevi, benign skin lesions that rarely progress to melanoma (Pollock et al. 2003). Furthermore, transfection of mutant BRAF into non-transformed human melanocytes has been shown to induce p16 expression, cell cycle arrest, and senescence (Michaloglou et al. 2005). As most melanomas are deficient in p16, these data suggest that concurrent inactivation of p16 may be one of several alterations that cooperate with oncogenic BRAF to promote melananomagenesis (Bennett 2003; Gray-Schopfer et al. 2006; Sviderskaya et al. 2003). Similarly, BRAF mutations are common in colonic polyps suggesting that BRAF mutation in colorectal cancer is an early lesion that requires additional cooperative events to induce transformation. Several candidate cooperative genetic alterations have been identified in melanoma, including *MITF* amplification, and mutation and/or deletion of the tumor suppressor genes *PTEN, TP53* and *CDKN2A* (Dankort et al. 2009, 2007; Garraway et al. 2005).

Studies in genetically engineered zebrafish and mouse models highlight the requirement for cooperative genetic events in ^{V600E}BRAF-driven melanomagenesis. In zebrafish, TP53 inactivation cooperates with ^{V600E}BRAF to induce melanocyte transformation (Patton et al. 2005). Zebrafish engineered to express ^{V600E}BRAF develop melanocytic nevi, whereas expression of ^{V600E}BRAF in TP53 deficient zebrafish results in formation of invasive tumors resembling those of human melanoma. Similarly, melanocyte-specific expression of ^{V600E}BRAF in mice results in melanocytic hyperplasia that fails to progress to invasive melanoma (Dankort et al. 2009). In the setting of a PTEN null background, however, melanocyte-specific ^{V600E}BRAF expression results in invasive melanoma formation with 100% penetrance in genetically engineered mice. In melanocytes, loss of IGFBP7 may also allow for escape from BRAF mediated senescence (Wajapeyee et al. 2008). Analogous results have also been observed in lung tissue, where expression of mutant BRAF at physiological levels in mice is associated with the development of benign lung tumors that only rarely progress to invasive adenocarcinoma (Dankort et al. 2007). Loss of Ink4a/Arf and TP53 function, however, promote cancer progression in this model (Dankort et al. 2007). In summary, these data suggest that multiple genetic changes likely cooperate with oncogenic BRAF to induce transformation and progression in human cancers. The extent to which lineage determines the complement of these additional genetic alterations remains unknown but may be critical. Whether any of these concurrent genetic changes leads to a reduced requirement for continued BRAF and MEK activity for tumor maintenance also remains to be determined.

3 Disabling Physiologic Feedback as a Requirement for RAS-MAPK Activation

Physiologic activation of RAS/RAF signaling is balanced by inhibitory regulators of the pathway which include sprouty proteins, MAP kinase phosphatases (DUSPs), KSR-1, and RKIP (Morrison and Cutler 1997), and by scaffolding proteins such as 14-3-3 which regulate RAF cellular localization and stability (Dougherty and Morrison 2004; Morrison 1994). Pathway activity is also regulated by cross talk with parallel signaling pathways, such as by AKT phosphorylation of inhibitory sites on RAF (Zimmermann and Moelling 1999) and through PI3K-dependent feedback (Carracedo et al. 2008). Under physiologic conditions, activation of the MAPK pathway is balanced by inhibitory signals, which dampen or limit the duration of pathway activity. In tumor cells, this normal feedback regulation is often disabled through mutation or decreased expression of feedback regulators thus allowing for unhindered pathway activation.

Sprouty proteins, encoded by one of four *SPRY* genes (*SPRY*1–4), negatively regulate RAS activity and may have direct inhibitory effects on RAF, by blocking its activation by protein kinase C-δ (PKCδ) (Kim and Bar-Sagi 2004; Sasaki et al. 2003; Yusoff et al. 2002). The inducible expression of sprouty family members by ERK activation follows the classic pattern of a negative feedback loop whereby the expression of the negative feedback regulator is controlled by the signaling pathways that it ultimately regulates (Hanafusa et al. 2002). The idea that disruption of this negative feedback loop is a prerequisite for sustained pathway activation is supported by the observation that expression of sprouty proteins is suppressed in a variety of cancers. For example, inactivation or loss of sprouty expression has been reported in breast, hepatocellular, lung, and prostate cancers. This suggests that activation of the RAS/MAPK pathway is mediated in part by disruption of its normal physiological feedback (Fong et al. 2006; Lee et al. 2008; Lo et al. 2004; Sutterluty et al. 2007).

In contrast, in melanoma, *SPRY*2 expression is higher in cells harboring a [V600E]BRAF mutation compared to cells that are wild-type for BRAF (Tsavachidou et al. 2004). Using an unbiased approach to identify MEK-ERK dependent transcriptional targets in [V600E]BRAF melanoma cells, *SPRY*2 transcription (along with other feedback regulators) was found to be profoundly and rapidly downregulated in response to MEK inhibition. Additionally, *SPRY*2 expression is significantly higher in cells harboring a BRAF mutation compared to cells in which the MAPK pathway is activated by RTKs (Pratilas et al. 2009). This seemingly paradoxical overexpression of feedback regulators of the pathway in the setting of high pathway activation in [V600E]BRAF tumors can be attributed to the inability of *SPRY*2 to inhibit the [V600E]BRAF mutant (Brady et al. 2009).

MAP kinase phosphatases (MKPs, or DUSPs) recognize dually phosphorylated proteins at threonine/tyrosine residues in a consensus–pTXpY-motif, found in several MAPK family members including ERK, SAPK/JNK, and p38 MAPK. Analogous to the loss of expression of sprouty proteins, loss of DUSP6 function may contribute to pancreatic cancer progression (Furukawa et al. 2005, 2003) and MAPK pathway activation in endometrial cancer (Ogawa et al. 2005). In melanomas with [V600E]BRAF mutation, the upstream feedback mediated by sprouty proteins is disrupted as outlined above, whereas the downstream feedback at the level of ERK, mediated by the MAP kinase phosphatases, remains intact. This pattern of feedback deregulation in [V600E]BRAF cancer cells leads to steady-state levels of phosphorylated ERK that are not strikingly high despite high levels of MEK phosphorylation and ERK pathway output. These data provide a mechanistic basis for the lack of correlation between phosphorylated ERK expression and MAPK pathway output and suggest that levels of phosphorylated ERK should not be used as a predictive biomarker in clinical trials of RAF and MEK inhibitors.

MAPK pathway activity is regulated not only by transcriptional targets of ERK but also by direct phosphorylation events. CRAF activation is regulated by its phosphorylation at S338 and other activating sites (Chong et al. 2001). CRAF also contains six ERK dependent phosphorylation sites through which its activity is negatively regulated (S29, S43, S289, S296, S301, and S642) (Dougherty et al. 2005). Highlighting the critical role of these feedback regulators in determining ERK pathway output, CRAF activation of MEK has been observed following treatment with MEK inhibitors (Alessi et al. 1995; Friday et al. 2008; Pratilas et al. 2009), in the setting of impaired ERK activation by dominant negative kinase suppressor of RAS (KSR) (Therrien et al. 1996), and in cells overexpressing IMP (Matheny et al. 2004). From a drug development perspective, these findings suggest that the clinical activity of selective inhibitors of BRAF and MEK may be attenuated by relief of feedback inhibition of CRAF. Consistent with this possibility, overexpression of CRAF has been demonstrated as a mechanism of acquired resistance to the selective RAF inhibitor AZ628 (Montagut et al. 2008).

4 MEK Kinase Inhibitors

Several strategies for inhibiting MAPK signaling are now being tested as cancer therapies (Table 2). These include selective inhibitors of the RAF and MEK kinases and inhibitors of the Hsp90 chaperone. We will focus first on selective inhibitors of the MEK kinases. CI-1040 (PD184352, Pfizer Oncology) was the first selective small molecule inhibitor of MEK to advance into clinical testing (Sebolt-Leopold et al. 1999). CI-1040 is non-ATP-competitive and inhibits MEK activation by binding to a pocket adjacent to the ATP binding site (Ohren et al. 2004). CI-1040 is highly selective for MEK1 and MEK2, with its only other known target being MEK5, whose inhibition occurs at a 100-fold greater concentration than that required to inhibit MEK1/2. Cell lines with BRAF mutation are selectively sensitive to CI-1040 (Solit et al. 2006). In BRAF mutant tumors, MEK inhibition results in downregulation of cyclin D1, upregulation of p27, hypophosphorylation of RB1 and growth arrest in G1 (Solit et al. 2006). MEK inhibition also induces differentiation and senescence of BRAF mutant tumors and apoptosis in some, but not all, [V600E]BRAF mutant models (Solit et al. 2006, 2007). Anti-tumor activity was observed in the phase I trial of CI-1040, with one patient demonstrating a partial response and 25% of patients exhibiting prolonged stable disease (Lorusso et al. 2005). Clinical activity was, however, disappointing in the phase 2 setting and therefore development of CI-1040 was halted in favor of a more potent second-generation compound (Rinehart et al. 2004). Notably, the clinical development of CI-1040 was initiated prior to the identification of BRAF mutations in human tumors and therefore this agent was not tested in tumor types, including melanoma, with the highest reported frequency of BRAF mutation.

PD0325901 (Pfizer Oncology) (Fig. 1) is a second-generation allosteric inhibitor of MEK1 and MEK2. PD0325901 is 50–100-fold more potent than CI-1040 and has improved oral bioavailability and increased metabolic stability (Brown et al. 2007; Sebolt-Leopold and Herrera 2004). BRAF mutant cell lines are also selectively sensitive to PD0325901 (Solit et al. 2006). In pharmacodynamic studies, the drug reduced the expression of phosphorylated ERK by more than 70%

Targeting Oncogenic BRAF in Human Cancer

Table 2 RAF and MEK kinase inhibitors

RAF inhibitors		
Sorafenib (Nexavar)	Bayer	FDA approved
PLX4032	Plexxikon/Roche	Phase 3 trial positive for survival
GSK2118436	GlaxoSmithKline	Phase 3 ongoing
XL281/BMS-908662	Exelixis/BMS	Phase 1/2
RAF265	Novartis	Phase 1
ARQ 680	ArQule	Phase 1
GDC-0879	Genentech	Pre-clinical testing
MEK inhibitors		
AZD6244	Array BioPharma/AstraZeneca	Phase 3
ARRY-704/AZD8330	Array BioPharma/AstraZeneca	Phase 1
PD0325901	Pfizer	Phase 1
CI-1040	Pfizer	Phase 2
XL518	Exelixis/Genentech	Phase 1
RDEA119	Ardea Biosciences	Phase 1
AS703026	Merck Serono	Phase 1
GSK1120212	GlaxoSmith Kline	Phase 1/2
CH5126766	Chugai/Roche	Phase 1

relative to baseline in the tumors of seven out of nine patients tested. Three patients with melanoma treated with PD0325901 had RECIST (Response Evaluation Criteria in Solid Tumors) partial responses on the phase 1 clinical trial, but development of this agent beyond the phase 1 setting has not been pursued due to concerns over neurological toxicity (Wang et al. 2007).

AZD6244 (AstraZeneca) is also an ATP non-competitive, allosteric inhibitor of MEK1 and MEK2. AZD6244 recently completed phase 2 testing in melanoma, lung and colorectal cancers (Dummer et al. 2008; Lang et al. 2008; Tzekova et al. 2008). In a phase 2 trial of AZD6244 in patients with melanoma, 200 patients were randomized to AZD6244 (100 mg BID) or temozolamide (200 mg/m^2 for 5 days, q28 days) (Dummer et al. 2008). Antitumor activity with AZD6244 was observed on the trial with partial responses in six patients, five of whom had tumors that expressed ^{V600E}BRAF. There was, however, no significant difference between the treatment arms for the primary endpoint of progression-free survival. In the NSCLC trial, MEK inhibition with AZD6244 was compared with pemetrexed (Tzekova et al. 2008). Two partial responses were observed in both arms, with no difference between the agents in time to progression. Similarly, in colorectal, AZD6244 was compared with capecitabine with no difference observed between the two arms in time to progression (Lang et al. 2008). In summary, the three randomized phase 2 trials of AZD6244 in melanoma, lung and colorectal cancer suggested that activity with this agent was comparable but not superior to disease-specific standard chemotherapy. In each case, enrichment for those patients most likely to respond to MEK inhibition as predicted by the preclinical data was not incorporated into the trial designs. On the basis of these clinical results and the preclinical data suggesting a correlation between BRAF mutation status and

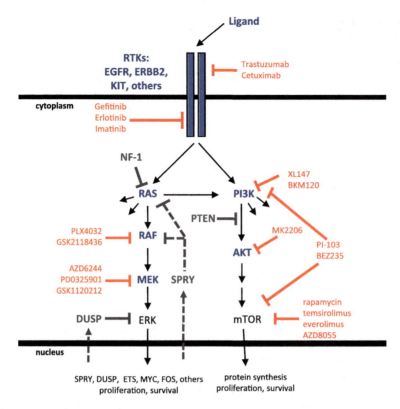

Fig. 1 The MAP kinase pathway. The MAP kinase pathway is activated in human tumors by the binding of ligand to receptor tyrosine kinases (RTKs), by constitutive activation of an RTK, by loss of NF-1 function, or by mutations in RAS, BRAF, and MEK1. Phosphorylation and thus activation of ERK regulates transcription of target genes which promote cell cycle progression and tumor survival. The ERK pathway contains a classical feedback loop in which the expression of feedback elements such as SPRY and DUSP family proteins are regulated by ERK (*dashed grey lines*). Selected agents that target the MAP kinase and PI3 kinase/AKT pathway are shown (*red*)

sensitivity to MEK inhibition, ongoing studies are testing the efficacy of AZD6244 in a subset of patients with mutational activation of the pathway (BRAF and RAS mutant only).

The importance of pretreatment stratification by mutational status is highlighted by the promising results recently reported with the MEK inhibitor GSK1120212. GSK1120212 is also a potent, non-ATP competitive MEK inhibitor (IC_{50}s for MEK1 and MEK2 of 0.7 and 0.9 nM, respectively) (Gilmartin et al. 2011). Preliminary results from the Phase 1 trial of GSK1120212 were reported at the 2010 American Society of Clinical Oncology Annual meeting. In twenty patients with BRAF mutant melanoma, two achieved complete responses with an additional six patients demonstrating partial responses for a total response rate of 40% (Infante et al. 2010). The GSK1120212 trial is the only trial of a MEK inhibitor reported to date to have stratified patients based upon BRAF mutational status.

It thus remains unknown whether the greater activity of this compound compared to others in the class was the result of enrichment for patients whose tumors harbored a BRAF mutation or to the compound's specific pharmacologic properties.

5 RAF Kinase Inhibitors

Sorafenib (BAY43-9006, Nexavar) was the first RAF kinase inhibitor to enter clinical testing. Sorafenib is now FDA approved for use in renal cell carcinoma and hepatocellular carcinoma. Although this compound was initially developed as a selective inhibitor of RAF, later studies revealed other targets of sorafenib, including VEGF receptor 2 and 3, PDGFR, Flt-3, c-KIT, and FGFR-1 (Wilhelm et al. 2004). Sorafenib has virtually no activity as a single-agent in melanoma, the tumor type with highest prevalence of BRAF mutations (Eisen et al. 2006). Phase 2 trials combining sorafenib with chemotherapy showed early promise in melanoma but the activity of this combination regimen did not correlate with BRAF mutational status (Flaherty et al. 2008). Furthermore, a Phase 3 trial of sorafenib in combination with carboplatin and paclitaxel in patients with advanced melanoma failed to meet its primary endpoint of improvement in progression-free survival (Hauschild et al. 2009). Overall, the data suggest that the primary basis for the anti-tumor activity of sorafenib in renal cancer is likely anti-angiogenic and that RAF inhibition contributes minimally, if at all, to its activity in patients with advanced cancer.

The limited activity of sorafenib in tumors with BRAF mutation prompted the development of second-generation RAF inhibitors with greater selectivity for BRAF and greater potency for the target in vivo. PLX4032 (vemurafenib) and its close analogue PLX4720 are selective RAF inhibitors developed by Plexxikon (Bollag et al. 2010; Tsai et al. 2008) (see also "Setting up a Kinase Discovery and Development Project"). These compounds were designed to bind to the active conformation of BRAF and show three-fold selectivity for ^{V600E}BRAF versus wild-type BRAF, good oral bioavailability, and little toxicity in pre-clinical models. The compounds demonstrate potent antiproliferative effects, but in contrast to sorafenib and MEK inhibitors, do so only in BRAF mutant cell lines (Joseph et al. 2010). The selective anti-tumor activity of PLX4032 for tumors with BRAF mutation is attributable to its mutant-selective inhibition of MAPK pathway activity. PLX4032 binds to all three RAF isoforms and exhibits only modest selectivity for mutant BRAF over wild-type BRAF. Despite binding to all three RAF isoforms at low nanomolar concentrations, the drug potently inhibits MAPK pathway activity only in cells expressing ^{V600E}BRAF, whereas it activates ERK in BRAF wild-type tumor and normal cells (Hatzivassiliou et al. 2010; Heidorn et al. 2010; Poulikakos et al. 2010). The basis for this activation of ERK activity lies in the formation of RAF homo- and heterodimers, a process regulated by RAS (Poulikakos et al. 2010). In BRAF wild-type tumor and normal cells, the current model suggests that PLX4032 induces ERK signaling by transactivating RAF dimers in a process that is RAS-dependent. At low concentrations, binding of PLX4032 to one protomer within a RAF dimer results in transactivation and thus activation of the non-drug bound RAF. At saturating concentrations, which are likely not achievable in patients, PLX4032 binds to both protomers within such dimers, thus inhibiting RAF activation (Poulikakos et al. 2010).

In the Phase 1 trial of PLX4032, 81% of patients with [V600E]BRAF mutant tumors treated at the recommended Phase II dose achieved a partial response (Flaherty et al. 2010). This level of clinical activity is significantly greater than that of the MEK1/2 inhibitors AZD6244 and GSK1120212, even when considering only the cohort of patients whose tumors express [V600E]BRAF. The most common toxicities of PLX4032 included skin rash, arthralgias, and fatigue. In addition, approximately one-third of patients developed squamous cell carcinomas (keratoacanthoma type) while on treatment (Flaherty et al. 2010). These toxicities have been attributed to the activation of ERK induced by RAF inhibitors such as PLX4032 in non-tumor cells that are BRAF wild-type. Consistent with the clinical profile of PLX4032, a second highly selective RAF inhibitor GSK2118436 (GlaxoSmithKline) also demonstrated a high response rate (63%) in BRAF mutant patients in a recently reported Phase I trial (Kefford et al. 2010).

The basis for the greater antitumor activity of PLX4032 as compared to the MEK inhibitors may be that the mutant selectivity for ERK pathway inhibition of the former allows for more potent and durable MAPK pathway inhibition. Whereas the MEK inhibitor downregulates ERK activity in all cells including normal tissues, the RAF inhibitor PLX4032 inhibits ERK activity only in tumor cells expressing oncogenic BRAF (Joseph et al. 2010). This mutant selectivity for pathway inhibition likely confers a broader therapeutic index, which allows for greater MAPK pathway inhibition with PLX4032 and thus increase anti-tumor efficacy in patients whose tumors harbor a sensitive BRAF mutation. Supporting this hypothesis, pharmacokinetic data from the Phase I trial suggests that the half-life of PLX4032 is long (~ 40–50 h) and steady-state plasma levels of over 40 μM can be achievable in patients (Flaherty et al. 2010). Alternatively, RAF inhibition may be superior to MEK inhibition in tumors with mutant BRAF due to inhibition of non-MEK effectors of RAF by the RAF inhibitor but not the MEK inhibitor. Although potential non-MEK effectors of CRAF have been reported, their biological significance remains controversial and their relevance in the setting of mutant BRAF unexplored. Additionally, differences in CNS penetration and thus a lower frequency of progression in brain may also have played a role in the greater activity observed with PLX4032 compared to inhibitors of MEK. The high level of activity observed with PLX4032 also supports the contention that sorafenib's lack of clinical activity in patients with BRAF mutant tumors is attributable to its low potency against the [V600E]BRAF mutation.

The promising Phase I results with PLX4032 prompted the initiation of a randomized Phase III study (BRIM3) comparing PLX4032 to dacarbazine in previously untreated patients with metastatic melanoma (clinicaltrials.gov identifier: NCT01006980). Eligibility for BRIM3 was restricted to treatment-naïve (no prior systemic anticancer therapy) patients with Stage IIIC and IV melanoma whose tumors were positive for the ^{V600E}BRAF mutation. The BRIM3 results have not yet been published but the study sponsors (Roche/Plexxikon) have announced that treatment with PLX4032 resulted in significant improvements in overall survival and progression-free survival. Future studies will be needed to address the mechanistic basis for the heterogeneity of responses observed with PLX4032 within the ^{V600E}BRAF cohort and the molecular basis for intrinsic and acquired resistance in patients who initially respond to this approach but then progress (Johannessen et al. 2010; Nazarian et al. 2010; Poulikakos et al. 2011; Villanueva et al. 2010). Novel RAF inhibitors that potently suppress ERK activation in BRAF mutant cells but lack the paradoxical activation of ERK noted with PLX4032 in BRAF wild-type cells are also in development on the presumption that such agents would exhibit a broader therapeutic index (Bollag 2011).

6 Future Perspective

Activation of the MAP kinase pathway is a frequent event in human cancer and pathway activity is often the result of activating mutations in RAS and BRAF. Drugs that target RAF and its primary downstream effector MEK are in clinical development. Preliminary results suggest that one such compound, the selective RAF inhibitor PLX4032, prolongs survival in patients with ^{V600E}BRAF mutant melanomas. As the activity of these agents correlates with the mechanisms responsible for pathway activation (BRAF mutation, RAS mutation or receptor tyrosine kinase activation), prospective genotyping of patients to enrich for those most likely to respond will be critical in the future clinical development of selective inhibitors of this pathway.

References

Alessi DR, Cuenda A, Cohen P, Dudley DT, Saltiel AR (1995) PD 098059 is a specific inhibitor of the activation of mitogen-activated protein kinase kinase in vitro and in vivo. J Biol Chem 270:27489–27494

Bennett DC (2003) Human melanocyte senescence and melanoma susceptibility genes. Oncogene 22:3063–3069

Bollag G (2011) Overcoming the paradoxical pathway activation of first-generation RAF kinase inhibitors. AACR annual meeting 2011, Orlando, FL

Bollag G, Hirth P, Tsai J, Zhang J, Ibrahim PN, Cho H, Spevak W, Zhang C, Zhang Y, Habets G, Burton EA, Wong B, Tsang G, West BL, Powell B, Shellooe R, Marimuthu A, Nguyen H, Zhang KY, Artis DR, Schlessinger J, Su F, Higgins B, Iyer R, D'Andrea K, Koehler A, Stumm M, Lin PS, Lee RJ, Grippo J, Puzanov I, Kim KB, Ribas A, McArthur GA, Sosman JA, Chapman PB, Flaherty KT, Xu X, Nathanson KL, Nolop K (2010) Clinical efficacy of a RAF inhibitor needs broad target blockade in BRAF-mutant melanoma. Nature 467:596–599

Brady SC, Coleman ML, Munro J, Feller SM, Morrice NA, Olson MF (2009) Sprouty2 association with B-RAF is regulated by phosphorylation and kinase conformation. Cancer Res 69:6773–6781

Brose MS, Volpe P, Feldman M, Kumar M, Rishi I, Gerrero R, Einhorn E, Herlyn M, Minna J, Nicholson A, Roth JA, Albelda SM, Davies H, Cox C, Brignell G, Stephens P, Futreal PA, Wooster R, Stratton MR, Weber BL (2002) BRAF and RAS mutations in human lung cancer and melanoma. Cancer Res 62:6997–7000

Brown AP, Carlson TC, Loi CM, Graziano MJ (2007) Pharmacodynamic and toxicokinetic evaluation of the novel MEK inhibitor, PD0325901, in the rat following oral and intravenous administration. Cancer Chemother Pharmacol 59:671–679

Carracedo A, Ma L, Teruya-Feldstein J, Rojo F, Salmena L, Alimonti A, Egia A, Sasaki AT, Thomas G, Kozma SC, Papa A, Nardella C, Cantley LC, Baselga J, Pandolfi PP (2008) Inhibition of mTORC1 leads to MAPK pathway activation through a PI3K-dependent feedback loop in human cancer. J Clin Invest 118:3065–3074

Catling AD, Schaeffer HJ, Reuter CW, Reddy GR, Weber MJ (1995) A proline-rich sequence unique to MEK1 and MEK2 is required for RAF binding and regulates MEK function. Mol Cell Biol 15:5214–5225

Chang EH, Furth ME, Scolnick EM, Lowy DR (1982) Tumorigenic transformation of mammalian cells induced by a normal human gene homologous to the oncogene of Harvey murine sarcoma virus. Nature 297:479–483

Chong H, Lee J, Guan KL (2001) Positive and negative regulation of RAF kinase activity and function by phosphorylation. Embo J 20:3716–3727

Dankort D, Filenova E, Collado M, Serrano M, Jones K, McMahon M (2007) A new mouse model to explore the initiation, progression, and therapy of BRAFV600E-induced lung tumors. Genes Dev 21:379–384

Dankort D, Curley DP, Cartlidge RA, Nelson B, Karnezis AN, Damsky WE Jr, You MJ, DePinho RA, McMahon M, Bosenberg M (2009) BRAF(V600E) cooperates with pten loss to induce metastatic melanoma. Nat Genet 41:544–552

Davies H, Bignell GR, Cox C, Stephens P, Edkins S, Clegg S, Teague J, Woffendin H, Garnett MJ, Bottomley W, Davis N, Dicks E, Ewing R, Floyd Y, Gray K, Hall S, Hawes R, Hughes J, Kosmidou V, Menzies A, Mould C, Parker A, Stevens C, Watt S, Hooper S, Wilson R, Jayatilake H, Gusterson BA, Cooper C, Shipley J, Hargrave D, Pritchard-Jones K, Maitland N, Chenevix-Trench G, Riggins GJ, Bigner DD, Palmieri G, Cossu A, Flanagan A, Nicholson A, Ho JW, Leung SY, Yuen ST, Weber BL, Seigler HF, Darrow TL, Paterson H, Marais R, Marshall CJ, Wooster R, Stratton MR, Futreal PA (2002) Mutations of the BRAF gene in human cancer. Nature 417:949–954

Der CJ, Krontiris TG, Cooper GM (1982) Transforming genes of human bladder and lung carcinoma cell lines are homologous to the RAS genes of Harvey and Kirsten sarcoma viruses. Proc Nat Acad Sci U S A 79:3637–3640

Dougherty MK, Morrison DK (2004) Unlocking the code of 14-3-3. J Cell Sci 117:1875–1884

Dougherty MK, Muller J, Ritt DA, Zhou M, Zhou XZ, Copeland TD, Conrads TP, Veenstra TD, Lu KP, Morrison DK (2005) Regulation of RAF-1 by direct feedback phosphorylation. Mol Cell 17:215–224

Dummer R, Robert C, Chapman PB, Sosman JA, Middleton M, Bastholt L, Kemsley K, Cantarini MV, Morris C, Kirkwood JM (2008) AZD6244 (ARRY-142886) vs temozolomide (TMZ) in patients (pts) with advanced melanoma: an open-label, randomized, multicenter, phase II study. J Clin Oncol 26:9033 (Meeting Abstracts)

Eisen T, Ahmad T, Flaherty KT, Gore M, Kaye S, Marais R, Gibbens I, Hackett S, James M, Schuchter LM, Nathanson KL, Xia C, Simantov R, Schwartz B, Poulin-Costello M, O'Dwyer PJ, Ratain MJ (2006) Sorafenib in advanced melanoma: a phase II randomised discontinuation trial analysis. Br J Cancer 95:581–586

Flaherty KT, Schiller J, Schuchter LM, Liu G, Tuveson DA, Redlinger M, Lathia C, Xia C, Petrenciuc O, Hingorani SR, Jacobetz MA, Van Belle PA, Elder D, Brose MS, Weber BL,

Albertini MR, O'Dwyer PJ (2008) A phase I trial of the oral, multikinase inhibitor sorafenib in combination with carboplatin and paclitaxel. Clin Cancer Res 14:4836–4842

Flaherty KT, Puzanov I, Kim KB, Ribas A, McArthur GA, Sosman JA, O'Dwyer PJ, Lee RJ, Grippo JF, Nolop K, Chapman PB (2010) Inhibition of mutated, activated BRAF in metastatic melanoma. N Engl J Med 363:809–819

Fong CW, Chua MS, McKie AB, Ling SH, Mason V, Li R, Yusoff P, Lo TL, Leung HY, So SK, Guy GR (2006) Sprouty 2, an inhibitor of mitogen-activated protein kinase signaling, is down-regulated in hepatocellular carcinoma. Cancer Res 66:2048–2058

Friday BB, Yu C, Dy GK, Smith PD, Wang L, Thibodeau SN, Adjei AA (2008) BRAF V600E disrupts AZD6244-induced abrogation of negative feedback pathways between extracellular signal-regulated kinase and RAF proteins. Cancer Res 68:6145–6153

Furukawa T, Sunamura M, Motoi F, Matsuno S, Horii A (2003) Potential tumor suppressive pathway involving DUSP6/MKP-3 in pancreatic cancer. Am J Pathol 162:1807–1815

Furukawa T, Fujisaki R, Yoshida Y, Kanai N, Sunamura M, Abe T, Takeda K, Matsuno S, Horii A (2005) Distinct progression pathways involving the dysfunction of DUSP6/MKP-3 in pancreatic intraepithelial neoplasia and intraductal papillary-mucinous neoplasms of the pancreas. Mod Pathol 18:1034–1042

Garraway LA, Widlund HR, Rubin MA, Getz G, Berger AJ, Ramaswamy S, Beroukhim R, Milner DA, Granter SR, Du J, Lee C, Wagner SN, Li C, Golub TR, Rimm DL, Meyerson ML, Fisher DE, Sellers WR (2005) Integrative genomic analyses identify MITF as a lineage survival oncogene amplified in malignant melanoma. Nature 436:117–122

Gilmartin AG, Bleam MR, Groy A, Moss KG, Minthorn EA, Kulkarni SG, Rominger CM, Erskine S, Fisher KE, Yang J, Zappacosta F, Annan R, Sutton D, Laquerre SG (2011) GSK1120212 (JTP-74057) is an inhibitor of MEK activity and activation with favorable pharmacokinetic properties for sustained in vivo pathway inhibition. Clin Cancer Res 17:989–1000

Gorden A, Osman I, Gai W, He D, Huang W, Davidson A, Houghton AN, Busam K, Polsky D (2003) Analysis of BRAF and N-RAS mutations in metastatic melanoma tissues. Cancer Res 63:3955–3957

Gray-Schopfer VC, Cheong SC, Chong H, Chow J, Moss T, Abdel-Malek ZA, Marais R, Wynford-Thomas D, Bennett DC (2006) Cellular senescence in naevi and immortalisation in melanoma: a role for p16? Br J Cancer 95:496–505

Hanafusa H, Torii S, Yasunaga T, Nishida E (2002) Sprouty1 and sprouty2 provide a control mechanism for the RAS/MAPK signalling pathway. Nat Cell Biol 4:850–858

Hatzivassiliou G, Song K, Yen I, Brandhuber BJ, Anderson DJ, Alvarado R, Ludlam MJ, Stokoe D, Gloor SL, Vigers G, Morales T, Aliagas I, Liu B, Sideris S, Hoeflich KP, Jaiswal BS, Seshagiri S, Koeppen H, Belvin M, Friedman LS, Malek S (2010) RAF inhibitors prime wild-type RAF to activate the MAPK pathway and enhance growth. Nature 464:431–435

Hauschild A, Agarwala SS, Trefzer U, Hogg D, Robert C, Hersey P, Eggermont A, Grabbe S, Gonzalez R, Gille J, Peschel C, Schadendorf D, Garbe C, O'Day S, Daud A, White JM, Xia C, Patel K, Kirkwood JM, Keilholz U (2009) Results of a phase III, randomized, placebo-controlled study of sorafenib in combination with carboplatin and paclitaxel as second-line treatment in patients with unresectable stage III or stage IV melanoma. J Clin Oncol 27:2823–2830

Heidorn SJ, Milagre C, Whittaker S, Nourry A, Niculescu-Duvas I, Dhomen N, Hussain J, Reis-Filho JS, Springer CJ, Pritchard C, Marais R (2010) Kinase-dead BRAF and oncogenic RAS cooperate to drive tumor progression through CRAF. Cell 140:209–221

Hingorani SR, Jacobetz MA, Robertson GP, Herlyn M, Tuveson DA (2003) Suppression of BRAF(V599E) in human melanoma abrogates transformation. Cancer Res 63:5198–5202

Hoeflich KP, Gray DC, Eby MT, Tien JY, Wong L, Bower J, Gogineni A, Zha J, Cole MJ, Stern HM, Murray LJ, Davis DP, Seshagiri S (2006) Oncogenic BRAF is required for tumor growth and maintenance in melanoma models. Cancer Res 66:999–1006

Infante JR, Fecher LA, Nallapareddy S, Gordon MS, Flaherty KT, Cox DS, DeMarini DJ, Morris SR, Burris HA, Messersmith WA (2010) Safety and efficacy results from the first-in-human study of the oral MEK 1/2 inhibitor GSK1120212. ASCO annual meeting 2010. J Clin Oncol 28:15s, (suppl; abstr 2503)

Johannessen CM, Boehm JS, Kim SY, Thomas SR, Wardwell L, Johnson LA, Emery CM, Stransky N, Cogdill AP, Barretina J, Caponigro G, Hieronymus H, Murray RR, Salehi-Ashtiani K, Hill DE, Vidal M, Zhao JJ, Yang X, Alkan O, Kim S, Harris JL, Wilson CJ, Myer VE, Finan PM, Root DE, Roberts TM, Golub T, Flaherty KT, Dummer R, Weber BL, Sellers WR, Schlegel R, Wargo JA, Hahn WC, Garraway LA (2010) COT drives resistance to RAF inhibition through MAP kinase pathway reactivation. Nature 468:968–972

Joseph EW, Pratilas CA, Poulikakos PI, Tadi M, Wang W, Taylor BS, Halilovic E, Persaud Y, Xing F, Viale A, Tsai J, Chapman PB, Bollag G, Solit DB, Rosen N (2010) The RAF inhibitor PLX4032 inhibits ERK signaling and tumor cell proliferation in a V600E BRAF-selective manner. Proc Natl Acad Sci U S A 107:14903–14908

Kefford R, Arkenau H, Brown MP, Millward M, Infante JR, Long GV, Ouellet D, Curtis M, Lebowitz PF, Falchook GS (2010) Phase I/II study of GSK2118436, a selective inhibitor of oncogenic mutant BRAF kinase, in patients with metastatic melanoma and other solid tumors. ASCO annual meeting 2010. J Clin Oncol 28:15s, (suppl; abstr 8503)

Kim HJ, Bar-Sagi D (2004) Modulation of signalling by sprouty: a developing story. Nat Rev Mol Cell Biol 5:441–450

Lang I, Adenis A, Boer K, Escudero P, Kim T, Valladares M, Sanders N, Pover G, Douillard J (2008) AZD6244 (ARRY-142886) versus capecitabine (CAP) in patients (pts) with metastatic colorectal cancer (mCRC) who have failed prior chemotherapy. J Clin Oncol 26:4114 (Meeting Abstracts)

Lee SA, Ho C, Roy R, Kosinski C, Patil MA, Tward AD, Fridlyand J, Chen X (2008) Integration of genomic analysis and in vivo transfection to identify sprouty 2 as a candidate tumor suppressor in liver cancer. Hepatology 47:1200–1210

Lo TL, Yusoff P, Fong CW, Guo K, McCaw BJ, Phillips WA, Yang H, Wong ES, Leong HF, Zeng Q, Putti TC, Guy GR (2004) The RAS/mitogen-activated protein kinase pathway inhibitor and likely tumor suppressor proteins, sprouty 1 and sprouty 2 are deregulated in breast cancer. Cancer Res 64:6127–6136

Lorusso PM, Adjei AA, Varterasian M, Gadgeel S, Reid J, Mitchell DY, Hanson L, DeLuca P, Bruzek L, Piens J, Asbury P, Van Becelaere K, Herrera R, Sebolt-Leopold J, Meyer MB (2005) Phase I and pharmacodynamic study of the oral MEK inhibitor CI-1040 in patients with advanced malignancies. J Clin Oncol 23:5281–5293

Malumbres M, Barbacid M (2003) RAS oncogenes: the first 30 years. Nat Rev Cancer 3:459–465

Matheny SA, Chen C, Kortum RL, Razidlo GL, Lewis RE, White MA (2004) RAS regulates assembly of mitogenic signalling complexes through the effector protein IMP. Nature 427:256–260

Michaloglou C, Vredeveld LC, Soengas MS, Denoyelle C, Kuilman T, van der Horst CM, Majoor DM, Shay JW, Mooi WJ, Peeper DS (2005) BRAFE600-associated senescence-like cell cycle arrest of human naevi. Nature 436:720–724

Montagut C, Sharma SV, Shioda T, McDermott U, Ulman M, Ulkus LE, Dias-Santagata D, Stubbs H, Lee DY, Singh A, Drew L, Haber DA, Settleman J (2008) Elevated CRAF as a potential mechanism of acquired resistance to BRAF inhibition in melanoma. Cancer Res 68:4853–4861

Moodie SA, Willumsen BM, Weber MJ, Wolfman A (1993) Complexes of RAS.GTP with RAF-1 and mitogen-activated protein kinase kinase. Science 260:1658–1661

Morrison D (1994) 14-3-3: modulators of signaling proteins? Science 266:56–57

Morrison DK, Cutler RE (1997) The complexity of RAF-1 regulation. Curr Opin Cell Biol 9:174–179

Nazarian R, Shi H, Wang Q, Kong X, Koya RC, Lee H, Chen Z, Lee MK, Attar N, Sazegar H, Chodon T, Nelson SF, McArthur G, Sosman JA, Ribas A, Lo RS (2010) Melanomas acquire resistance to B-RAF(V600E) inhibition by RTK or N-RAS upregulation. Nature 468:973–977

Ogawa K, Sun C, Horii A (2005) Exploration of genetic alterations in human endometrial cancer and melanoma: distinct tumorigenic pathways that share a frequent abnormal PI3K/AKT cascade. Oncol Rep 14:1481–1485

Ohren JF, Chen H, Pavlovsky A, Whitehead C, Zhang E, Kuffa P, Yan C, McConnell P, Spessard C, Banotai C, Mueller WT, Delaney A, Omer C, Sebolt-Leopold J, Dudley DT, Leung IK, Flamme C, Warmus J, Kaufman M, Barrett S, Tecle H, Hasemann CA (2004) Structures of human MAP kinase kinase 1 (MEK1) and MEK2 describe novel noncompetitive kinase inhibition. Nat Struct Mol Biol 11:1192–1197

Patton EE, Widlund HR, Kutok JL, Kopani KR, Amatruda JF, Murphey RD, Berghmans S, Mayhall EA, Traver D, Fletcher CD, Aster JC, Granter SR, Look AT, Lee C, Fisher DE, Zon LI (2005) BRAF mutations are sufficient to promote nevi formation and cooperate with p53 in the genesis of melanoma. Curr Biol 15:249–254

Pollock PM, Harper UL, Hansen KS, Yudt LM, Stark M, Robbins CM, Moses TY, Hostetter G, Wagner U, Kakareka J, Salem G, Pohida T, Heenan P, Duray P, Kallioniemi O, Hayward NK, Trent JM, Meltzer PS (2003) High frequency of BRAF mutations in nevi. Nat Genet 33:19–20

Poulikakos PI, Zhang C, Bollag G, Shokat KM, Rosen N (2010) RAF inhibitors transactivate RAF dimers and ERK signalling in cells with wild-type BRAF. Nature 464:427–430

Poulikakos P, Persaud Y, Gabay M, Janakiraman M, Joseph EW, Pratilas CA, Chapman PA, Rosen N, DB S (2011) An in-frame deletion in the N-terminal regulatory domain of BRAF(V600E) causes resistance to the RAF inhibitor PLX4032. AACR annual meeting, 2011. Orlando FL Abstract # LB–419

Pratilas CA, Taylor BS, Ye Q, Viale A, Sander C, Solit DB, Rosen N (2009) (V600E)BRAF is associated with disabled feedback inhibition of RAF-MEK signaling and elevated transcriptional output of the pathway. Proc Natl Acad Sci U S A 106:4519–4524

Repasky GA, Chenette EJ, Der CJ (2004) Renewing the conspiracy theory debate: does RAF function alone to mediate RAS oncogenesis? Trends Cell Biol 14:639–647

Rinehart J, Adjei AA, Lorusso PM, Waterhouse D, Hecht JR, Natale RB, Hamid O, Varterasian M, Asbury P, Kaldjian EP, Gulyas S, Mitchell DY, Herrera R, Sebolt-Leopold JS, Meyer MB (2004) Multicenter phase II study of the oral MEK inhibitor, CI-1040, in patients with advanced non-small-cell lung, breast, colon, and pancreatic cancer. J Clin Oncol 22:4456–4462

Sasaki A, Taketomi T, Kato R, Saeki K, Nonami A, Sasaki M, Kuriyama M, Saito N, Shibuya M, Yoshimura A (2003) Mammalian sprouty4 suppresses RAS-independent ERK activation by binding to RAF1. Nat Cell Biol 5:427–432

Sebolt-Leopold JS, Herrera R (2004) Targeting the mitogen-activated protein kinase cascade to treat cancer. Nat Rev Cancer 4:937–947

Sebolt-Leopold JS, Dudley DT, Herrera R, Van Becelaere K, Wiland A, Gowan RC, Tecle H, Barrett SD, Bridges A, Przybranowski S, Leopold WR, Saltiel AR (1999) Blockade of the MAP kinase pathway suppresses growth of colon tumors in vivo. Nat Med 5:810–816

Shimizu K, Goldfarb M, Suard Y, Perucho M, Li Y, Kamata T, Feramisco J, Stavnezer E, Fogh J, Wigler MH (1983) Three human transforming genes are related to the viral RAS oncogenes. Proc Natl Acad Sci U S A 80:2112–2116

Solit DB, Garraway LA, Pratilas CA, Sawai A, Getz G, Basso A, Ye Q, Lobo JM, She Y, Osman I, Golub TR, Sebolt-Leopold J, Sellers WR, Rosen N (2006) BRAF mutation predicts sensitivity to MEK inhibition. Nature 439:358–362

Solit DB, Santos E, Pratilas CA, Lobo J, Moroz M, Cai S, Blasberg R, Sebolt-Leopold J, Larson S, Rosen N (2007) 3'-deoxy-3'-[18F] fluoro thymidine positron emission tomography is a sensitive method for imaging the response of BRAF-dependent tumors to MEK inhibition. Cancer Res 67:11463–11469

Sutterluty H, Mayer CE, Setinek U, Attems J, Ovtcharov S, Mikula M, Mikulits W, Micksche M, Berger W (2007) Down-regulation of sprouty2 in non-small cell lung cancer contributes to tumor malignancy via extracellular signal-regulated kinase pathway-dependent and -independent mechanisms. Mol Cancer Res 5:509–520

Sviderskaya EV, Gray-Schopfer VC, Hill SP, Smit NP, Evans-Whipp TJ, Bond J, Hill L, Bataille V, Peters G, Kipling D, Wynford-Thomas D, Bennett DC (2003) p16/cyclin-dependent kinase inhibitor 2A deficiency in human melanocyte senescence, apoptosis, and immortalization: possible implications for melanoma progression. J Natl Cancer Inst 95:723–732

Therrien M, Michaud NR, Rubin GM, Morrison DK (1996) KSR modulates signal propagation within the MAPK cascade. Genes Dev 10:2684–2695

Tsai J, Lee JT, Wang W, Zhang J, Cho H, Mamo S, Bremer R, Gillette S, Kong J, Haass NK, Sproesser K, Li L, Smalley KS, Fong D, Zhu YL, Marimuthu A, Nguyen H, Lam B, Liu J, Cheung I, Rice J, Suzuki Y, Luu C, Settachatgul C, Shellooe R, Cantwell J, Kim SH, Schlessinger J, Zhang KY, West BL, Powell B, Habets G, Zhang C, Ibrahim PN, Hirth P, Artis DR, Herlyn M, Bollag G (2008) Discovery of a selective inhibitor of oncogenic B-RAF kinase with potent antimelanoma activity. Proc Natl Acad Sci U S A 105:3041–3046

Tsavachidou D, Coleman ML, Athanasiadis G, Li S, Licht JD, Olson MF, Weber BL (2004) SPRY2 is an inhibitor of the RAS/extracellular signal-regulated kinase pathway in melanocytes and melanoma cells with wild-type BRAF but not with the V599E mutant. Cancer Res 64:5556–5559

Tzekova V, Cebotaru C, Ciuleanu TE, Damjanov D, Ganchev H, Kanarev V, Stella PJ, Sanders N, Pover G, Hainsworth JD (2008) Efficacy and safety of AZD6244 (ARRY-142886) as second/third-line treatment of patients (pts) with advanced non-small cell lung cancer (NSCLC). J Clin Oncol 26:8029 (Meeting Abstracts)

Villanueva J, Vultur A, Lee JT, Somasundaram R, Fukunaga-Kalabis M, Cipolla AK, Wubbenhorst B, Xu X, Gimotty PA, Kee D, Santiago-Walker AE, Letrero R, D'Andrea K, Pushparajan A, Hayden JE, Brown KD, Laquerre S, McArthur GA, Sosman JA, Nathanson KL, Herlyn M (2010) Acquired resistance to BRAF inhibitors mediated by a RAF kinase switch in melanoma can be overcome by cotargeting MEK and IGF-1R/PI3K. Cancer Cell 18:683–695

Wajapeyee N, Serra RW, Zhu X, Mahalingam M, Green MR (2008) Oncogenic BRAF induces senescence and apoptosis through pathways mediated by the secreted protein IGFBP7. Cell 132:363–374

Wan PT, Garnett MJ, Roe SM, Lee S, Niculescu-Duvaz D, Good VM, Jones CM, Marshall CJ, Springer CJ, Barford D, Marais R (2004) Mechanism of activation of the RAF-ERK signaling pathway by oncogenic mutations of B-RAF. Cell 116:855–867

Wang D, Boerner SA, Winkler JD, LoRusso PM (2007) Clinical experience of MEK inhibitors in cancer therapy. Biochim Biophys Acta 1773:1248–1255

Wellbrock C, Ogilvie L, Hedley D, Karasarides M, Martin J, Niculescu-Duvaz D, Springer CJ, Marais R (2004) V599EB-RAF is an oncogene in melanocytes. Cancer Res 64:2338–2342

Wilhelm SM, Carter C, Tang L, Wilkie D, McNabola A, Rong H, Chen C, Zhang X, Vincent P, McHugh M, Cao Y, Shujath J, Gawlak S, Eveleigh D, Rowley B, Liu L, Adnane L, Lynch M, Auclair D, Taylor I, Gedrich R, Voznesensky A, Riedl B, Post LE, Bollag G, Trail PA (2004) BAY 43–9006 exhibits broad spectrum oral antitumor activity and targets the RAF/MEK/ERK pathway and receptor tyrosine kinases involved in tumor progression and angiogenesis. Cancer Res 64:7099–7109

Yusoff P, Lao DH, Ong SH, Wong ES, Lim J, Lo TL, Leong HF, Fong CW, Guy GR (2002) Sprouty2 inhibits the RAS/MAP kinase pathway by inhibiting the activation of RAF. J Biol Chem 277:3195–3201

Zimmermann S, Moelling K (1999) Phosphorylation and regulation of RAF by AKT (protein kinase B). Science 286:1741–1744

Beyond BRAF in Melanoma

Adil Daud and Boris C. Bastian

Abstract Recent progress in the analysis of genetic alterations in melanoma has identified recurrent mutations that result in the activation of critical signaling pathways promoting growth and survival of tumors cells. Alterations in the RAS-RAF-MAP kinase and PI3-kinase signaling pathways are commonly altered in melanoma. Mutations in *BRAF*, *NRAS*, *KIT*, and *GNAQ* occur in a mutually exclusive pattern and lead to MAP-kinase activation. Loss of PTEN function, primarily by deletion, is the most common known genetic alteration in the PI3-kinase cascade, and is commonly associated with BRAF mutations (Curtin et al., N Engl J Med 353:2135–2147, 2005; Tsao et al., Cancer Res 60:1800–1804, 2000, J Investig Dermatol 122:337–341, 2004). The growth advantage conveyed by the constitutive activation of these pathways leads to positive selection of cells that have acquired the mutations and in many instances leads to critical dependency of the cancer cells on their activation. This creates opportunities for therapeutic interventions targeted at signaling components within these pathways that are amenable for pharmacological inhibition. This concept follows the paradigm established by the landmark discovery that inhibition of the fusion kinase BCR-ABL can be used to treat chronic myelogenous leukemia (Druker et al., N Engl J Med 344:1031–037, 2001). The review will focus primarily on kinases involved in signaling that are currently being evaluated for therapeutic intervention in melanoma.

A. Daud
University of California, San Francisco,
CA 94143, USA

B. C. Bastian (✉)
Memorial Sloan-Kettering Cancer Center,
New York, NY 10021, USA
e-mail: bastianb@mskcc.org

Current Topics in Microbiology and Immunology (2012) 355: 99–117
DOI: 10.1007/82_2011_163
© Springer-Verlag Berlin Heidelberg 2011
Published Online: 9 August 2011

Contents

1   Introduction 100
2   Melanoma Pathogenesis 101
3   KIT Mutations 102
4   Mutations in G-Protein-Coupled Receptors 104
5   Mutations in RAS and RAF Family Members 104
6   Mutations at the G1-Checkpoint 106
7   The EGF Receptor Family 107
8   The PI(3)K-MTOR Pathway in Melanoma 109
9   Other Growth Factor Receptor Pathways 110
     9.1   MET 110
     9.2   Fibroblast Growth Factor Receptor Family 111
10 Future Perspectives 112
References 112

1 Introduction

The incidence of melanoma is in the midst of a sustained rapid increase worldwide. While melanoma was an uncommon malignancy in the early part of the twentieth century, in 2009 it is estimated to be the fifth most common cancer in males and the sixth most common in females in the United States (Jemal et al. 2009). While the increase can be in part attributed to the changed diagnostic criteria and an increase in the number of skin biopsies, a simultaneous increase in deeper melanoma indicates that the melanoma burden has increased (Linos et al. 2009). Melanoma on the sun-exposed skin primarily affects fair-skinned people living in regions with a high level of ambient sunlight. Epidemiologic studies have shown association with a previous history of blistering sunburns, especially in childhood, and to a lesser extent with total ultraviolet exposure from all sources, including tanning beds. The risk of developing melanoma is also increased in subjects who have many melanocytic nevi (moles), i.e. benign proliferations of neoplastic melanocytes, and those with freckles and red hair, traits associated with germline polymorphisms in the gene encoding melanocortin receptor 1 (*MC1R*).

While melanoma can be cured if the primary lesion is removed surgically before metastasis has occurred, the treatment of metastatic disease is challenging. Standard cytotoxic chemotherapy benefits only a small minority of patients with metastatic melanoma. The methylating agent, 5 (dimethyl triazeno) imidazole 4-carboxamide (DTIC, Dacarbazine) and its chemical congener temozolomide are the mainstay of melanoma therapy with objective response rates around 15% (Khan et al. 2006). Other common therapies of metastatic melanoma include modulators of the immune system. These include cytokines such as interferon-α 2B and interleukin-2 which have shown modest benefit in early and late stage melanomas, respectively, but are associated with very marked toxicity. To summarize the current state of melanoma therapy, for the vast majority of patients, neither immunotherapy nor cytotoxic chemotherapy produces even transient shrinkage of tumor, much less sustained responses or complete remission (Gogas et al. 2007). As outlined below, deregulated signal transduction pathways represent a rich area for drug development in melanoma.

2 Melanoma Pathogenesis

Melanoma arises from transformed melanocytes. These long-lived pigment-producing cells are derived from progenitor cells originating from the embryonic neural crest and colonize the epidermis during development. A complex network of signaling pathways including the KIT-, WNT-, and endothelin-signaling pathways, govern the migration and homing process and once the process is completed, melanocytes are found in the basilar epidermis of the skin, where they provide neighboring keratinocytes with melanin pigment through the extension of dendrites. Pigment production gets stimulated upon exposure of the skin to DNA damage-inducing agents such as UV irradiation. DNA damage in epidermal keratinocytes leads to the transcription of pro-opiomelanocortin, a precursor polypeptide cleaved into several biologically important peptides, including alpha-melanocyte stimulating hormone (α-MSH). α-MSH binds and activates the melanocortin receptor 1 (MC1R) on melanocytes and induces pigment synthesis and subsequent delivery of melanin to the neighboring keratinocytes. Inherited polymorphisms affecting components of this "tanning response", most prominently germ line variants of MC1R, are associated with light skin, inability to tan, and increased risk to skin cancer, including melanoma. As opposed to these germline alterations which are common but have a low penetrance, inherited mutations in *CDKN2A* (coding for p16 and p14), and rarely of the *CDK4* locus (which encodes a cyclin dependent kinase inhibited by p16), represent high-penetrance alterations associated with familial melanoma.

The clinical and histopathological presentation of melanoma varies with the anatomic site in which it originates, which has led to the distinction of "histo-genetic" subtypes of melanoma (McGovern et al. 1986). Data from genetic analyses have confirmed the existence of distinct subtypes with characteristic genetic alterations depending on anatomic site and degree of sun-exposure (Curtin et al. 2005; Viros et al. 2008). In addition to the skin, melanocytes are also present in leptomeninges, mucous membranes, and in the uvea of the eye and can occasionally give rise to melanoma. In contradistinction to melanomas on the sun-exposed skin, which are most common in Caucasians, melanomas arising from sites such as the palms, soles, and nail beds (acral melanomas) and melanomas originating from mucous membranes of the oropharynx, nasopharynx, the anogenital region, or rectum (mucosal melanoma) show similar incidence in Asians, Africans, and Caucasians. In addition to their anatomic location in sun-protected sites which makes UV-radiation an unlikely etiologic factor, acral and mucosal melanomas show distinct genetic features indicating that they are distinct categories (Bastian et al. 2000a; Curtin et al. 2005; van Dijk et al. 2003). Uveal melanoma arises from melanocytes in the choroid, the iris, or the ciliary body (uveal melanoma) and also has unique genetic and clinical features (Ehlers and Harbour 2006; Van Raamsdonk et al. 2009).

3 KIT Mutations

KIT is a receptor tyrosine kinase encoded by the c-kit proto-oncogene (Besmer et al. 1986) [see also "Gastrointestinal stromal tumors (GISTs)"]. Upon binding to its ligand stem cell factor (SCF) (Zsebo et al. 1990), also known as steel factor or c-kit ligand, KIT dimerizes, autophosphorylates, and activates downstream pathways (Matsui et al. 1990). KIT signaling is essential for melanoblast viability. While complete loss of function of KIT or SCF is lethal, loss of function alleles lead to defects involving the pigmentation, hematopoesis, and fertility. SCF is composed of extracellular, transmembrane, and cytoplasmic domains and exists in soluble and membrane-bound forms (Ashman 1999). In the skin the majority of SCF exist in membrane-bound form on the surface of keratinocytes (Longley et al. 1993). Mice with the so-called Steel-Dickie mutation of SCF, which lacks the transmembrane and cytoplasmic domains of SCF, are unpigmented (black–eyed white), deficient in mast cells, anemic and sterile (Brannan et al. 1991), indicating an important role of membrane-bound SCF in the skin and other tissues. Epidermal SCF promotes the survival, proliferation, and migration of intraepidermal melanocytes through its activation of KIT (Kunisada et al. 1998).

Despite these effects on normal melanocytes, KIT was initially regarded as a potential tumor suppressor gene in melanoma because melanomas were found to frequently lose KIT expression while progressing to more advanced stages (Lassam and Bickford 1992; Montone et al. 1997; Natali et al. 1992). The discovery of distinct patterns of genetic alterations in melanoma (Curtin et al. 2005) led to a reappraisal of the role of KIT in specific disease subsets in which it was found to be amplified. Mutations, copy-number increases, or both were found in 30% of CSD, and 40% of acral and mucosal melanomas (Curtin et al. 2006), a distribution confirmed in independent studies (Beadling et al. 2008). The majority of the mutations occur in the juxtamembrane domain of KIT and are likely to be inhibited by imatinib.

Several trials with imatinib have been carried out in *unselected melanoma* patients:

- A Phase II trial of Imatinib, given at 400 mg po BID in 8 week cycles and conducted at two centers in Europe, found no responses in 16 evaluable patients (Ugurel et al. 2005). Of 12 patients whose tumors were examined for KIT expression by immunohistochemistry one patient had strong staining, two intermediate, and the rest had minimal or no c-kit expression. None of the three patients with high expression had a KIT mutation.

- Another multicenter trial with similar doses of imatinib also showed no responses in 18 evaluable patients (Wyman et al. 2006a). Immunohistochemistry was performed on 17 patients and no patients had strong KIT expression, three had moderate expression, and the remainder had weak or no expression. No mutation analysis was performed.
- A third more recently reported trial with imatinib at similar dosage enrolled 21 stage IV melanoma patients (Kim et al. 2008). One sustained partial response (>12 months) in cutaneous, lymph node and lung disease was observed. Interestingly, the responder had an acral melanoma, i.e. a melanoma type with frequent KIT mutations or copy-number increases. Sequencing of KIT revealed splice site mutation in exon 15.

Two other responders of *KIT mutant melanomas* that responded dramatically to imatinib have been reported as case reports:

- The first was a 79-year-old man with a metastatic melanoma originating from a primary of the rectal mucosa which by sequencing had a seven-codon duplication in exon 11 of KIT and who had a pronounced response to 400 mg of imatinib daily (Hodi et al. 2008).
- The second patient had a mucosal melanoma of the anus with extensive locoregional metastasis and a KIT mutation in exon 13. She had a complete response to 400 mg of imatinib daily. Interestingly, a transient dose reduction to 200 mg daily that was necessary because of pancytopenia led to rapid recurrence of the metastases. A subsequent dose increase to 600 mg led to complete remission, which now sustained under ongoing therapy for over three years later (Lutzky et al. 2008).

Recently, the first results of a multicenter trial for melanoma patients with *KIT mutations or amplifications* were reported (Carvajal et al. 2009). Eighty-eight patients were screened for mutations or amplifications of KIT to be enrolled in this trial. At the time of the interim report, of 12 patients who went on treatment, all with KIT mutations, two had a complete response, two a partial response, and six had stable disease. Only two progressed under treatment. The experience to date indicates that KIT expression by immunohistochemistry is not a reliable predictor of response to treatment with KIT inhibitors. By contrast, melanoma patients with mutations in KIT appear to respond to drugs that inhibit the specific mutants. Little information exists to date on whether patient with amplification of KIT without mutations will also respond to therapies targeted at KIT. While overall these data are very encouraging, significantly more information needs to be gathered to learn about predictors of response and primary resistance as well as mechanisms of secondary resistance. Generalizing from these data, it is reasonable to assert that trials with targeted inhibitors in unselected patients using a conventional Phase II trial design in melanoma may well appear to be "negative" even if the agent is actually active and the target is valid.

4 Mutations in G-Protein-Coupled Receptors

The G-protein alpha subunits, GNAQ and GNA11, which are involved in mediating signals between G-protein coupled receptors (GPCRs) and the MAP-kinase and PI3-kinase signal transduction cascades also appear to be mutational hotspots in specific subtypes of melanoma. Van Raamsdonk et al. (2009) reported that 46% of uveal melanomas showed mutations in codon 209, which is in the RAS-like domain of GNAQ, conferring constitutive activation of this pathway. Subsequently, mutations in a highly homologous gene, GNA11, were observed in a further 32% of uveal melanomas, accounting for 83% of all uveal melanomas examined having mutations in either of the two genes (Van Raamsdonk et al. 2010). GNAQ and GNA11 mutation occur in a mutually exclusive pattern so that only one of the two genes is mutated in a given tumor.

Melanoma cells with the GNAQ Q209L mutation were highly sensitive to MEK inhibitors, suggesting that these could be employed against uveal melanoma (Van Raamsdonk et al. 2009). A clinical trial with the MEK inhibitor in uveal melanoma with GNAQ or GNA11 mutations is currently underway (ClinicalTrials.gov NCT01143402).

5 Mutations in RAS and RAF Family Members

RAS proteins are a family of intracellular GTPases that are crucial intermediaries in signaling through multiple signaling cascades including the MAP-kinase and PI3-kinase pathways. The three RAS proteins, KRAS, HRAS, and NRAS are frequently mutated in human malignancies. The first mutations discovered in melanoma were in NRAS (Padua et al. 1985). They most frequently occur at codon 61 and in 15–20% of melanomas. Different from BRAF mutations (see below), mutations in NRAS are found with similar frequencies in different melanoma types, but are absent in uveal melanoma (Curtin et al. 2005; Wong et al. 2005). NRAS mutations are also found in benign melanocytic nevi, in particular large congenital nevi (Bauer et al. 2007), and thus are not sufficient to fully transform melanocytes. Mutations in KRAS appear to be very rare in melanoma (Curtin et al. 2005). By contrast, mutations in HRAS are found in a small minority of melanomas (<1%), but are found in up to 20% of Spitz nevi, a benign nevus that can have histomorphologic similarities to melanoma (Bastian et al. 2000b). RAS has proved to be a difficult therapeutic target, because the mutations lead to loss of the enzymatic activity of the GTPase, which locks the enzyme in its activated, GTP-bound state. As RAS proteins need to be anchored to the inner leaflet of membranes for activation by fatty acid modification (mostly farnesylation), therapeutic inhibition of farnesyl transferase has been evaluated to treat RAS-mutant cancers. Unfortunately, inhibitors of farnesyl transferase have not been successful against RAS-dependent cancers, as additional enzymes exist that add alternative lipid moieties to RAS family members (Sousa et al. 2008).

RAF proteins are a family of serine/threonine protein kinases that are activated by RAS and in turn phosphorylate MEK (MAP-kinase-kinase). There are three RAF proteins: ARAF, BRAF, and CRAF (RAF-1). Only BRAF is commonly mutated in cancer, including melanoma. BRAF mutations most frequently (over 90%) affect codon V600E in exon 15 and result in a glutamic acid for valine substitution (Davies et al. 2002). This mutation causes aberrant activation of BRAF and increased signaling through MEK. BRAF mutations are very common (up to 70%) in melanomas that arise on the non-chronically sun-damaged skin, i.e. the trunk and proximal extremities of individuals younger than 55 years of age (Curtin et al. 2005; Maldonado et al. 2003; Viros et al. 2008) but are less frequent in melanomas arising on the chronically sun-damaged skin of older individuals, acral, and mucosal melanomas, and are not found in uveal melanoma. Melanomas with BRAF mutations also have distinct morphological features suggesting that they may represent a biological entity (Viros et al. 2008). The common BRAF mutation results in increased kinase activity and subsequent increase of the downstream MAP-kinase cascade. Similar to NRAS, BRAF is frequently mutated in benign melanocytic nevi, indicating that it by itself is not sufficient for melanoma formation. In contrast to the attempts of targeting mutant RAS, inhibition of mutant BRAF with highly specific inhibitors has met with great success and is described in detail elsewhere in this volume ("Setting up a Kinase Discovery and Development Project" and "Targeting Oncogenic BRAF in Human Cancer").

MEK, the MAP-kinase-kinase downstream of RAF proteins is also under evaluation as a therapeutic target in melanoma. A phase I trial with the MEK inhibitor AZD6244 suggested activity in melanoma, with six out of eleven melanoma patients showing some tumor shrinkage. One patient with an NRAS mutant melanoma showed a 70% tumor reduction after three cycles of treatment, but then progressed in the brain. Additionally, a patient with uveal melanoma had stable disease over 22 cycles of treatment (Adjei et al. 2008). A maculopapular skin rash was the most frequent and dose limiting toxicity; the maximal concentration, C_{max} reached was 1,016 ng/mL (2.2 nM) at day 22, which is several orders of magnitude lower than the inhibitory concentration required in vitro. Based on these data, a subsequent larger randomized Phase II trial of 200 patients with metastatic melanoma showed no advantage compared against temozolomide (Dummer et al. 2008). Specifically, there was no difference in overall survival between the two treatment arms in the overall population (HR 1.07; 80% CI 0.86, 1.34), nor in the BRAF mutant subgroup (HR 0.85; 80% CI 0.58, 1.24). However, of the six patients receiving AZD6244 who had a confirmed PR, five carried a BRAF mutation. By contrast, of the nine patients receiving TMZ with confirmed PR, only three had BRAF mutant melanomas. More potent MEK inhibitors have been tested recently and these have had markedly higher response rates both in BRAF mutant and BRAF wild-type melanoma. GSK1120212, a potent allosteric MEK1/2 inhibitor, was tested in a Phase I/II study in patients with melanoma as well as in other tumor types (Infante et al. 2010). The most common side effects were rash and diarrhea. The levels of pERK and KI-67 were reduced by 90% in melanoma patients. In 11 BRAF mutant patients, 3 PRs and 5 SDs were observed. More surprisingly, among nine patients without BRAF mutations, 2 PRs and 1 SD were observed. Of these, one patient had a GNAQ mutation, raising the possibility that MAP-kinase pathway inhibition could suppress tumor growth in this group of melanomas. Larger trials in melanoma are ongoing and further data are expected with this drug. The MEK1/2 inhibitor AS703026 has also been tested recently in a Phase I trial (Delord et al. 2010). While mutation status was not reported, 2 PRs were observed, both observed in previously treated patients with melanoma. While BRAF inhibitors and MEK inhibitors have not been compared directly, at present it appears that MEK inhibitors may have a wider spectrum of activity while BRAF inhibitors may be more effective in *BRAF* mutant melanoma, with the caveat that considerable inter- and intra- trial variation exists.

6 Mutations at the G1-Checkpoint

The cyclin-dependent kinases (CDKs) are a large evolutionarily conserved family of serine/threonine protein kinases that form multisubunit complexes that play critical roles in the cell cycle. Multiple genes encoding CDKs and CDK-like proteins have been identified in humans. The CDKs can be divided into two groups, a core group that controls cell cycle progression and a second group that regulates transcription initiation and elongation. Enzymatic activation of CDKs requires binding of a regulatory 'cyclin' subunit, which acts as a co-enzyme. Within the core group of cell cycle regulatory CDKs, CDKs 4 and 6 control entry into the G1 phase of the cell cycle, CDK2 controls G1/S transition and CDK1 controls G2/M transition. When bound to cyclin D family members, CDK4 and 6 phosphorylate retinoblastoma family proteins (pRB). pRBs act as pocket proteins by binding and sequestering members of the E2F transcription factors of family. Thus, pRBs act as pivotal sup pressors of cellular proliferation by forming a restriction point for cell cycle entry. Phosphorylation of pRb by complexes of CDK4/6 and cyclin D at specific sites followed by additional phosphorylations by a complex of CDK2 and cyclin E leads to the release of E2F proteins. The liberated E2F transcription factors lead to the transcription of critical factors of DNA synthesis such as PCNA, a cofactor for DNA polymerase, enabling the initiation of S phase. Because of the critical role of CDKs in cell cycle initiation and orchestration their activity is tightly regulated by a family of cyclin-dependent kinase inhibitors (CDKNs) (Sherr and Roberts 1999). Most prominently, the gene CDKN2A encodes two distinct proteins of critical importance in melanoma and cancer in general: p16 (transcribed from exons 1α, 2, and 3) and p14 (transcribed from exons 1β and 2 in an alternate reading frame to p16). p16 binds and inhibits CDK4/6 and acts as a negative regulator of cell proliferation (Serrano et al. 1996), and p14 helps in stabilizing p53 by inhibiting its ubiquitin ligase HDM2.

The G1 entry checkpoint at the level of CDK4/6, cyclin D, and p16 are of critical importance in melanoma as evidenced by common mutations affecting these genes. Germline mutations of CDKN2A, mostly affecting the p16 reading frame, occur in 25–40% of familial melanoma cases. Rare kindreds have germline mutations of CDK4. In addition to germline alterations, somatic mutations affecting these genes also occur frequently in melanoma. The CDKN2A locus on chromosome 9p21 is the most commonly deleted region in primary melanomas and cyclin D1 and CDK4 are amplified in specific subsets of melanomas (Curtin et al. 2005). Amplification of cyclin D1 is found primarily in melanomas without mutations in upstream kinases, suggesting that it may act as an independent oncogene in melanoma (Sauter et al. 2002) and possibly convey resistance to inhibitors targeted at upstream kinases (Curtin et al. 2005). This notion has been confirmed experimentally in BRAF mutant cell lines with concomitant cyclin D1 amplification (Smalley et al. 2008).

The potential of CDKs as a drug target in cancer has been controversial, as they are of critical importance in normal cell division and therefore may provide little selective advantage. Drug discovery programs have produced potent small molecule CDK inhibitors from a variety of chemical classes, including purine and pyrimidine analogues, indenopyrazoles, pyridopyrimidines, pyrazolopyridines, indolocarbazoles, pyrrolocarbazoles, oxindoles, and aminothiazoles. First generation compounds such as flavopiridol and UCN-01 (7-hydroxystaurosporine) have not been successful in clinical trials in solid tumors (Shapiro 2006) and these compounds are hampered by their promiscuous CDK inhibitory profile. As expected, many of these compounds are notably myelosuppressive. More selective CDK inhibitors have been developed that target CDK4 and 6. These include PD-0332991 (Fry et al. 2001) and CINK4 (Soni et al. 2001). The principal and dose limiting toxicity of PD-0332991 in a phase I dose-escalation trial was myelosuppression (O'Dwyer et al. 2007). No responses were seen among melanoma patients enrolled in this trial. Several trials are ongoing looking at this agent in combination with other chemotherapy drugs. In general, the responses to CDK inhibitors in solid tumors have been disappointing. Targeting the clinical studies at patients with specific genetic alterations such as amplifications of cyclin D1 or CDK4 may result in a higher response rate.

7 The EGF Receptor Family

The EGFR family comprises four distinct receptors: EGFR/ErbB-1, HER2/ErbB-2, HER3/ErbB-3, and HER4/ErbB-4. Similar to KIT these transmembrane receptors are composed of an extracellular ligand-binding domain and a cytoplasmic region with enzymatic activity (Yarden 2001). A number of different ligands, including EGF-like molecules, transforming growth factor (TGF)-α, and neuregulins, activate the receptors by binding to the extracellular domain and inducing the formation of receptor homodimers or heterodimers. With the exception of HER3, which does not have kinase activity, the dimerized receptors cross-phosphorylate the other member of the receptor pair, which creates binding sites for signaling complexes which relay the signal towards the MAP-kinase and PI3-kinase pathways.

ErbB1 is expressed, albeit at low level in up to 96% of primary melanomas and in 90% of metastatic lesions (Sparrow and Heenan 1999). The EGFR gene resides on chromosome 7, which is gained in about 50% of melanomas. Increased copy-number of chromosome 7 has been found to be associated with poor prognosis in some studies (Rákosy et al. 2007; Trent et al. 1990). However, the gains typically involve large chromosomal regions or the entire chromosome 7 (Bastian et al. 2003; Maldonado et al. 2003) so that a direct implication of EGFR is difficult to make. In particular, BRAF is situated on chromosome 7 as well and has been demonstrated to be a major driver of chromosome 7 copy-number increases as they preferentially affect the chromosome harboring the mutant copy of BRAF, indicating selection for increased gene dosage of mutant BRAF during melanoma progression (Maldonado et al. 2003; Willmore-Payne et al. 2006).

By contrast, overexpression of ErB2 or targeted amplifications of the ErB2 region on chromosome 17 are not common in melanoma (Curtin et al. 2005; Inman et al. 2003; Kluger et al. 2004; Potti et al. 2004). However, ErbB3 is frequently expressed in primary melanomas and in the majority of metastatic lesions and has been associated with melanoma progression and worse prognosis (Buac et al. 2009; Djerf et al. 2009; Ueno et al. 2008). In a B16 melanoma model, heregulin activation of erbB3 increased tumor growth and metastasis, which could be inhibited by the EGFR inhibitor PD153035, implicating heterodimerization of ErbB3 and EGFR in melanoma growth (Ueno et al. 2008). Additional evidence implicating EGFR signaling in melanocytic neoplasia comes from the Xiphophorus fish in which an oncogenic variant of the Xmrk gene, a receptor tyrosine kinase related to the EGFR family in mammals, causes a hereditable tumor of pigment cells with similarities to human melanoma (Wellbrock et al. 1997).

Most recently, a screen for somatic mutations in receptor tyrosine kinases revealed recurring mutations in the fourth EGFR family member ErbB4 (Prickett et al. 2009). In a first study, 19% of 79 tissues of metastatic melanoma showed somatic mutations in ErbB4. Different from other mutations in receptor tyrosine kinases, the mutations were scattered across all domains of the protein, instead of clustering to specific regions. The majority of mutations occurred in tumors that also harbored mutations in BRAF or NRAS, other receptor tyrosine kinases, metalloproteinases (Palavalli et al. 2009), and transcription factors (Cronin et al. 2009), indicating an unusually high mutation frequency in these samples, possibly pointing to an increased mutation frequency due to chemotherapy as described in glioma (2008). Additional studies are warranted to determine the frequency of ErbB4 mutations in untreated melanoma samples. If confirmed, mutant ErbB4 would offer another opportunity for targeted therapy for melanoma.

Several types of ErbB inhibitors are already in the clinic, including monoclonal antibodies that interfere with ligand binding (trastuzumab) and receptor dimerization (pertumumab) and small molecule inhibitors such as the ErbB1 receptor tyrosine kinase inhibitor, gefitinib and erlotinib and the dual ErbB1 and ErbB2 inhibitor lapatinib. These compounds have primarily been tested in NSCLCA and breast cancer. Single agent erlotinib has been evaluated in a phase II trial in melanoma with no objective responses, but four of 14 patients showed disease stabilization (Wyman et al. 2006b). Single agent gefitinib has also been tested in melanoma in a prospective single arm Phase II trial (Patel et al. 2011). Two out of 50 evaluable patients had a partial response; interestingly one was of choroidal origin. It was concluded that gefitinib was well tolerated, but had minimal clinical efficacy as a single-agent therapy for metastatic melanoma of cutaneous origin. A second trial at the Vanderbilt-Ingram Cancer Center evaluated a combination of bevacizumab and erlotinib. Here, two of 23 patients had partial responses and five were stable for at least 6 months (Wyman et al. 2006a). Unfortunately, the toxicity was also more significant; one patient each had a myocardial infarction and a bowel perforation.

8 The PI(3)K-MTOR Pathway in Melanoma

The PI3-kinase/AKT/mTOR pathway conveys signals that result in decreased apoptosis, increased proliferation, and metabolic activity of cells and is frequently activated in cancer. PI3-kinase acts downstream of receptor tyrosine kinases and RAS and phosphorylates phosphatidylinositol-4,5-biphosphate (PIP2) to phosphatidylinositol-3,4,5-triphosphate (PIP3), leading to activation of downstream effectors including AKT and PDK1, which relay signals through the mTOR complex 1 (mTORC1) to p70 S6 kinase. The mammalian target of rapamycin (mTOR) is a serine/threonine protein kinase with a catalytic domain closely related to the PI3-kinases. It belongs to the family of PI3 K-related protein kinases that includes ataxia–telangiectasia mutated (ATM), ATM- and Rad3-related (ATR), DNA-dependent protein kinase (DNA-PK). mTOR also has an FRB (FKBP12/rapamycin-binding) domain that binds the drug rapamycin in complex with its intracellular receptor protein FKBP12. mTOR integrates growth factor-activated signals with inputs from the metabolic state of the cell to ascertain the presence of sufficient nutrients and energy for cell growth, proliferation, and survival. It has been shown recently that mTOR binds to different regulatory subunits to produce complexes with distinct signaling properties. mTOR is involved in two different multiprotein complexes, mTORC1, which is rapamycin-sensitive, and mTORC2, which is insensitive to rapamycin. The mTORC1 complex (containing mTOR, Raptor, and mLST8) activates translation by phosphorylation and activation of ribosomal S6 kinase (S6 K) and by inactivating the translation repressor 4EBP1 (Ma and Blenis 2009). Other biological processes regulated by mTORC1 include ribosome biogenesis, autophagy, glucose metabolism, and the cellular response to hypoxia (Guertin and Sabatini 2005). mTORC1 is activated primarily through inactivation of its negative regulator tuberous sclerosis complex 2 (TSC2) via phosphorylation by upstream kinases such as AKT, ERK. TSC2 acts as GTPase-activating protein for Rheb, a small GTP-binding protein related to RAS. The activation processes involved for the mTORC2 complex (containing mTOR, Rictor, mLST8, and mSin1) are less well understood. Interestingly, mTORC2 phosphorylates and activates AKT, placing some of its activities upstream of mTORC1.

Activation of the PI3-kinase pathway as evidenced by expression of phosphorylated AKT is found in a high proportion of melanomas and increases with progression (Dhawan et al. 2002). The most common genetic alterations in this path way in melanoma known to date are inactivation of the lipid phosphatase PTEN, frequently occurring together with mutations in BRAF (Curtin et al. 2005; Tsao et al. 2000, 2004; Druker et al. 2001). In about 50% of melanomas PTEN is deleted and mutations or epigenetic silencing is also found in a smaller proportion (Birck et al. 2000; Guldberg et al. 1997; Reifenberger et al. 2000; Zhou et al. 2000). PTEN is a negative regulator of the pathway as it dephosphorylates PIP3 so that inactivation results in increased pathway activity. In a minority of cases amplification of AKT family members has been reported and AKT3 appears to be the dominant player in melanoma (Chudnovsky et al. 2005; Stahl et al. 2004; Tran et al. 2008). Recently, mutations in AKT3 and AKT1 have been found in a small proportion of melanoma cell lines (Davies et al. 2008). Increased phospho-Akt expression in melanoma is associated with tumor progression and shorter survival (Dai et al. 2005; Dhawan et al. 2002).

While AKT and PI3 kinase inhibitors are in active development, no data are available for their effectiveness in melanoma. Several rapamycin analogs (rapalogs) are in clinical trial. Rad001 (everolimus), CC1-779 (sirolimus), and AP 23,573 (deferolimus) have been tested in phase I clinical trials in solid tumors (Mita et al. 2008), and in melanoma (Margolin et al. 2005). While the drug was well tolerated, only one of 33 melanoma patients had a partial response to treatment. More recently, molecules combining mTOR + PI3-kinase inhibition (BEZ 238) have been synthesized. These appear to have more activity in preclinical melanoma models and are currently in phase I testing (Maira et al. 2008).

9 Other Growth Factor Receptor Pathways

9.1 MET

Met is a receptor tyrosine kinase that has been known to stimulate the invasive growth of cancer cells, increase their metastatic potential, and to be expressed and/ or mutated in a variety of solid tumors. It consists of a disulfide-linked heterodimer with a molecular weight of 190 kDa. The ligand, hepatocyte growth factor (HGF), also known as scatter factor, is a multifunctional cytokine acting as a trophic factor, for many epithelial cells. HGF is physiologically secreted by cells of mesenchymal origin and acts on neighboring epithelial cells through a paracrine loop. In normal skin, Met is expressed on epithelial cells and melanocytes, whereas HGF is produced mainly by mesenchymal cells and, consequently, interacts with its receptor in a paracrine manner (Hsu et al. 2002). Overexpression of c-Met correlates with the invasive growth phase of melanoma cells and many melanomas actively secrete HGF, which can induce sustained activation of its receptor in an autocrine manner (Economou et al. 2008; Hsu et al. 2002). Ectopic expression of HGF in epidermal keratinocytes leads to increased epidermal melanocytes and pigmentation (Kunisada et al. 2000; Takayama et al. 1997). In these mice, UV radiation early in life induces melanoma with histopathological features closely mimicking human melanoma (Noonan et al. 2000). The small molecule met inhibitor SU11274 or c-Met specific siRNA led to decreased cell growth and viability of melanoma cells in a preclinical study (Puri et al. 2007). A novel MET mutation was identified in the juxtamembranous domain of one of fourteen melanomas in the study. Met inhibitors are actively being evaluated for melanoma in the clinic. The c-Met inhibitor, XL184, is currently being explored in a randomized discontinuation trial in several cancers including melanoma. A second MET inhibitor, XL880, which also inhibits VEGFR2 activity, has shown activity in renal cancer and melanoma in a phase I clinical trial (Eder et al. 2011).

9.2 Fibroblast Growth Factor Receptor Family

The fibroblast growth factor (FGF) family contains at least 22 growth factors involved in diverse processes such as development, angiogenesis, and wound healing. The FGF ligands bind to four different FGF receptors designated FGFR1-4. The common structure of the receptors consists of an extracellular region containing three immunoglobulin-like domains, a transmembrane domain, and a cytoplasmic region comprising the tyrosine kinase domain. Multiple secreted and membrane-bound receptor isoforms with different ligand specificities can be generated by alternative splicing events. FGF2 or basic FGF (bFGF) is important for melanocyte survival and is produced in the skin by keratinocytes and fibroblasts. While bFGF is not expressed by normal melanocytes, it has been shown to be expressed by melanoma cells (Halaban et al. 1988b) and acts as strong mitogen for human melanocytes, endothelial cells and fibroblasts in vitro (Halaban et al. 1988a; Nesbit et al. 1999; Sauter et al. 2001) bFGF binds to low-affinity receptors on the cell surface, mainly FGFR-1. Interestingly, by immunohistochemistry, bFGF is strongly expressed in melanocytic nevi and in melanoma, while FGFR1 is only expressed in melanoma (Ahmed et al. 1997; Giehl et al. 2007; Ueda et al. 1994). Co- expression of FGFR-1 and bFGF in melanoma cells was associated with increased microvessel density (Straume and Akslen 2002). In an in vivo model of melanoma, antisense targeting of bFGF or FGFR-1 resulted in blockage of angiogenesis and tumor growth (Wang and Becker 1997). The multi-kinase inhibitor TKI258 with activity against FGF receptors 1, 2, and 3 has been tested in melanoma in a phase I trial, without notable antitumor activity (Sarker et al. 2008). Interestingly, FGFR2 shows apparent loss of function in approximately 10% of melanomas, indicating that FGF signaling does not invariably stimulate melanoma growth, but may have opposite effects as well (Gartside et al. 2009).

10 Future Perspectives

Melanoma treatment is undergoing fundamental changes. While chemotherapy and immunotherapy have been tested and sometimes produce durable remission in a small subset of patients, for most patients these treatments are ineffective. In the last 5 years, there has been a drastic change in our understanding of melanoma. It has become clear that melanoma comprises biologically distinct subtypes with characteristic patterns of mutations in genes feeding into the MAP-kinase pathway, which vary depending on the site of the primary, age of the patient, and degree of sun-exposure of the site of the primary.

Extrapolating from this development and from data from the most recent clinical trials, it is becoming clear that each patient with metastatic melanoma will have to undergo an analysis of the specific mutations underlying the disease and have the treatment strategy determined based on this mutation pattern. This approach is a sea change compared to the standard oncologic practice of even a few years ago, where a given pathology falls into a given therapeutic space and patient performance status, disease velocity, and patient preference perhaps are the most significant modifying factors. While the pathway inhibitors have shown a high degree of activity, very few patients are actually cured and resistance develops often within a few months of treatment. Additionally, once resistance develops, it is not clear, whether salvage will be possible with a downstream inhibitor. Once the precise mechanism of resistance has been uncovered, combinatorial treatment approaches can be conceived that are expected to result in more durable responses. Furthermore, specific pathway inhibitors may work better with orthogonal treatment approaches such as immune-, radio-, chemo-, or anti-angiogenic therapy.

References

Adjei AA, Cohen RB, Franklin W et al (2008) Phase I pharmacokinetic and pharmacodynamic study of the oral, small-molecule mitogen-activated protein kinase kinase 1/2 inhibitor AZD6244 (ARRY-142886) in patients with advanced cancers. J Clin Oncol 26:2139–2146. doi:10.1200/JCO.2007.14.4956

Ahmed NU, Ueda M, Ito A et al (1997) Expression of fibroblast growth factor receptors in naevus-cell naevus and malignant melanoma. Melanoma Res 7:299–305

Ashman LK (1999) The biology of stem cell factor and its receptor C-kit. Int J Biochem Cell Biol 31:1037–1051. doi:10.1016/S1357-2725(99)00076-X

Bastian BC, Kashani-Sabet M, Hamm H et al (2000a) Gene amplifications characterize acral melanoma and permit the detection of occult tumor cells in the surrounding skin. Cancer Res 60:1968–1973

Bastian BC, LeBoit PE, Pinkel D (2000b) Mutations and copy number increase of HRAS in Spitz nevi with distinctive histopathological features. Amn J Pathol 157:967–972

Bastian BC, Olshen AB, LeBoit PE, Pinkel D (2003) Classifying melanocytic tumors based on DNA copy number changes. Am J Pathol 163:1765–1770

Bauer J, Curtin JA, Pinkel D, Bastian BC (2007) Congenital melanocytic nevi frequently harbor NRAS mutations but no BRAF mutations. J Invest Dermatol 127:179–182

Beadling C, Jacobson-Dunlop E, Hodi FS et al (2008) KIT gene mutations and copy number in melanoma subtypes. Clin Cancer Res 14:6821–6828. doi:14/21/6821

Besmer P, Murphy JE, George PC et al (1986) A new acute transforming feline retrovirus and relationship of its oncogene v-kit with the protein kinase gene family. Nature 320:415–421. doi:10.1038/320415a0

Birck A, Ahrenkiel V, Zeuthen J et al (2000) Mutation and allelic loss of the PTEN/MMAC1 gene in primary and metastatic melanoma biopsies. J Invest Dermatol 114:277–280

Brannan CI, Lyman SD, Williams DE et al (1991) Steel-Dickie mutation encodes a c-kit ligand lacking transmembrane and cytoplasmic domains. Proc Natl Acad Sci U S A 88:4671–4674

Buac K, Xu M, Cronin J et al (2009) NRG1/ERBB3 signaling in melanocyte development and melanoma: inhibition of differentiation and promotion of proliferation. Pigment Cell Melanoma Res 22:773–784. doi:10.1111/j.1755-148X.2009.00616.x

Carvajal R, Chapman P, Wolchok J et al (2009) A phase II study of imatinib mesylate (IM) for patients with advanced melanoma harboring somatic alterations of KIT. J Clin Oncol (Meeting Abstracts) (15S):9001

Chudnovsky Y, Adams AE, Robbins PB et al (2005) Use of human tissue to assess the oncogenic activity of melanoma-associated mutations. Nat Genet 37:745–749. doi:ng1586

Cronin JC, Wunderlich J, Loftus SK et al (2009) Frequent mutations in the MITF pathway in melanoma. Pigment Cell Melanoma Res 22:435–444. doi:10.1111/j.1755-148X.2009.00578.x

Curtin JA, Fridlyand J, Kageshita T et al (2005) Distinct sets of genetic alterations in melanoma. N Engl J Med 353:2135–2147

Curtin JA, Busam K, Pinkel D, Bastian BC (2006) Somatic activation of KIT in distinct subtypes of melanoma. J Clin Oncol 24:4340–4346

Dai DL, Martinka M, Li G (2005) Prognostic significance of activated Akt expression in melanoma: a clinicopathologic study of 292 cases. J Clin Oncol 23:1473–1482. doi:10.1200/JCO.2005.07.168

Davies H, Bignell GR, Cox C et al (2002) Mutations of the BRAF gene in human cancer. Nature 417:949–954. doi:10.1038/nature00766

Davies MA, Stemke-Hale K, Tellez C et al (2008) A novel AKT3 mutation in melanoma tumours and cell lines. Br J Cancer 99:1265–1268. doi:10.1038/sj.bjc.6604637

Delord J, Houede N, Awada A et al (2010) First-in-human phase I safety, pharmacokinetic (PK), and pharmacodynamic (PD) analysis of the oral MEK-inhibitor AS703026 [two regimens (R)] in patients (pts) with advanced solid tumors. J Clin Oncol 28

Dhawan P, Singh AB, Ellis DL, Richmond A (2002) Constitutive activation of Akt/protein kinase B in melanoma leads to up-regulation of nuclear factor-kappaB and tumor progression. Cancer Res 62:7335–7342

Djerf EA, Trinks C, Abdiu A et al (2009) ErbB receptor tyrosine kinases contribute to proliferation of malignant melanoma cells: inhibition by gefitinib (ZD1839). Melanoma Res 19:156–166. doi:10.1097/CMR.0b013e32832c6339

Druker BJ, Talpaz M, Resta DJ et al (2001) Efficacy and safety of a specific inhibitor of the BCR-ABL tyrosine kinase in chronic myeloid leukemia. N Engl J Med 344:1031–1037. doi:10.1056/NEJM200104053441401

Dummer R, Robert C, Chapman PB et al (2008) AZD6244 (ARRY-142886) vs temozolomide (TMZ) in patients (pts) with advanced melanoma: An open-label, randomized, multicenter, phase II study. J Clin Oncol 26

Economou MA, All-Ericsson C, Bykov V et al (2008) Receptors for the liver synthesized growth factors IGF-1 and HGF/SF in uveal melanoma: intercorrelation and prognostic implications. Acta Ophthalmol 86(Thesis 4):20–25. doi:10.1111/j.1755-3768.2008.01182.x

Eder JP, Appleman L, Heath E et al (2011) A phase I study of a novel spectrum selective kinase inhibitor (SSKI), XL880, administered orally in patients (pts) with advanced solid tumors (STs).–ASCO. http://www.asco.org/ascov2/Meetings/Abstracts?&vmview=abst_detail_view&confID=40&abstractID=32125. Accessed 3 Jun 2011

Ehlers JP, Harbour JW (2006) Molecular pathobiology of uveal melanoma. Int Ophthalmol Clin 46:167–180

Fry DW, Bedford DC, Harvey PH et al (2001) Cell cycle and biochemical effects of PD 0183812. A potent inhibitor of the cyclin D-dependent kinases CDK4 and CDK6. J Biol Chem 276:16617–16623. doi:10.1074/jbc.M008867200

Gartside MG, Chen H, Ibrahimi OA et al (2009) Loss-of-function fibroblast growth factor receptor-2 mutations in melanoma. Mol Cancer Res 7:41–54. doi:10.1158/1541-7786.MCR-08-0021

Giehl KA, Nägele U, Volkenandt M, Berking C (2007) Protein expression of melanocyte growth factors (bFGF, SCF) and their receptors (FGFR-1, c-kit) in nevi and melanoma. J Cutan Pathol 34:7–14. doi:10.1111/j.1600-0560.2006.00569.x

Gogas HJ, Kirkwood JM, Sondak VK (2007) Chemotherapy for metastatic melanoma: time for a change? Cancer 109:455–464. doi:10.1002/cncr.22427

Guertin DA, Sabatini DM (2005) An expanding role for mTOR in cancer. Trends Mol Med 11:353–361. doi:10.1016/j.molmed.2005.06.007

Guldberg P, Straten PT, Birck A et al (1997) Disruption of the mmac1/pten gene by deletion or mutation is a frequent event in malignant melanoma. Cancer Res 57:3660–3663

Halaban R, Langdon R, Birchall N et al (1988a) Basic fibroblast growth factor from human keratinocytes is a natural mitogen for melanocytes. J Cell Biol 107:1611–1619

Halaban R, Kwon BS, Ghosh S et al (1988b) bFGF as an autocrine growth factor for human melanomas. Oncogene Res 3:177–186

Hodi FS, Friedlander P, Corless CL et al (2008) Major response to imatinib mesylate in KIT-mutated melanoma. J Clin Oncol 26:2046–2051

Hsu M-Y, Meier F, Herlyn M (2002) Melanoma development and progression: a conspiracy between tumor and host. Differentiation 70:522–536. doi:10.1046/j.1432-0436.2002.700906.x

Infante JR, Fecher LA, Nallapareddy S et al (2010) Safety and efficacy results from the first-in-human study of the oral MEK 1/2 inhibitor GSK1120212. J Clin Oncol 28

Inman JL, Kute T, White W et al (2003) Absence of HER2 overexpression in metastatic malignant melanoma. J Surg Oncol 84:82–88. doi:10.1002/jso.10297

Jemal A, Siegel R, Ward E et al (2009) Cancer statistics, 2009. CA Cancer J Clin 59:225–249. doi:10.3322/caac.20006

Khan MA, Andrews S, Ismail-Khan R et al (2006) Overall and progression-free survival in metastatic melanoma: analysis of a single-institution database. Cancer Control 13:211–217

Kim KB, Eton O, Davis DW et al (2008) Phase II trial of imatinib mesylate in patients with metastatic melanoma. Br J Cancer 99:734–740. doi:10.1038/sj.bjc.6604482

Kluger HM, DiVito K, Berger AJ et al (2004) Her2/neu is not a commonly expressed therapeutic target in melanoma–a large cohort tissue microarray study. Melanoma Res 14:207–210

Kunisada T, Yoshida H, Yamazaki H et al (1998) Transgene expression of steel factor in the basal layer of epidermis promotes survival, proliferation, differentiation and migration of melanocyte precursors. Development 125:2915–2923

Kunisada T, Yamazaki H, Hirobe T et al (2000) Keratinocyte expression of transgenic hepatocyte growth factor affects melanocyte development, leading to dermal melanocytosis. Mech Dev 94:67–78

Lassam N, Bickford S (1992) Loss of C-Kit expression in cultured melanoma-cells. Oncogene 7:51–56

Linos E, Swetter SM, Cockburn MG et al (2009) Increasing burden of melanoma in the United States. J Invest Dermatol 129:1666–1674. doi:10.1038/jid.2008.423

Longley BJ Jr, Morganroth GS, Tyrrell L et al (1993) Altered metabolism of mast-cell growth factor (c-kit ligand) in cutaneous mastocytosis. N Engl J Med 328:1302–1307. doi:10.1056/NEJM199305063281803

Lutzky J, Bauer J, Bastian BC (2008) Dose-dependent, complete response to imatinib of a metastatic mucosal melanoma with a K642E KIT mutation. Pigment Cell Melanoma Res 21(4):492–495

Ma XM, Blenis J (2009) Molecular mechanisms of mTOR-mediated translational control. Nat Rev Mol Cell Biol 10:307–318. doi:10.1038/nrm2672

Maira S-M, Stauffer F, Brueggen J et al (2008) Identification and characterization of NVP-BEZ235, a new orally available dual phosphatidylinositol 3-kinase/mammalian target of rapamycin inhibitor with potent in vivo antitumor activity. Mol Cancer Ther 7:1851–1863. doi:10.1158/1535-7163.MCT-08-0017

Maldonado JL, Fridlyand J, Patel H et al (2003) Determinants of BRAF mutations in primary melanoma. J Natl Cancer Inst 95:1878–1890

Margolin K, Longmate J, Baratta T et al (2005) CCI-779 in metastatic melanoma: a phase II trial of the California Cancer consortium. Cancer 104:1045–1048. doi:10.1002/cncr.21265

Matsui Y, Zsebo KM, Hogan BL (1990) Embryonic expression of a haematopoietic growth factor encoded by the Sl locus and the ligand for c-kit. Nature 347:667–669. doi:10.1038/347667a0

McGovern VJ, Cochran AJ, Van der Esch EP et al (1986) The classification of malignant melanoma, its histological reporting and registration: a revision of the 1972 Sydney classification. Pathology 18:12–21

Mita MM, Mita AC, Chu QS et al (2008) Phase I trial of the novel mammalian target of rapamycin inhibitor deforolimus (AP23573; MK-8669) administered intravenously daily for 5 days every 2 weeks to patients with advanced malignancies. J Clin Oncol 26:361–367. doi:10.1200/JCO.2007.12.0345

Montone KT, Belle P, Elder DE (1997) Proto-oncogene c-kit expression in malignant melanoma: protein loss with tumor progression. Mod Pathol 10(9):939–944

Natali PG, Nicotra MR, Winkler AB et al (1992) Progression of human cutaneous melanoma is associated with loss of expression of C-Kit protooncogene receptor. Int J Cancer 52:197–201

Nesbit M, Nesbit HK, Bennett J et al (1999) Basic fibroblast growth factor induces a transformed phenotype in normal human melanocytes. Oncogene 18:6469–6476. doi:10.1038/sj.onc.1203066

Noonan FP, Otsuka T, Bang S et al (2000) Accelerated ultraviolet radiation-induced carcinogenesis in hepatocyte growth factor/scatter factor transgenic mice. Cancer Res 60:3738–3743

O'Dwyer PJ, LoRusso P, DeMichele A et al (2007) A phase I dose escalation trial of a daily oral CDK 4/6 inhibitor PD-0332991. J Clin Oncol 2007 ASCO Ann Meet Proc 25

Padua RA, Barrass NC, Currie GA (1985) Activation of N-ras in a human melanoma cell line. Mol Cell Biol 5:582–585

Palavalli LH, Prickett TD, Wunderlich JR et al (2009) Analysis of the matrix metalloproteinase family reveals that MMP8 is often mutated in melanoma. Nat Genet 41:518–520. doi:10.1038/ng.340

Patel S, Bedikian A, Kim K et al (2011) A phase II study of gefitinib in patients with metastatic melanoma.–ASCO. http://www.asco.org/ascov2/Meetings/Abstracts?&vmview=abst_detail_view&confID=65&abstractID=34308. Accessed 3 Jun 2011

Potti A, Moazzam N, Langness E et al (2004) Immunohistochemical determination of HER-2/neu, c-Kit (CD117), and vascular endothelial growth factor (VEGF) overexpression in malignant melanoma. J Cancer Res Clin Oncol 130:80–86

Prickett TD, Agrawal NS, Wei X et al (2009) Analysis of the tyrosine kinome in melanoma reveals recurrent mutations in ERBB4. Nat Genet 41:1127–1132. doi:10.1038/ng.438

Puri N, Ahmed S, Janamanchi V et al (2007) c-Met is a potentially new therapeutic target for treatment of human melanoma. Clin Cancer Res 13:2246–2253. doi:10.1158/1078-0432.CCR-06-0776

Rákosy Z, Vízkeleti L, Ecsedi S et al (2007) EGFR gene copy number alterations in primary cutaneous malignant melanomas are associated with poor prognosis. Int J Cancer 121:1729–1737. doi:10.1002/ijc.22928

Reifenberger J, Wolter M, Bostrom J et al (2000) Allelic losses on chromosome arm 10q and mutation of the PTEN (MMAC1) tumour suppressor gene in primary and metastatic malignant melanomas. Virchows Arch 436:487–493

Sarker D, Molife R, Evans TRJ et al (2008) A phase I pharmacokinetic and pharmacodynamic study of TKI258, an oral, multitargeted receptor tyrosine kinase inhibitor in patients with advanced solid tumors. Clin Cancer Res 14:2075–2081. doi:10.1158/1078-0432.CCR-07-1466

Sauter ER, Nesbit M, Tichansky D et al (2001) Fibroblast growth factor-binding protein expression changes with disease progression in clinical and experimental human squamous epithelium. Int J Cancer 92:374–381

Sauter ER, Yeo UC, Von Stemm A et al (2002) Cyclin D1 is a candidate oncogene in cutaneous melanoma. Cancer Res 62:3200–3206

Serrano M, Lee H, Chin L et al (1996) Role of the INK4a locus in tumor suppression and cell mortality. Cell 85:27–37

Shapiro GI (2006) Cyclin-dependent kinase pathways as targets for cancer treatment. J Clin Oncol 24:1770–1783. doi:10.1200/JCO.2005.03.7689

Sherr CJ, Roberts JM (1999) CDK inhibitors: positive and negative regulators of G1-phase progression. Genes Dev 13:1501–1512

Smalley KSM, Lioni M, Dalla Palma M et al (2008) Increased cyclin D1 expression can mediate BRAF inhibitor resistance in BRAF V600E-mutated melanomas. Mol Cancer Ther 7:2876–2883. doi:10.1158/1535-7163.MCT-08-0431

Soni R, O'Reilly T, Furet P et al (2001) Selective in vivo and in vitro effects of a small molecule inhibitor of cyclin-dependent kinase 4. J Natl Cancer Inst 93:436–446

Sousa SF, Fernandes PA, Ramos MJ (2008) Farnesyltransferase inhibitors: a detailed chemical view on an elusive biological problem. Curr Med Chem 15:1478–1492

Sparrow LE, Heenan PJ (1999) Differential expression of epidermal growth factor receptor in melanocytic tumours demonstrated by immunohistochemistry and mRNA in situ hybridization. Australas J Dermatol 40:19–24

Stahl JM, Sharma A, Cheung M et al (2004) Deregulated Akt3 activity promotes development of malignant melanoma. Cancer Res 64:7002–7010

Straume O, Akslen LA (2002) Importance of vascular phenotype by basic fibroblast growth factor, and influence of the angiogenic factors basic fibroblast growth factor/fibroblast growth factor receptor-1 and ephrin-A1/EphA2 on melanoma progression. Am J Pathol 160:1009–1019. doi:10.1016/S0002-9440(10)64922-X

Takayama H, LaRochelle WJ, Sharp R et al (1997) Diverse tumorigenesis associated with aberrant development in mice overexpressing hepatocyte growth factor/scatter factor. Proc Natl Acad Sci U S A 94:701–706

Tran MA, Gowda R, Sharma A et al (2008) Targeting V600EB-Raf and Akt3 using nanoliposomal-small interfering RNA inhibits cutaneous melanocytic lesion development. Cancer Res 68:7638–7649. doi:10.1158/0008-5472.CAN-07-6614

Trent JM, Meyskens FL, Salmon SE et al (1990) Relation of cytogenetic abnormalities and clinical outcome in metastatic melanoma. N Engl J Med 322:1508–1511

Tsao H, Zhang X, Fowlkes K, Haluska FG (2000) Relative reciprocity of NRAS and PTEN/MMAC1 alterations in cutaneous melanoma cell lines. Cancer Res 60:1800–1804

Tsao H, Goel V, Wu H et al (2004) Genetic interaction between NRAS and BRAF mutations and PTEN/MMAC1 inactivation in melanoma. J Investig Dermatol 122:337–341

Ueda M, Funasaka Y, Ichihashi M, Mishima Y (1994) Stable and strong expression of basic fibroblast growth factor in naevus cell naevus contrasts with aberrant expression in melanoma. Br J Dermatol 130:320–324

Ueno Y, Sakurai H, Tsunoda S et al (2008) Heregulin-induced activation of ErbB3 by EGFR tyrosine kinase activity promotes tumor growth and metastasis in melanoma cells. Int J Cancer 123:340–347. doi:10.1002/ijc.23465

Ugurel S, Hildenbrand R, Zimpfer A et al (2005) Lack of clinical efficacy of imatinib in metastatic melanoma. Br J Cancer 92:1398–1405

van Dijk M, Sprenger S, Rombout P et al (2003) Distinct chromosomal aberrations in sinonasal mucosal melanoma as detected by comparative genomic hybridization. Genes Chromosom Cancer 36:151–158

Van Raamsdonk CD, Bezrookove V, Green G et al (2009) Frequent somatic mutations of GNAQ in uveal melanoma and blue naevi. Nature 457:599–602. doi:10.1038/nature07586

Van Raamsdonk CD, Griewank KG, Crosby MB et al (2010) Mutations in GNA11 in uveal melanoma. N Engl J Med 363:2191–2199. doi:10.1056/NEJMoa1000584

Viros A, Fridlyand J, Bauer J et al (2008) Improving melanoma classification by integrating genetic and morphologic features. PLoS Med 5:e120

Wang Y, Becker D (1997) Antisense targeting of basic fibroblast growth factor and fibroblast growth factor receptor-1 in human melanomas blocks intratumoral angiogenesis and tumor growth. Nat Med 3:887–893

Wellbrock C, Gomez A, Schartl M (1997) Signal transduction by the oncogenic receptor tyrosine kinase Xmrk in melanoma formation of Xiphophorus. Pigment Cell Res 10:34–40

Willmore-Payne C, Holden JA, Hirschowitz S, Layfield LJ (2006) BRAF and c-kit gene copy number in mutation-positive malignant melanoma. Hum Pathol 37:520–527

Wong CW, Fan YS, Chan TL et al (2005) BRAF and NRAS mutations are uncommon in melanomas arising in diverse internal organs. J Clin Pathol 58:640–644

Wyman K, Atkins MB, Prieto V et al (2006a) Multicenter Phase II trial of high-dose imatinib mesylate in metastatic melanoma: significant toxicity with no clinical efficacy. Cancer 106:2005–2011

Wyman K, Kelley M, Puzanov I et al (2006b) Phase II study of erlotinib given daily for patients with metastatic melanoma (MM). J Clin Oncol 24

Yarden Y (2001) The EGFR family and its ligands in human cancer. Signalling mechanisms and therapeutic opportunities. Eur J Cancer 37(Suppl 4):S3–S8

Zhou XP, Gimm O, Hampel H et al (2000) Epigenetic PTEN silencing in malignant melanomas without PTEN mutation [In process citation]. Am J Pathol 157:1123–1128

Zsebo KM, Williams DA, Geissler EN et al (1990) Stem cell factor is encoded at the Sl locus of the mouse and is the ligand for the c-kit tyrosine kinase receptor. Cell 63:213–224. doi:10.1016/0092-8674(90)90302-U

JAK-Mutant Myeloproliferative Neoplasms

Ross L. Levine

Abstract Although the Janus family of kinases (JAK1, JAK2, JAK3, and TYK2) has been extensively characterized and investigated, the role of Janus kinase activation in the pathogenesis and therapy of human malignancies was not fully appreciated until recently when multiple studies identified a recurrent somatic mutation in the JAK2 tyrosine kinase (JAK2V617F) in the majority of patients with BCR-ABL-negative myeloproliferative neoplasms (MPN), polycythemia vera, essential thrombocytosis, and primary myelofibrosis. Other mutations that activate the JAK-STAT signaling pathway have since been identified in JAK2V617F-negative MPN patients and in a subset of patients with acute myeloid leukemia and acute lymphoid leukemia. In addition, dysregulated JAK-STAT signaling has been implicated in the pathogenesis of a spectrum of epithelial neoplasms. In this chapter, we will review the recent studies that identified genetic alterations that activate JAK signaling in different malignancies, and discuss the recent efforts aimed at developing small-molecule inhibitors of JAK kinase activity for the treatment of MPNs and other malignancies.

Contents

1	Introduction	120
2	Myeloproliferative Neoplasms	122
3	Discovery of JAK2V617F Mutations	122
4	JAK2V617F-Negative MPN	124
5	Additional Somatic Mutations in MPN	125

R. L. Levine (✉)
Memorial Sloan Kettering Cancer Center,
New York, NY 10021, USA
e-mail: leviner@mskcc.org

Current Topics in Microbiology and Immunology (2012) 355: 119–133
DOI: 10.1007/82_2011_170
© Springer-Verlag Berlin Heidelberg 2011
Published Online: 7 August 2011

6	Evidence for Germline Mutations in MPN	127
7	Role of JAK-STAT Signaling in Other Malignancies	127
8	JAK2 Inhibitor Therapy	128
9	Future Perspectives	130
References		130

1 Introduction

JAK1, *JAK2*, *JAK3*, and *TYK2* belong to the Janus family of non-receptor tyrosine kinases. They were initially identified using PCR-based strategies designed to identify novel protein tyrosine kinases (Harpur et al. 1992). Investigators subsequently demonstrated that the Janus kinases specifically associate with cytokine receptors and transmit signals from cytokine receptors. Cytokine receptors themselves lack catalytic activity and thus JAK kinase signaling serves as the intracellular mechanism by which cytokines can activate signaling pathways (Fig. 1, panel A). For example, it has been shown that ligand binding to the growth hormone receptor (Argetsinger et al. 1993) and to the erythropoietin receptor (EPOR) (Witthuhn et al. 1993) results in JAK2 autophosphorylation and activation of downstream signaling. Elegant in vitro and in vivo studies have demonstrated that the distinct effects of different cytokines on different cell populations is due, at least in part, to the affinity of specific cytokine receptors to one or more members of the JAK kinase family. In most cases, cytokine receptors associate with multiple members of the JAK family of kinases, but this is not always the case. In particular, genetic studies using JAK2-deficient mice have demonstrated that erythropoietin signaling is abrogated in JAK2-deficient hematopoietic cells, and *JAK2* deficiency results in complete absence of erythropoiesis (Parganas et al. 1998).

JAK1, JAK2, JAK3, and TYK2 each possess seven JAK homology domains (Fig. 1, panel B). Starting with the C-terminus, the first homology domain, known as the JH1 domain, possesses the kinase domain. Importantly, the JH2 domain, which is proximal to the JH1 kinase domain, is thought to be a pseudokinase domain without intrinsic catalytic activity. The JH7 domain at the N-terminus contains the FERM domain, which is required for interaction with specific cytokine receptors. The crystal structure of the JH1 domains of JAK2 and JAK3 has been solved by crystallizing the catalytic domains in complex with ATP-competitive small-molecule inhibitors (Boggon et al. 2005; Lucet et al. 2006). However, the full length structure of any of the JAK kinases, or of the JH1 and JH2 domains of any of the Janus kinases, has not been solved. Despite the lack of structural insight, given that deletion of the JAK2 JH2 pseudokinase domain results in constitutive JAK2 kinase activity (Saharinen and Silvennoinen 2002), investigators predict that the JH2 domain negatively regulates JH1 kinase activity, similar to the autoinhibitory role of juxtamembrane domains in receptor tyrosine kinases. This is particularly important given that the JAK2V617F mutation which predominates in MPN patients (James et al. 2005; Baxter et al. 2005; Kralovics

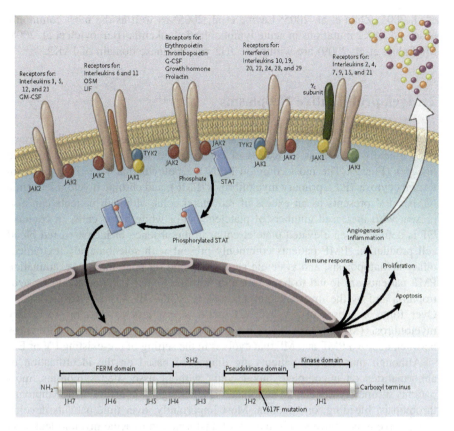

Fig. 1 The Janus kinase (JAK)-STAT pathway. a JAK activation. Transmembrane cytokine receptors lack intrinsic kinase activity. After engagement of the receptor by a cognate cytokine, they associate with the JAK family of tyrosine kinases. JAKs undergo transphosphorylation and in turn phosphorylate critical residues in the receptor and downstream signaling molecules, including the signal transducers and activators of transcription (STAT) family of DNA-binding proteins. Phosphorylated STATs (*blue rectangles* with *red dots*) dimerize and relocalize to the nucleus, where they regulate the expression of many genes. Different cytokine receptors preferentially use one or more JAKs. Thus, a great pleomorphism of effects is produced by inhibition of JAK1 and JAK2. On the contrary, JAK3 is activated only by cytokine receptors containing the γc subunit (in *green* on the *right*). G-CSF granulocyte colony-stimulating factor, GM-CSF granulocyte–macrophage colony-stimulating factor, LIF leukemia inhibitory factor, OSM oncostatin M. b Structure of JAK kinases. The JAK family of tyrosine kinases consists of four members [JAK1, JAK2, JAK3, and tyrosine kinase 2 (TYK2)] which share structural and functional homologies defined by seven JAK homology (JH) domains. These seven domains may be categorized into the JH1 kinase domain, the JH2 pseudokinase domain, the SRC homology 2 (SH2)-like domain (that mediates binding to phosphorylated tyrosine residues), and the FERM (protein 4.1, ezrin, radixin, and moesin) domain (required for JAK interaction with cytokine receptors). The myeloproliferative neoplasm-associated V617F mutation in JAK2 is located in the JH2 autoregulatory domain (*red line*) (from Vannuchi et al. NEJM Sept 2010)

et al. 2005; Zhao et al. 2005; Levine et al. 2005) as well as the most commonly observed JAK2 mutations in acute lymphoblastic leukemia (Bercovich et al. 2008; Mullighan et al. 2009) are within the JH2 pseudokinase domain of JAK2.

2 Myeloproliferative Neoplasms

Myeloproliferative neoplasms (MPN) are clonal hematopoietic stem cell disorders that clinically present as an excess of cells derived from one or more myeloid lineages (Fig. 2). The most common MPN are polcythemia vera (PV), essential thrombocytosis (ET), primary myelofibrosis (PMF), and chronic myeloid leukemia (CML). PV presents as an excess of red blood cells, although patients can also present with increased numbers of platelets and/or white blood cells. In contrast, ET is defined as an elevated platelet count in the absence of increased red blood cell production. PMF patients commonly present with splenomegaly, extramedullary hematopoiesis, and systemic symptoms, and on bone marrow examination PMF patients are found to have reticulin fibrosis. CML is characterized by neutrophilia and by the invariant presence of the BCR-ABL fusion tyrosine kinase. Over time, a subset of PV and ET patients progress to develop secondary myelofibrosis (MF). It is not known whether there are biologic or clinical differences between de novo PMF and MF that evolves in the setting of pre-existing PV or ET.

Although many MPN patients are diagnosed based on the identification of abnormalities on a complete blood count without associated symptoms, most patients ultimately develop symptomatic splenomegaly, constitutional symptoms, thrombosis, bleeding, or infection. Most importantly, over time patients develop progressive bone marrow failure and/or transformation to acute myeloid leukemia (AML); AML transformation is specifically associated with a dismal overall prognosis (Mesa et al. 2005). The shared clinical features of PV, ET, and PMF illustrate their biologic and clinical overlap, and the discovery of *JAK2V617F* mutations in these disorders provided a common genetic alteration in the majority of patients with these MPN.

3 Discovery of JAK2V617F Mutations

The genetic basis for these disorders remained elusive until 2005 when several groups identified somatic *JAK2V617F* mutations in MPN patients (James et al. 2005; Baxter et al. 2005; Kralovics et al. 2005; Zhao et al. 2005; Levine et al. 2005). William Vainchenker and colleagues used small-molecule inhibition and shRNA-mediated knockdown approaches to investigate signaling pathways required for endogenous erythroid colony (EEC) formation in PV patients. They found that JAK2 inhibition inhibited PV EEC formation, which led them to identify the *JAK2V617F* allele (James et al. 2005). Anthony Green's group performed sequence analysis of genes in oncogenic signaling pathways to discover

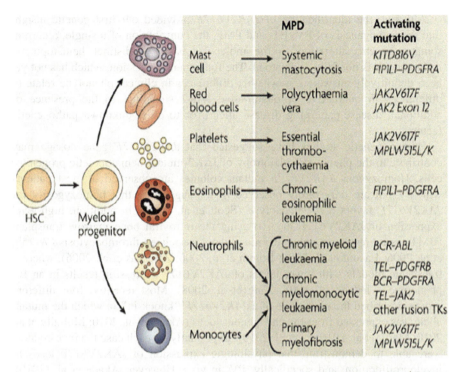

Fig. 2 MPN classification/molecular alterations (from Harpur et al. 1992)

the *JAK2V617F* mutation (Baxter et al. 2005). Kralovics, Skoda, and their colleagues sequenced the genes in the minimal region of acquired uniparental disomy (UPD), previously described by Prchal (Kralovics et al. 2002), to identify the *JAK2V617F* allele. Gilliland and colleagues performed a systematic mutational survey of the tyrosine kinome to identify the recurrent mutation in *JAK2* in MPN.

The mutation in *JAK2* is a somatic guanine to thymidine substitution; this mutation results in a change from valine to phenylalanine at codon 617. Sensitive, specific assays for *JAK2V617F* demonstrate that 90–95% of PV patients and 50–60% of ET/PMF patients are *JAK2V617F*-positive. The JAK2V617F mutation is the only mutation seen at this codon. This observation is quite surprising in light of the recent work which has demonstrated that substitution of either tryptophan, methionine, isoleucine, or leucine for valine at codon 617 also results in activation of JAK2 signaling and cellular transformation (Dusa et al. 2008); however, these mutations to date have not been observed in patients with MPNs or other human malignancies. Although alternate activating mutations that activate JAK2, including the less common *JAK2* exon 12 mutations in *JAK2V617F*-negative PV (Scott et al. 2007) and *JAK2* mutations in high-risk ALL (Bercovich et al. 2008; Mullighan et al. 2009) have been observed in patient samples, JAK2V617F is by far the most common mutation reported to date in human malignancies.

Although the identification of *JAK2V617F* provided our first genetic insight into the pathogenesis of PV, ET, and PMF, the contribution of a single, recurrent somatic genetic alteration to the molecular basis of distinct hematopoietic malignancies is not fully understood. The fundamental question, which has not yet been definitively answered, is whether differences in clinical phenotype relate to differences in qualitative or quantitative JAK2 signaling, to the presence of additional, disease-patterning disease alleles, or to other unknown pathogenetic factors.

Human genetic studies have suggested that *JAK2V617F* gene dosage may contribute to the phenotypic pleiotropy of JAK2-mutant hematopoietic progenitor cells. Homozygous *JAK2V617F* mutant colonies are observed in most patients with PV but are only rarely observed in ET suggesting that homozygosity for *JAK2V617F* favors a PV phenotype (Scott et al. 2006). In addition, high-level expression of JAK2V617F in vivo using the retroviral bone marrow transplant (BMT) assay results in polycythemia without associated thrombocytosis (Wernig et al. 2006; Lacout et al. 2006; Bumm et al. 2006; Zaleskas et al. 2006), whereas transgenic models with lower levels of JAK2V617F expression results in an ET phenotype (Tiedt et al. 2008, Xing et al. 2008). Most recently, four different groups described the phenotype of a *JAK2V617F* "knock-in" in which the mutant allele was expressed from the endogenous locus (Akada et al. 2010; Mullally et al. 2010; Marty et al. 2010; Li et al. 2010). Importantly, in each case the investigators were able to demonstrate that physiologic expression of JAK2V617F leads to myeloproliferation, and specifically, PV, in vivo. However, Akada et al. (2010), who were able to generate homozygous and heterozygous knock-in mice, did not observe differences in phenotype (other than disease severity) based on mutant gene dosage. Most recently, Green and colleagues used expression profiling to suggest that differences in STAT1 signaling might distinguish between homozygous mutant erythroid progenitors and heterozygous mutant progenitors, suggesting that there may be differences in signaling based on JAK2V617F gene dosage (Chen et al. 2010). Future studies in murine models and in primary cells will need to elucidate whether differences in *JAK2V617F* gene dosage and expression levels are relevant to the phenotype of JAK2-mutant hematopoietic progenitor cells.

4 JAK2V617F-Negative MPN

Although the *JAK2V617F* allele is present in the majority of MPN patients, there are MPN patients with these disorders who are *JAK2V617F*-negative. Differences in clinical/laboratory parameters between JAK2-mutant and JAK2-wildtype ET patients (Campbell et al. 2005), are small in magnitude and do not allow investigators to separate ET patients into distinct biologic subtypes. It was therefore hypothesized that there must be somatic mutations that activate JAK2 signaling in *JAK2V617F*-negative MPN patients. Scott et al. (2007) sequenced all exons of the

JAK kinases in *JAK2V617F*-negative PV and identified somatic missense mutations, deletions, and insertions involving residues 538–543 in exon 12 of *JAK2*. The pleoitropic nature of *JAK2* exon 12 mutations is in stark contrast to the single recurrent mutation seen at codon 617 in MPN patients. In vitro and in vivo studies demonstrate that JAK2 exon 12 mutations activate JAK-STAT signaling and lead to hematopoietic transformation. To date, exon 12 mutations have only been identified in patients with *JAK2V617F*-negative PV (and not in ET and PMF), and in most cases are observed in patients with erythrocytosis without thrombocytosis or leukocytosis; the genetic and biologic basis for the specificity of exon 12 mutations for PV has not yet been delineated.

Somatic mutations in JAK kinases have not been identified in *JAK2*-negative ET and MF. Pikman and colleagues therefore performed mutational analysis of myeloid-specific cytokine receptors that normally bind and activate JAK2 signaling and identified a somatic point mutation at codon 515 of *MPL* in 10% of JAK2V617F-negative PMF patients (Pardanani et al. 2006; Pikman et al. 2006). Different mutations at codon 515 have been identified in ET and PMF patients that result in substitution of leucine, lysine, or alanine for tryptophan (Pardanani et al. 2006; Pikman et al. 2006), and mutational analysis of the PT-1 cohort has identified somatic MPL mutations (including mutations at codon 515 and at codon 505) in 4% of all ET patients, including 8.5% of *JAK2V617F*-negative ET patients (Ding et al. 2004). MPLW515L expression results in activation of JAK2 and of downstream signaling pathways in an analogous manner similar to *JAK2V617F*. However, expression of MPLW515L in the murine bone marrow transplant assay results in a distinct MPN phenotype notable for short latency disease characterized by thrombocytosis and marked MF. These studies demonstrate that somatic alterations in the JAK-STAT signaling pathway occur in the majority of MPN patients. Despite these important genetic insights, many questions remain regarding the role of *JAK2/MPL* mutations in MPN pathogenesis. Most importantly, the biologic basis for the association of specific disease alleles with specific clinical phenotypes is not yet understood. Most recently, loss-of-function mutations in LNK, an adapter protein which negatively regulates JAK2 signaling, were identified in patients with JAK2/MPL-negative MPN (Oh et al. 2010), providing further genetic data implicating the JAK2 pathway in MPN pathogenesis.

5 Additional Somatic Mutations in MPN

Although the discovery of mutations in *JAK2* and *MPL* was extremely enlightening, several lines of evidence suggested that additional mutations contribute to MPN pathogenesis. Analysis of patients with a clonogenic cytogenetic abnormality in conjunction with the *JAK2V617F* mutation has allowed investigators to identify cytogenetically abnormal clones with and without the *JAK2V617F* allele (Beer et al. 2009). In addition, subsets of JAK2-mutant MPN patients who transform into AML have leukemic blasts that are *JAK2* wildtype (Campbell et al. 2006;

Theocharides et al. 2007). This suggests that an ancestral clone bearing an abnormality preceding the *JAK2V617F* mutation could be present giving rise to both MPN and AML. Based on these data, investigators have used candidate gene and genome-wide approaches to identify disease alleles that cooperate with, and may even precede, acquisition of the *JAK2V617F* allele.

In 2010, two groups identified somatic mutations in *TET2* in patients with MPN and other myeloid malignancies (Langemeijer et al. 2009; Delhommeau et al. 2009). Mutations in *TET2* have been found in all coding regions and can appear as missense, nonsense, or frameshift mutations consistent with a loss-of-function genomic alteration. Preliminary evidence of the functional importance of *TET2* myelopoiesis came from xenograft studies showing that TET2-mutant cells efficiently engraft in NOD-SCID mice, whereas TET2-wild-type cells poorly engraft in a xenotransplant assay (Delhommeau et al. 2009). Subsequent studies have shown that TET2, and its homologs TET1 and TET3, catalyze the conversion of methylcytosine into hydroxymethylcytosine, implicating TET2 in regulation of the epigenetic state (Tahiliani et al. 2009). Most recently it has been shown that leukemia patients with TET2 mutations are characterized by reduced DNA hydroxymethylation (Ko et al. 2010) and by increased DNA methylation (Figueroa et al. 2010), and that TET2 loss leads to impaired myeloid differentiation, increased hematopoietic stem-progenitor function, and to CMML in vivo (Moran-Crusio et al. 2011, Quivoron et al. 2011). However, the functional role of TET2 mutations in MPN pathogenesis and the therapeutic relevance of mutations in TET2 to the response to JAK inhibitors and to epigenetic therapies remains to be delineated.

Shortly after the discovery of *TET2* mutations in myeloid cancers, somatic mutations were identified in the Additional Sex Combs Like 1 (*ASXL1*) gene at a similar frequency and spectrum of myeloid malignancies as *TET2* mutations (Carbuccia et al. 2009a, b; Gelsi-Boyer et al. 2009). These mutations are also presumed to result in loss-of-function given that the majority of these alleles are either nonsense or frameshift mutations. *ASXL1* is one of three mammalian homologs of the *Additional sex combs* gene in *Drosophilia*; notably these genes regulate the expression of both polycomb group (PcG) and Trithorax group (TxG) proteins in *Drosophilia* and mammals (Cho et al. 2006; Fisher et al. 2010). However, as with TET2, the functional consequences of *ASXL1* mutations, and the contribution of *ASXL1* mutations to MPN pathogenesis remains to be delineated. Moreover, it remains to be seen whether *ASXL1*-mutant MPN patients respond differently to JAK2-targeted therapies.

Most recently, a series of studies have identified recurrent somatic mutations in a spectrum of genes in patients with myeloid malignancies, including IDH1/2 mutations (Mardis et al. 2009; Ward et al. 2010; Marcucci et al. 2010; Gross et al. 2010), EZH2 mutations (Ernst et al. 2010; Nikoloski et al. 2010), and DNMT3A mutations (Yan et al. 2011; Ley et al. 2010). In each case these mutations can be observed in a subset of MPN patients (Abdel-Wahab et al. 2011a, b); however, these mutations are not specific to MPN as they are observed in patients with MDS and AML. In addition, a subset of these disease alleles, including IDH1/2, TET2, and DNMT3A mutations may be most common in MPN patients who undergo leukemic transformation (Abdel-Wahab et al. 2010). These data indicate that a set of novel disease alleles can contribute to the pathogenesis of myeloid malignancies, including MPN, and that these mutations may contribute to transformation by corrupting the epigenetic state of hematopoietic cells.

6 Evidence for Germline Mutations in MPN

The existence of families with MPNs has long suggested the presence of germline susceptibility genes that predispose to MPN development. The single largest report of the familial aggregation of MPNs comes from a population-based study in Sweden which found that first-degree relatives of MPN patients were at five to seven-fold increased risk of developing a subsequent MPN (Landgren et al. 2008). These epidemiologic data suggested the presence of one or more common MPN predisposition loci. In 2009, three groups reported the presence of a germline haplotype block, which includes *JAK2* itself associated with the development of both *JAK2V617F* mutation and MPN. This haplotype block is markedly enriched in MPN patients and tagged by an SNP (rs10974944) located within an intron of *JAK2* (Jones et al. 2009; Kilpivaara et al. 2009; Olcaydu et al. 2009). Heterozygotes for this haplotype were significantly more likely to acquire the *JAK2V617F* mutation in *cis* with the predisposition SNP allele than on the other chromosome. The genetic data is most consistent with the risk allele functioning as a dominant MPN predisposition allele and increasing the likelihood of developing an MPN to three- to fourfold (Jones et al. 2009; Kilpivaara et al. 2009; Olcaydu et al. 2009). Although these reports represent the first identification of a common MPN risk allele, the mechanism by which this germline allele predisposes to MPN development and the clinical/therapeutic relevance of this allele remains unknown.

7 Role of JAK-STAT Signaling in Other Malignancies

Thus far, the most compelling genetic data implicating the JAK-STAT signaling pathway in transformation has emerged from the MPN field. Nonetheless, there is abundant data from many groups suggesting that JAK-STAT signaling is relevant to a broad spectrum of other human malignancies and may represent a tractable therapeutic target in hematopoietic and non-hematopoietic neoplasms (Table 1). Genetic data from acute lymphoblastic leukemia (ALL) and AML has identified somatic mutations in JAK kinases in a subset of patients with these malignancies. Specifically, systematic mutational profiling of the tyrosine kinome in AML patients has identified rare, somatic activating mutations in JAK1 and JAK2 (Tomasson et al. 2008). More recently, a number of reports have identified somatic, recurrent activating mutations in JAK1, JAK2, and JAK3 in high-risk

Table 1 Genetic and functional evidence of JAK-STAT activation in different malignancies

Myeloproliferative disorders	JAK2, MPL, LNK mutations
Acute myeloid leukemia	JAK1, JAK2 mutations
Acute lymphoblastic leukemia	JAK1, JAK2, JAK3, IL-7 receptor, CRLF2 mutations
Hodgkin lymphoma	JAK2 amplification, SOCS1 mutations/methylation
Lung/breast cancer	Autocrine/paracrine IL-6 signaling
Hepatocellular adenomas	GP130 cytokine receptor mutations

ALL. The first reports emerged from mutational studies in Down syndrome-associated ALL, where recurrent somatic mutations at codon 683 (also within the pseudokinase domain) were identified in a significant proportion of patients (Bercovich et al. 2008). Subsequently, investigators identified somatic JAK1, JAK2, and JAK3 mutations in ALL (Mullighan et al. 2009; Flex et al. 2008). Of note, these mutations are most commonly identified in patients with high-risk disease, and as such are associated with a poor overall prognosis. Most recently, activating mutations in the IL-7 receptor and in the CRLF2 cytokine receptor have been identified in ALL (Yoda et al. 2009; Shochat et al. 2011), suggesting that activated JAK-STAT signaling is a common pathogenetic event in lymphoid malignancies.

In addition, several studies have identified alternate, non-mutational mechanisms of JAK-STAT activation in different malignancies, including in epithelial neoplasms. These include reports of somatic mutations in the GP130 cytokine receptor in hepatocellular adenoma (Rebouissou et al. 2009), providing the first instance of a somatic mutation which activates the JAK-STAT pathway in epithelial malignancies. Many studies have identified increased phosphorylation of STAT3 and/or STAT5 in primary tumor samples (Hedvat et al. 2009), but until recently the basis for constitutive activation of this pathway in epithelial tumors was not known. Recently, investigators have found that autocrine and/or paracrine IL-6 secretion by tumor and/or stromal cells can lead to potent JAK-STAT activation and to in vitro and in vivo sensitivity to JAK kinase inhibitors (Gao et al. 2007). These data suggest that additional genetic (mutation, amplification), epigenetic, and cell-extrinsic factors can lead to JAK-STAT pathway activation in vivo, and that JAK kinase inhibitors might have therapeutic efficacy outside of JAK-mutant hematopoietic neoplasms.

8 JAK2 Inhibitor Therapy

The remarkable efficacy of tyrosine kinase inhibitors for CML and other MPNs (Druker et al. 2001) and the identification of *JAK2/MPL* mutations in PV, ET, and PMF led to the development of JAK2 kinase inhibitors. Different JAK inhibitors have been developed and characterized in preclinical studies (Table 2) (Hedvat et al. 2009; Pardanani et al. 2007; Wernig et al. 2008; Hexner et al. 2008; Koppikar

JAK-Mutant Myeloproliferative Neoplasms

Table 2 JAK kinase inhibitors in clinical development

INCB18424	Phase III trials in MF completed, phase III in PV/ET ongoing, phase II in other diseases
TG101348	Phase II in MF
CYT787	Phase I in MF
AZD1480	Phase I in MF
EXL019	Phase I in MF (discontinued due to neurologic toxicity)

et al. 2010). JAK2 kinase signaling contributes to a myriad of cellular functions including normal erythropoiesis and thrombopoiesis (Parganas et al. 1998). Hence, it might be expected that JAK kinase inhibitor therapy results in on-target, JAK2-related mechanism-based toxicities, particularly within the hematopoietic compartment. This has borne out to be the case in early clinical trials with JAK2 inhibitors in which anemia and/or thrombocytopenia have been dose-limiting toxicities. Given that loss-of-function mutations in JAK3 and TYK2 result in immune deficiencies (Abdel-Wahab et al. 2010, 2011a, b), inhibition of JAK1, JAK3, and TYK2 should be minimized when using JAK2 inhibitors for MPN patients where there is evidence for mutation-dependent JAK2 activation. In contrast, for patients with mutations in other JAK kinases or with JAK-STAT activation due to IL-6 secretion by tumor and stromal cells, JAK kinase inhibitors with more broad activity or with specific activity against JAK1 and/or JAK3 might be of value.

JAK2 inhibitors have now entered the early phase clinical development initially, for the treatment of PMF and post-PV/ET myelofibrosis (Verstovsek et al. 2010; Pardanani et al. 2011). These trials have shown that JAK2 inhibitor therapy results in marked reductions in spleen size and significant improvement in constitutional symptoms in PMF patients. However, to date there have been modest effects on *JAK2V617F* allele burden and on peripheral blood cytopenias in the majority of myelofibrosis patients. Moreover, JAK2 inhibitor treatment has resulted in hematopoietic toxicities that are presumed (but not proven) to result from JAK2 inhibition in normal cells, specifically anemia and thrombocytopenia which is easily managed with dose alterations. Importantly, it has not been definitely assessed whether chronic, potent JAK2 inhibition is tolerated in vivo, and future studies will need to include pharmacodynamic measurements of target inhibition and pathway suppression to determine whether toxicity, efficacy, or both limit the efficacy of JAK kinase inhibitors. Importantly, JAK inhibition in MF patients is associated with reduction in the elevated levels of inflammatory cytokines characteristic of MF patients (Verstovsek et al. 2010), suggesting that, at least in part the clinical benefits of JAK inhibitors at clinically tolerated doses relate to suppression of systemic inflammation and not from complete inhibition of constitutive signaling in MPN cells. Alternatively, it is possible that JAK2 inhibitor treatment in vivo results in selection of resistant clones; to date putative mechanisms for JAK2 inhibitor resistance have not been delineated. If this turns out to be the case, additional therapies that can specifically target pathways downstream of JAK signaling may prove to be more effective, either alone or in combination with JAK kinase inhibitors, such as HSP90 inhibition or HDAC inhibition (Marubayashi et al. 2010; Wang et al. 2009). Alternatively, it is possible that the genetic diversity of MPN and other malignancies will necessitate the development of combination therapeutic strategies which target oncogenic pathways that are dysregluated in concert with the JAK-STAT pathway.

9 Future Perspectives

In the past decade, genetic and functional studies have demonstrated the importance of the JAK kinase signaling pathway to a spectrum of human malignancies, and early efforts have begun to assess whether JAK kinases have a specific role in the treatment of hematopoietic and epithelial neoplasms. It is expected that subsequent studies will further elucidate the mechanistic basis by which JAK signaling contributes to oncogenic transformation, the specific contexts in which JAK kinase inhibitors may be of value, and the efficacy of JAK kinase inhibitors, alone and in combination with other therapies in different human malignancies.

References

Abdel-Wahab O et al (2010) Genetic analysis of transforming events that convert chronic myeloproliferative neoplasms to leukemias. Cancer Res 70:447–452

Abdel-Wahab O et al (2011a) Concomitant analysis of EZH2 and ASXL1 mutations in myelofibrosis, chronic myelomonocytic leukemia and blast-phase myeloproliferative neoplasms. Leukemia 19(5):769–780

Abdel-Wahab O et al (2011b) DNMT3A mutational analysis in primary myelofibrosis, chronic myelomonocytic leukemia and advanced phases of myeloproliferative neoplasms. Leukemia 25:1219–1220

Akada H et al (2010) Conditional expression of heterozygous or homozygous JAK2V617F from its endogenous promoter induces a polycythemia vera-like disease. Blood 115(17):3589–3597

Argetsinger LS et al (1993) Identification of JAK2 as a growth hormone receptor-associated tyrosine kinase. Cell 74:237–244

Baxter EJ et al (2005) Acquired mutation of the tyrosine kinase JAK2 in human myeloproliferative disorders. Lancet 365:1054–1061

Beer PA et al (2009) Clonal diversity in the myeloproliferative neoplasms: independent origins of genetically distinct clones. Br J Haematol 144:904–908

Bercovich D et al (2008) Mutations of JAK2 in acute lymphoblastic leukaemias associated with Down's syndrome. Lancet 372:1484–1492

Boggon TJ, Li Y, Manley PW, Eck MJ (2005) Crystal structure of the JAK3 kinase domain in complex with a staurosporine analog. Blood 106:996–1002

Bumm TG et al (2006) Characterization of murine JAK2V617F-positive myeloproliferative disease. Cancer Res 66:11156–11165

Campbell PJ et al (2005) Definition of subtypes of essential thrombocythaemia and relation to polycythaemia vera based on JAK2 V617F mutation status: a prospective study. Lancet 366:1945–1953

JAK-Mutant Myeloproliferative Neoplasms

Campbell PJ et al (2006) Mutation of JAK2 in the myeloproliferative disorders: timing, clonality studies, cytogenetic associations, and role in leukemic transformation. Blood 108:3548–3555

Carbuccia N et al (2009a) Mutual exclusion of ASXL1 and NPM1 mutations in a series of acute myeloid leukemias. Leukemia 24(2):469–473

Carbuccia N et al (2009b) Mutations of ASXL1 gene in myeloproliferative neoplasms. Leukemia 23:2183–2186

Chen E et al (2010) Distinct clinical phenotypes associated with JAK2V617F reflect differential STAT1 signaling. Cancer Cell 18:524–535

Cho YS, Kim EJ, Park UH, Sin HS, Um SJ (2006) Additional sex comb-like 1 (ASXL1), in cooperation with SRC-1, acts as a ligand-dependent coactivator for retinoic acid receptor. J Biol Chem 281:17588–17598

Delhommeau F et al (2009) Mutation in TET2 in myeloid cancers. N Engl J Med 360:2289–2301

Ding J et al (2004) Familial essential thrombocythemia associated with a dominant-positive activating mutation of the c-MPL gene, which encodes for the receptor for thrombopoietin. Blood 103:4198–4200

Druker BJ et al (2001) Efficacy and safety of a specific inhibitor of the BCR-ABL tyrosine kinase in chronic myeloid leukemia. N Engl J Med 344:1031–1037

Dusa A et al (2008) Substitution of pseudokinase domain residue Val-617 by large non-polar amino acids causes activation of JAK2. J Biol Chem 283:12941–12948

Ernst T et al (2010) Inactivating mutations of the histone methyltransferase gene EZH2 in myeloid disorders. Nat Genet 42:722–726

Figueroa ME et al (2010) Leukemic IDH1 and IDH2 mutations result in a hypermethylation phenotype, disrupt TET2 function, and impair hematopoietic differentiation. Cancer Cell 18:553–567

Fisher CL et al (2010) Additional sex combs-like 1 belongs to the enhancer of trithorax and polycomb group and genetically interacts with Cbx2 in mice. Dev Biol 337:9–15

Flex E et al (2008) Somatically acquired JAK1 mutations in adult acute lymphoblastic leukemia. J Exp Med 205:751–758

Gao SP et al (2007) Mutations in the EGFR kinase domain mediate STAT3 activation via IL-6 production in human lung adenocarcinomas. J Clin Invest 117:3846–3856

Gelsi-Boyer V et al (2009) Mutations of polycomb-associated gene ASXL1 in myelodysplastic syndromes and chronic myelomonocytic leukaemia. Br J Haematol 145:788–800

Gross S et al (2010) Cancer-associated metabolite 2-hydroxyglutarate accumulates in acute myelogenous leukemia with isocitrate dehydrogenase 1 and 2 mutations. J Exp Med 207:339–344

Harpur AG, Andres AC, Ziemiecki A, Aston RR, Wilks AF (1992) JAK2, a third member of the JAK family of protein tyrosine kinases. Oncogene 7:1347–1353

Hedvat M et al (2009) The JAK2 inhibitor AZD1480 potently blocks Stat3 signaling and oncogenesis in solid tumors. Cancer Cell 16:487–497

Hexner EO et al (2008) Lestaurtinib (CEP701) is a JAK2 inhibitor that suppresses JAK2/STAT5 signaling and the proliferation of primary erythroid cells from patients with myeloproliferative disorders. Blood 111:5663–5671

James C et al (2005) A unique clonal JAK2 mutation leading to constitutive signalling causes polycythaemia vera. Nature 434:1144–1148

Jones AV et al (2009) JAK2 haplotype is a major risk factor for the development of myeloproliferative neoplasms. Nat Genet 41:446–449

Kilpivaara O et al (2009) A germline JAK2 SNP is associated with predisposition to the development of JAK2(V617F)-positive myeloproliferative neoplasms. Nat Genet 41:455–459

Ko M et al (2010) Impaired hydroxylation of 5-methylcytosine in myeloid cancers with mutant TET2. Nature 468:839–843

Koppikar P et al (2010) Efficacy of the JAK2 inhibitor INCB16562 in a murine model of MPLW515L-induced thrombocytosis and myelofibrosis. Blood 115(14):2919–2927

Kralovics R, Guan Y, Prchal JT (2002) Acquired uniparental disomy of chromosome 9p is a frequent stem cell defect in polycythemia vera. Exp Hematol 30:229–236

Kralovics R et al (2005) A gain-of-function mutation of JAK2 in myeloproliferative disorders. N Engl J Med 352:1779–1790

Lacout C et al (2006) JAK2V617F expression in murine hematopoietic cells leads to MPD mimicking human PV with secondary myelofibrosis. Blood 108:1652–1660

Landgren O et al (2008) Increased risks of polycythemia vera, essential thrombocythemia, and myelofibrosis among 24, 577 first-degree relatives of 11, 039 patients with myeloproliferative neoplasms in Sweden. Blood 112:2199–2204

Langemeijer SM et al (2009) Acquired mutations in TET2 are common in myelodysplastic syndromes. Nat Genet 41:838–842

Levine RL et al (2005) Activating mutation in the tyrosine kinase JAK2 in polycythemia vera, essential thrombocythemia, and myeloid metaplasia with myelofibrosis. Cancer Cell 7:387–397

Ley TJ et al (2010) DNMT3A mutations in acute myeloid leukemia. N Engl J Med 363:2424–2433

Li J et al (2010) JAK2 V617F impairs hematopoietic stem cell function in a conditional knock-in mouse model of JAK2 V617F-positive essential thrombocythemia. Blood 30(24):5741–5751

Lucet IS et al (2006) The structural basis of janus kinase 2 inhibition by a potent and specific pan-janus kinase inhibitor. Blood 107:176–183

Marcucci G et al (2010) IDH1 and IDH2 gene mutations identify novel molecular subsets within de novo cytogenetically normal acute myeloid leukemia: a cancer and leukemia group B study. J Clin Oncol 28:2348–2355

Mardis ER et al (2009) Recurring mutations found by sequencing an acute myeloid leukemia genome. N Engl J Med 361:1058–1066

Marty C et al (2010) Myeloproliferative neoplasm induced by constitutive expression of JAK2V617F in knock-in mice. Blood 116:783–787

Marubayashi S et al (2010) HSP90 is a therapeutic target in JAK2-dependent myeloproliferative neoplasms in mice and humans. J Clin Invest 120:3578–3593

Mesa RA et al (2005) Leukemic transformation in myelofibrosis with myeloid metaplasia: a single-institution experience with 91 cases. Blood 105:973–977

Moran-Crusio K et al (2011) Tet2 loss leads to increased hematopoietic stem cell self-renewal and myeloid transformation. Cancer Cell 20(1):11–24

Mullally A et al (2010) Physiological JAK2V617F expression causes a lethal myeloproliferative neoplasm with differential effects on hematopoietic stem and progenitor cells. Cancer Cell 17:584–596

Mullighan CG et al (2009) JAK mutations in high-risk childhood acute lymphoblastic leukemia. Proc Natl Acad Sci USA 106:9414–9418

Nikoloski G et al (2010) Somatic mutations of the histone methyltransferase gene EZH2 in myelodysplastic syndromes. Nat Genet 42:665–667

Oh ST et al (2010) Novel mutations in the inhibitory adaptor protein LNK drive JAK-STAT signaling in patients with myeloproliferative neoplasms. Blood 116:988–992

Olcaydu D et al (2009) A common JAK2 haplotype confers susceptibility to myeloproliferative neoplasms. Nat Genet 41:450–454

Pardanani AD et al (2006) MPL515 mutations in myeloproliferative and other myeloid disorders: a study of 1,182 patients. Blood 108:3472–3476

Pardanani A et al (2007) TG101209, a small molecule JAK2-selective kinase inhibitor potently inhibits myeloproliferative disorder-associated JAK2V617F and MPLW515L/K mutations. Leukemia 21:1658–1668

Pardanani A et al (2011) Safety and efficacy of TG101348, a selective JAK2 inhibitor, in myelofibrosis. J Clin Oncol 29(7):789–796

Parganas E et al (1998) JAK2 is essential for signaling through a variety of cytokine receptors. Cell 93:385–395

Pikman Y et al (2006) MPLW515L is a novel somatic activating mutation in myelofibrosis with myeloid metaplasia. PLoS Med 3:e270

Quivoron C et al (2011) TET2 inactivation results in pleiotropic hematopoietic abnormalities in mouse and is a recurrent event during human lymphomagenesis. Cancer Cell 19(6):805–813

Rebouissou S et al (2009) Frequent in-frame somatic deletions activate gp130 in inflammatory hepatocellular tumours. Nature 457:200–204

Saharinen P, Silvennoinen O (2002) The pseudokinase domain is required for suppression of basal activity of JAK2 and JAK3 tyrosine kinases and for cytokine-inducible activation of signal transduction. J Biol Chem 277:47954–47963

Scott LM, Scott MA, Campbell PJ, Green AR (2006) Progenitors homozygous for the V617F mutation occur in most patients with polycythemia vera, but not essential thrombocythemia. Blood 108:2435–2437

Scott LM et al (2007) JAK2 exon 12 mutations in polycythemia vera and idiopathic erythrocytosis. N Engl J Med 356:459–468

Shochat C et al (2011) Gain-of-function mutations in interleukin-7 receptor-alpha (IL7R) in childhood acute lymphoblastic leukemias. J Exp Med 208:901–908

Tahiliani M et al (2009) Conversion of 5-methylcytosine to 5-hydroxymethylcytosine in mammalian DNA by MLL partner TET1. Science 324:930–935

Theocharides A et al (2007) Leukemic blasts in transformed JAK2–V617F-positive myeloproliferative disorders are frequently negative for the JAK2–V617F mutation. Blood 110:375–379

Tiedt R et al (2008) Ratio of mutant JAK2–V617F to wild-type JAK2 determines the MPD phenotypes in transgenic mice. Blood 111:3931–3940

Tomasson MH et al (2008) Somatic mutations and germline sequence variants in the expressed tyrosine kinase genes of patients with de novo acute myeloid leukemia. Blood 111:4797–4808

Verstovsek S et al (2010) Safety and efficacy of INCB018424, a JAK1 and JAK2 inhibitor, in myelofibrosis. N Engl J Med 363:1117–1127

Wang Y et al (2009) Cotreatment with panobinostat and JAK2 inhibitor TG101209 attenuates JAK2V617F levels and signaling and exerts synergistic cytotoxic effects against human myeloproliferative neoplastic cells. Blood 114:5024–5033

Ward PS et al (2010) The common feature of leukemia-associated IDH1 and IDH2 mutations is a neomorphic enzyme activity converting alpha-ketoglutarate to 2-hydroxyglutarate. Cancer Cell 17:225–234

Wernig G et al (2006) Expression of JAK2V617F causes a polycythemia vera-like disease with associated myelofibrosis in a murine bone marrow transplant model. Blood 107:4274–4281

Wernig G et al (2008) Efficacy of TG101348, a selective JAK2 inhibitor, in treatment of a murine model of JAK2V617F-induced polycythemia vera. Cancer Cell 13:311–320

Witthuhn BA et al (1993) JAK2 associates with the erythropoietin receptor and is tyrosine phosphorylated and activated following stimulation with erythropoietin. Cell 74:227–236

Xing S et al (2008) Transgenic expression of JAK2V617F causes myeloproliferative disorders in mice. Blood 111:5109–5117

Yan XJ et al (2011) Exome sequencing identifies somatic mutations of DNA methyltransferase gene DNMT3A in acute monocytic leukemia. Nat Genet 43(4):309–315

Yoda A et al (2009) Functional screening identifies CRLF2 in precursor B-cell acute lymphoblastic leukemia. Proc Natl Acad Sci USA 107(1):252–257

Zaleskas VM et al (2006) Molecular pathogenesis and therapy of polycythemia induced in mice by JAK2 V617F. PLoS ONE 1:e18

Zhao R et al (2005) Identification of an acquired JAK2 mutation in polycythemia vera. J Biol Chem 280:22788–22792

Will Kinase Inhibitors Make it as Glioblastoma Drugs?

Ingo K. Mellinghoff, Nikolaus Schultz, Paul S. Mischel
and Timothy F. Cloughesy

Abstract Kinase inhibitors have emerged as effective cancer therapeutics in a variety of human cancers. Glioblastoma (GBM), the most common malignant brain tumor in adults, represents a compelling disease for kinase inhibitor therapy because the majority of these tumors harbor genetic alterations that result in aberrant activation of growth factor signaling pathways. Attempts to target the Ras—Phosphatidylinositol 3-kinase (PI3K)—mammalian Target of Rapamycin (mTOR) axis in GBM with first generation receptor tyrosine kinase (RTK) inhibitors and rapalogs have been disappointing. However, there is reason for renewed optimism given the now very detailed knowledge of the cancer genome in GBM and a wealth of novel compounds entering the clinic, including next generation RTK inhibitors, class I PI3K inhibitors, mTOR kinase inhibitors (TORKinibs), and dual PI3(K)/mTOR inhibitors. This chapter reviews common

---

I. K. Mellinghoff (✉)
Human Oncology and Pathogenesis Program, Department and Neurology,
Memorial Sloan-Kettering Cancer Center, New York, NY, USA
e-mail: mellingi@mskcc.org

N. Schultz
Computational Biology Program, Memorial Sloan-Kettering Cancer Center,
New York, NY, USA

P. S. Mischel
Department of Pathology, University of California Los Angeles,
Los Angeles, CA, USA

T. F. Cloughesy
Department of Neurology, University of California Los Angeles,
Los Angeles, CA, USA

Current Topics in Microbiology and Immunology (2012) 355: 135–169
DOI: 10.1007/82_2011_178
© Springer-Verlag Berlin Heidelberg 2011
Published Online: 21 October 2011

genetic alterations in growth factor signaling pathways in GBM, their validation as therapeutic targets in this disease, and strategies for future clinical development of kinase inhibitors for high grade glioma.

Contents

1	Introduction	136
2	Mutations in Growth Factor Receptors	138
	2.1 Epidermal Growth Factor Receptor (EGFR)	138
	2.2 Platelet-Derived Growth Factor Receptor (PDGFR)	141
	2.3 MET Tyrosine Kinase Receptor	142
3	Mutations in the Ras-Raf Axis	142
	3.1 Mutations in KRAS, NRAS, HRAS	142
	3.2 Mutations in NF1	143
	3.3 Mutations in BRAF	143
4	Mutations in PI3K and PTEN	144
	4.1 Mutations in PIK3CA	146
	4.2 Mutations in PIK3R1	147
	4.3 Mutations in PTEN	147
5	Experience with First-Generation RTK Inhibitors	148
6	Clinical Experience with Rapalogs	150
7	New Approaches to Target the PI(3)K-mTOR Axis	151
8	Leveraging the Cancer Genome Atlas for Clinical Drug Development	152
9	Future Perspective	153
	References	155

1 Introduction

Gliomas represent a spectrum of primary brain tumors which are classified by the World Health Organization (WHO) into low grade and high grade tumors based on the degree of tumor cell proliferation, cellular atypia, and microvascular proliferation (Louis et al. 2007). The median survival for patients with GBM has remained below 2 years despite multimodality therapy, including surgery, radiation, chemotherapy (Stupp et al. 2005), and most recently the anti-VEGF antibody bevacizumab (Friedman et al. 2009; Kreisl et al. 2009a). The term "low-grade" glioma (WHO grade II) refers to a group of tumors with histopathologically less aggressive features. However, many patients with these tumors also succumb to their disease within 3–10 years due to tumor "transformation" to an anaplastic glioma (WHO grade III) or GBM (WHO grade IV). GBMs that have evolved from a clinically overt, low-grade precursor lesion are referred to as "secondary" GBMs in contrast to de novo or "primary" GBMs. Primary and secondary GBMs differ substantially in their molecular pathogenesis (Lai et al. 2011; Ohgaki and Kleihues 2007).

The histopathological appearance of GBM is particularly diverse and has earned it the moniker "multi-forme" (multiformis [Latin]: many shapes) (Louis

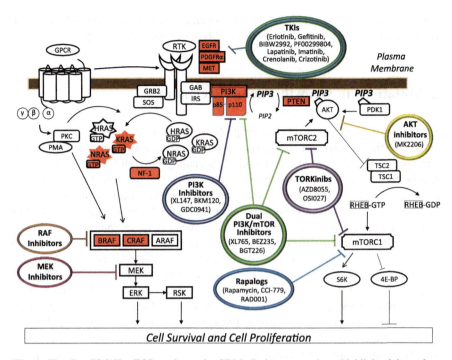

Fig. 1 The Ras-PI(3)K-mTOR pathway in GBM. Pathway members highlighted in *red* are mutated in human GBM tumor samples. Pathway inhibitors that have been or will be explored as therapeutics for GBM are indicated

et al. 2007). This morphological heterogeneity of GBM is often viewed as a reflection of the exceptional genetic heterogeneity of this cancer. Recent genomic studies provide a perhaps more encouraging view of GBM with a finite number of highly recurrent gene copy number alterations (Beroukhim et al. 2009) and missense mutations (TCGA 2005; Parsons et al. 2008). Genome wide RNA expression profiling identifies distinct disease subgroups (Phillips et al. 2006) each of which is enriched for particular mutations (Verhaak et al. 2010).

One key result of the extensive profiling of human glioma samples (Beroukhim et al. 2007; Kotliarov et al. 2006; McLendon et al. 2008; Misra et al. 2005; Parsons et al. 2008) is the *re-*appreciation that nearly all human GBMs harbor genetic alterations in three "core" pathways, namely the RTK/RAS/PI3K signaling axis, the p53-ARF-MDM2/MDM4 pathway, and the RB-CDK4-INK4A pathway. Many of the genetic lesions most consistently found in human tumors have been shown to cooperate in glioma formation in mice (Chow et al. 2011; Reilly et al. 2000; Zheng et al. 2008; Zhu et al. 2005a) and represent the currently most "actionable" drug targets (Fig. 1). This chapter highlights genetic alterations in growth factor signaling pathways in GBM and discusses new directions to develop kinase inhibitors as glioma therapeutics. Our comments largely focus on the adult patient population as genetic alterations (Bax et al. 2010; Paugh et al. 2010) and considerations regarding clinical drug development differ considerably for pediatric glioma patients.

2 Mutations in Growth Factor Receptors

Receptor tyrosine kinases (RTKs) are proteins which transmit signals from the cell surface to the nucleus and participate in most fundamental aspects of cell growth, survival, differentiation, and metabolism. Signaling through RTKs is initiated by ligand binding and terminated by receptor internalization from the cell surface, dissociation of the receptor-ligand complex, receptor dephosphorylation, and degradation of the receptor protein (Lemmon and Schlessinger 2010). The RTK family of proteins includes the epidermal growth factor receptor family (EGFR, HER2, ERBB3, and ERBB4), the platelet-derived growth factor receptor family (PDGFR-α and PDGFR-β), the MET receptor tyrosine kinase, the Vascular-Endothelial Growth Factor Receptor family (VEGFR1/FLT1, VEGFR2/KDR/FLK1, and VEGFR3/FLT4), and others. Many human cancers harbor mutations in RTKs which relieve auto-inhibitory constraints on the kinase activity or impair the downregulation of the ligand-activated receptor protein (Blume-Jensen and Hunter 2001). Within the RTK family, mutations in the genes encoding EGFR, PDGFR-α, and MET are the most common in high grade gliomas (Table 1 and Fig. 2).

2.1 Epidermal Growth Factor Receptor (EGFR)

Genetic alterations that result in uncontrolled EGFR kinase activity were amongst the first to be associated with human cancer (Gschwind et al. 2004). A number of alterations involving the *EGFR* gene have been described in GBM. These include: (a) *EGFR* gene amplification in $\sim 40\%$ of primary GBMs (Libermann et al. 1985; Wong et al. 1987); extra gene copies reside on double-minutes and are easily detected by fluorescence-in situ hybridization (FISH) (Jansen et al. 2010); (b) In-frame deletions affecting the 5' end of the *EGFR* gene (Malden et al. 1988; Yamazaki et al. 1988); these are found mostly, but not exclusively, in tumors with *EGFR* gene amplification. The most common EGFR variant IIII (or EGFRvIII) is a deletion of exons 2–7, resulting in an 801 amino acid in-frame deletion within the EGFR extracellular domain (Sugawa et al. 1990). The EGFRvIII mutant does not bind the ligands EGF or TGF-α, but is constitutively active (Ekstrand et al. 1994); (c) truncations affecting the C-terminus of the EGFR protein. These alterations are seen in 15–25% of high grade gliomas with *EGFR* gene amplification (Ekstrand et al. 1992; Eley et al. 1998; Frederick et al. 2000). The EGFR C-terminus encodes receptor portions that are required for ligand-induced receptor internalization (Chen et al. 1989; Decker et al. 1992) and (d) missense mutations in the *EGFR* extracellular domain in about 10% of primary GBMs (Lee et al. 2006b).

Will Kinase Inhibitors Make it as Glioblastoma Drugs? 139

Table 1 Mutations in Growth Factor Signaling Pathways in GBM (adult patients)

Gene	Alteration	Frequency in GBM %
EGFR	Amplification	35–40
	EGFR-variant III (EGFRvIII)	~20
	Nonsynonymous Mutations	10–15
	other in-frame deletions/truncations	5–10
PDGFRA	Amplification	5–15
	delta-8,9 truncation	2–5
	Nonsynonymous Mutations	<2
MET	Amplification	2–5
	Nonsynonymous Mutations	<2
KRAS	Nonsynonymous Mutations	<2
NRAS	Nonsynonymous Mutations	<2
NF1	Homozygous Deletion	2–5
	Hemizygous Deletion	5–10
	Nonsynonymous Mutations	~15
BRAF	V600E BRAF	<2 (2–5 in PA)
	KIAA1549-BRAF fusions	n.d. (60–70 in PA)
	p.A598_T599insT BRAF	n.d. (1–3 in PA)
	FAM131B-BRAF fusion	n.d. (1–3 in PA)
CRAF	SRGAP3-CRAF fusion	n.d. (1–3 in PA)
PIK3CA	Nonsynonymous Mutations	5–10
	Amplification	~2
PIK3R1	Nonsynonymous Mutations	5–10
PTEN	Homozygous Deletion	5–10
	Hemizygous Deletion	~70
	Nonsynonymous Mutations	15–25

Please see text for references
n.d not detected, *PA* Pilocytic Astrocytoma

Most EGFR alterations found in human GBM have been shown to represent gain-of-function events. Expression of a truncated EGF receptor lacking the extracellular ligand binding domain induces transformation of immortalized rodent fibroblasts (Haley et al. 1989). Expression of the EGFRvIII mutant enhances the tumorigenicity of GBM cells (Nishikawa et al. 1994) and is able to transform mouse NIH-3T3 fibroblasts in the absence of ligand (Batra et al. 1995). In mice, low grade oligodendrogliomas develop when the retroviral oncogene *v-erb-B*, encoding a truncated version of EGFR (Schatzman et al. 1986), is expressed under the control of the $S100\beta$ promoter (Weiss et al. 2003). Expression of the EGFRvIII mutant is not sufficient to induce glioma formation in mice but cooperates with mutant *H-RAS* or inactivation of *CDKN2A* in glioma formation (Bachoo et al. 2002; Ding et al. 2003; Holland et al. 1998; Zhu et al. 2009). A C-terminal EGFR truncation mutant has been shown to confer anchorage-independent growth and tumorigenicity to NIH-3T3 cells (Wells et al. 1990; Masui et al. 1991). Several of the extracellular *EGFR* missense mutations (R108K, T263P, A289V, G598V) have been shown to transform NIH3T3 cells

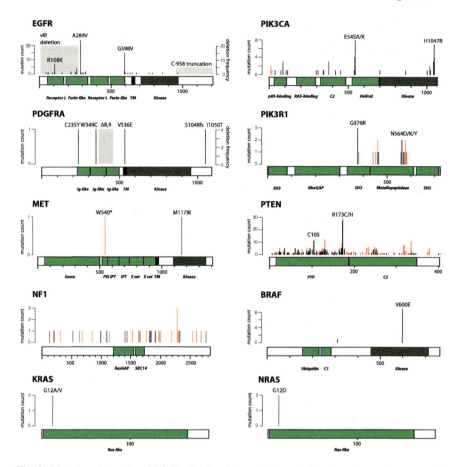

Fig. 2 Mutations in the Ras-PI(3)K-mTOR axis in WHO grade IV astrocytoma. Shown are all confirmed somatic or previously reported mutations that have been listed in COSMIC v54 under astrocytoma grade IV. The y-axis indicates the number of times a particular mutant has been observed in a primary tumor sample, xenograft tumor, or cell line. Missense mutations are shown in *black*; nonsense and frameshift mutations as well as small in-frame insertions and deletions are shown in *red*. Recurrent deletions/truncations in the coding regions of *EGFR* and *PDGFRA* are indicated in shaded *gray* and their estimated frequency is shown as percent of all GBMs (*right y*-axis)

and confer tumorigenicity (Lee et al. 2006b). In contrast to the *EGFR* mutants described above, overexpression of wild-type EGFR does not transform mouse NIH3T3 in the absence of exogenous EGF (Di Fiore et al. 1987). In mice, overexpression of wild-type EGFR induces glioma formation only in the presence of *CDKN2A* deletion and, even then, with very low efficiency (Zhu et al. 2009).

The role of mutant EGFR for tumor maintenance needs to be defined more extensively, but current data suggests that at least a subset of *EGFR* mutant gliomas require EGFR signals for maintenance of the malignant phenotype (Eller et al. 2002; Martens et al. 2008; Sarkaria et al. 2007).

2.2 Platelet-Derived Growth Factor Receptor (PDGFR)

Platelet-derived growth factor (PDGF) is a potent mitogen for glia-derived cells (Richardson et al. 1988) and consists of five dimeric isoforms. These include homodimers of A-, B-, C-, and D-polypeptide chains (i.e., PDGF-AA, -BB, -CC, and –DD) and a PDGF-AB heterodimer. PDGF dimers bind to the RTKs PDGFR-α and PDGFR-β and activate the receptors by inducing receptor dimerization. Different types of receptor dimers are induced by different ligands: A-, B-, and C-chains of PDGF bind to PDGFR-α, whereas B-and D-chains bind to PDGFR-β. PDGF ligands and receptors are frequently co-expressed in human gliomas, perhaps reflecting the presence of an autocrine signaling loop (Hermanson et al. 1992; Lokker et al. 2002).

Mutations in genes encoding PDGF ligands or receptors have been found in a variety of human cancers, including Dermatofibrosarcoma Protuberans (*PDGFB*), Chronic Myelomonocytic Leukemia (*PDGFR-β*), and Gastrointestinal Stromal Tumors (*PDGFR-α*). Many of these cancers respond to PDGFR kinase inhibitors such as imatinib (Ostman and Heldin 2007). Kumabe et al. first reported amplification of the *PDGFR-α* gene locus in 1/9 (11%) human gliomas. Interestingly, the one case with *PDGFR-α* gene amplification also harbored an in-frame deletion of exons 8 and 9 of *PDGFR-α* (Kumabe et al. 1992). Subsequent studies reported *PDGFR-α* gene amplification in 8–11% of primary human GBMs (Beroukhim et al. 2009; Fleming et al. 1992). Functional characterization of the *PDGFR-α-Δ8,9* mutant by Peter Dirk's laboratory showed that the 243 base pairs deletion results in a constitutively active receptor with greater transforming and tumorigenic ability than wild-type PDGFR-α (Clarke and Dirks 2003). Other *PDGFR-α* mutations reported in GBM include a two basepair deletion in exon 23, resulting in a truncation of the C-terminus of the receptor (Rand et al. 2005) and an oncogenic gene fusion between the $5'$ end of the *kinase insert domain receptor* (*KDR*) and the kinase domain and $3'$ portion of *PDGFR-α* (Ozawa et al. 2010) (Table 1).

The contribution of PDGF signaling toward glioma formation in mice has been well documented. Injection of a PDGF-B chain-encoding retrovirus into the brain of newborn C57B16 mice induced brain tumor formation in 40% of animals (Uhrbom et al. 1998). This result has been confirmed by somatic cell type-specific gene transfer experiments in which targeted expression of PDGF-B in nestin-expressing neural progenitors or GFAP-expressing astrocytes induced gliomas in 60 and 40% of mice, respectively (Dai et al. 2001). Retroviral infection of adult white matter progenitor cells similarly resulted in glioma formation (Assanah et al. 2006) and expression of doxycycline-regulated PDGF-B in the spinal cord produced mixed oligoastrocytomas (Hitoshi et al. 2008).

2.3 MET Tyrosine Kinase Receptor

The MET tyrosine kinase is the cell surface receptor for hepatocyte growth factor (HGF). Aberrant activation of MET in human cancers results from amplification of the *MET* gene (e.g., gastric/esophageal carcinoma, medulloblastoma), missense mutations in the *MET* gene (e.g., papillary renal cancer), and transcriptional upregulation of MET and its ligand HGF (Comoglio et al. 2008; Koochekpour et al. 1997). While missense mutations in *MET* are rare in human GBM, focal amplification of the *MET* gene occurs in about 5% of primary human GBMs (Beroukhim et al. 2009). Amplification of MET has been linked with increased sensitivity to MET kinase inhibition in a panel of human cancer cell lines (McDermott et al. 2007) and radiographic regression of a *MET*-amplified GBM was recently reported in a patient treated with the MET/ALK kinase inhibitor crizotinib (PF-02341066) (Chi et al. 2011).

3 Mutations in the Ras-Raf Axis

The family of RAS GTPases (HRAS, NRAS, and KRAS) are proteins which cycle between a GTP-bound active form and a GDP-bound inactive form. Guanine nucleotide exchange factors (GEFs) promote formation of GTP-bound RAS, whereas GTPase-activating proteins (GAPs) stimulate the hydrolysis of GTP on RAS. The first critical effector of Ras to be identified in mammalian cells was the RAF-MEK-ERK pathway. Serine/threonine kinases of the RAF family (C-Raf or Raf-1, A-Raf, and B-Raf) bind to RAS-GTP and then relocalize to the plasma membrane where they are phosphorylated. Once activated, they phosphorylate and activate mitogen-activated protein kinase kinase (MAPKK or MEK) that, in turn, phosphorylates and activates extracellular signal-regulated kinases 1 and 2 (ERK1/2) (Castellano and Downward 2011; Shaw and Cantley 2006). The RAS-RAF axis is activated in glioma through several mechanisms, including mutations in *NRAS* and *KRAS*, inactivating mutations in the neurofibromatosis gene (*NF1*), and mutations involving *BRAF* and *CRAF* (Table 1 and Fig. 2).

3.1 Mutations in KRAS, NRAS, HRAS

Mutations in *KRAS*, and *NRAS* are rare in human gliomas and particularly rare in WHO grade III and IV gliomas in adult patients. Sequencing of 94 high grade gliomas for mutations in *NRAS* (entire coding region), *KRAS* (entire coding region) and the first exon of *HRAS* identified 2 cases (2/94 = 2%) with *G12D-NRAS* mutation (Knobbe et al. 2004). Another study examined 93 gliomas for "hotspot" mutations in *HRAS* (exon 2/3), *KRAS* (exon 2/3), and *NRAS* (exon 2/3) and reported one *NRAS* mutation (G10E-*NRAS*) (Jeuken et al. 2007). Mutations in *KRAS* have been reported in 5–10% of pediatric gliomas (Cin et al. 2011; Forshew et al. 2009; Janzarik et al. 2007; Maltzman et al. 1997; Schiffman et al. 2010; Sharma et al. 2005). Based on the effects of mutant *RAS* on glioma formation and maintenance in genetically engineered mouse models (de Vries et al. 2010; Ding et al. 2001; Holland et al. 2000; Holmen and Williams 2005; Marumoto et al. 2009; Uhrbom et al. 2002), Ras mutations are likely relevant for the biology and drug response of the (rare) gliomas in which they are found.

3.2 Mutations in NF1

Neurofibromin, the protein product of the neurofibromatosis gene (*NF1*) gene, is a $p21^{ras}$-GTPase activating protein (RasGAP) which critically regulates Ras signal output (Buday and Downward 2008; Shaw and Cantley 2006). Somatic missense mutations in the NF1 gene were first reported in astrocytoma many years ago (Li et al. 1992; Thiel et al. 1995). More complete sequencing of the *NF1* coding sequence in a larger number of tumors has uncovered missense mutations in *NF1* in ~15% of GBM patients (McLendon et al. 2008; Parsons et al. 2008). Other mechanisms of *NF1* silencing in GBM include heterozygous or homozygous *NF1* copy loss and posttranslational modifications that result in destabilization of the NF1 protein (McGillicuddy et al. 2009). There is strong evidence for a role of NF1 in gliomagenesis. Patients with neurofibromatosis type I, a genetic disorder caused by germline mutations in *NF1*, are at increased risk to develop high grade gliomas (Listernick et al. 1999; Rodriguez et al. 2008) and these gliomas often show inactivation of the second NF1 allele (Gutmann et al. 2003). Mice with targeted disruption of the *NF1* locus develop astrocytosis and *NF1* inactivation cooperates with *TP53* inactivation and *PTEN* inactivation to produce high grade gliomas with rapid onset and high penetrance (Alcantara Llaguno et al. 2009; Bajenaru et al. 2003; Reilly et al. 2000; Zhu et al. 2005a, b).

3.3 Mutations in BRAF

The frequency and type of *BRAF* alterations in glioma varies substantially between adults and children and between distinct glioma subtypes. *V600E-BRAF* or *V600M-BRAF* mutations are rare in WHO grade III/IV gliomas in adults, ranging from 0 to 3% in most studies (Basto et al. 2005; El-Habr et al. 2010; Hagemann et al. 2009; Jeuken et al. 2007; Knobbe et al. 2004; Schindler et al. 2011). The frequency of *V600E-BRAF* mutations is substantially higher in pediatric gliomas. One series reported *V600E-BRAF* in 23% (7/31) of WHO grade II–IV pediatric astrocytomas (Schiffman et al. 2010); another series observed *V600E-BRAF* mutations in 9% (4/42) of WHO grade III/IV pediatric gliomas (Schindler et al. 2011). *V600E BRAF* mutations are particularly common in the two glioma subtypes *pleomorphic xanthoastrocytoma* (60–70%) and *gangliogliomas* (20–60%) (Dougherty et al. 2010; MacConaill et al. 2009; Schindler et al. 2011).

The majority (50–70%) of *pilocytic astrocytomas (PAs)*, the most common central nervous system tumor in children, show low-level copy gain at the *BRAF* gene locus at 7q34 (Bar et al. 2008; Deshmukh et al. 2008; Pfister et al. 2008). Detailed characterization of this genomic alteration in 44 human PAs by Peter Collins' group uncovered a tandem duplication that produces fusion proteins between *KIAA1549* and *BRAF* in 66% (29/44) of pilocytic astrocytomas. The most common event fuses *KIAA1549* exon 16 and *BRAF* exon 9. KIAA1549-BRAF fusions generate proteins that lack the BRAF autoregulatory domain and exhibit enhanced BRAF kinase activity (Jones et al. 2008). Further examination of PAs without 7q34 duplication identified alternative mechanisms for activation of the RAF-MEK axis. These included *NF1* inactivation (family history of neurofibromatosis type I) (3/44 cases), *V600E BRAF* mutation (2/44 cases), a tandem duplication at 3p25 fusing *SLIT-ROBO Rho GTPase Activating Protein 3 (SRGAP3)* and *CRAF/RAF1* (1/44 cases), and a 3 bp insertion at codon 598 in *BRAF* (1/44 cases). The *SRGAP3-RAF1* fusion protein and the *p.A598_T599insT BRAF* mutant both increased the kinase activity of RAF1 and BRAF, respectively. Altogether, 82% (36/44) of pilocytic astrocytomas in this series showed mutational activation of the RAS/RAF axis (Jones et al. 2008, 2009).

Profiling of human pilocytic astrocytomas by other groups confirmed near-universal activation of the RAS/RAF/MEK signaling axis in this disease through *KIAA1549-BRAF* fusions ($\sim$70%), *V600E BRAF* mutations (5–10%), *BRAF* codon 598 insertions (1–3%), *NF1* inactivation (1–3%), *KRAS* mutations (1–3%), the *SRGAP3-RAF1* fusion (1–3%), and a recently described fusion involving *BRAF* and *Family with sequence similarity 131, member B (FAM131B)* (2%) (Cin et al. 2011; Eisenhardt et al. 2010; Forshew et al. 2009; Jacob et al. 2009; Pfister et al. 2008; Schindler et al. 2011; Sievert et al. 2009; Yu et al. 2009). Functional studies support a role of glioma-related *BRAF* mutants and activated Raf-1 in transformation and gliomagenesis, in particular in combination with *CDKN2A* inactivation (Gronych et al. 2011; Jones et al. 2008, 2009; Lyustikman et al. 2008; Robinson et al. 2010, 2011).

4 Mutations in PI3K and PTEN

Phosphatidyloinositide 3-kinases (PI3K) belong to a family of lipid kinases that phosphorylate the 3-hydroxyl group of the inositol ring of phosphatidylinositol (PtdIns), PtdIns4P, and PtdIns $(4, 5)P_2$. PI3Ks have been assigned to different classes based on substrate preference and structural features. Class I PI(3)Ks are activated by receptor tyrosine kinases and G-protein coupled receptors and use PtdIns$(4, 5)P_2$ as substrate to generate phosphoinositide 3,4,5 trisphosphate (PIP$_3$). Other classes are class II and class II PI3Ks (Fig. 3a) and the family of

Will Kinase Inhibitors Make it as Glioblastoma Drugs?

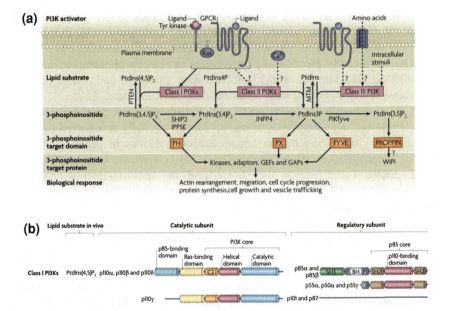

Fig. 3 The 3-phosphoinositide lipid network. (a) Following activation by upstream agonists, phosphoinositide 3-kinases (PI3Ks) generate phosphatidylinositol-3,4,5-trisphosphate (PtdIns(3,4,5)P3), PtdIns-3,4-bisphosphate (PtdIns(3,4)P2) and PtdIns-3-phosphate (PtdIns3P). These lipids interact with lipid binding domains in PI3K effector proteins and change their localization and/or activity. Lipid phosphatases degrade or interconvert 3-phosphoinositides. These include lipid phosphatases for PtdIns(3,4,5)P3, such as phosphatase and tensin homologue deleted on chromosome 10 (PTEN), inositol polyphosphate-5-phosphatase E (IPP5E), and SH2 domain-containing inositol 5-phosphatase type 2 (SHIP2). GAP, GTPase-activating protein; GEF, guanine nucleotide exchange factor; GPCR, G protein-coupled receptor. (b) Classification and domain structure of mammalian Class I PI3Ks. All PI3K catalytic subunits have a PI3K core structure consisting of a C2 domain, a helical domain and a catalytic domain. Class I PI3Ks exist in complex with a regulatory subunit, either a p85 isoform (for p110α, p110β and p110δ) or p101 or p87 (for p110γ). All p85 isoforms have two Src homology 2 (SH2) domains and are encoded by either PIK3R1 (which encodes p85α, p55α and p50α), PIK3R2 (which encodes p85β) and PIK3R3 (which encodes p55γ). Figure modified from (Vanhaesebroeck et al. 2010)

PI3K-related protein kinases (PIKKs) which include mammalian Target of Rapamycin (mTOR), ATM, ATR, DNA-PK, and hSMG1 (Vanhaesebroeck et al. 2010).

PI(3)Ks are composed of a catalytic subunit and a regulatory subunit (Fig. 3b). Catalytic subunits include p110α (encoded by *PIK3CA*), p110β (encoded by *PIK3CB*), p110γ (encoded by *PIK3CG*), and p110δ (encoded by *PIK3CD*). Regulatory subunits include p85α, p55α, and p50α (all encoded by *PIK3R1*), p85β (encoded by *PIK3R2*), p55γ (encoded by *PIK3R3*), p101 and p87. p110 subunits share a five-domain structure, which includes an N-terminal adaptor binding domain (ABD domain), a Ras binding domain (RBD domain), a C2 (Protein kinase C homology-2) domain, a helical domain, and a catalytic domain. All p85 isoforms (p85α, p55α, p50α, p85β, p55γ) have two Src homology domains 2 (SH2) domains and an intervening domain (iSH2) that binds to the adapter binding domain in p110 (Vanhaesebroeck et al. 2010). P85 isoforms provide at least three functions to p110 proteins: (i) they stabilize the intrinsically unstable p110 protein, (ii) they recruit p110 proteins to pTyr residues in receptor and adaptor molecules (through the SH2 domains of p85 isoforms) upon activation, and (iii) they restrain the kinase activity of p110 proteins in their un-activated state.

PI3K were first linked to cancer through the study of oncogenic viruses. Their critical role in the pathogenesis of human cancer was fully recognized following the discovery that many human tumors harbor mutations in genes whose gene products regulate levels of the lipid molecule PIP_3 (Shaw and Cantley 2006; Vogt et al. 2009). These include the phosphatase and tensin homolog deleted on chromosome 10 (*PTEN*) (Li et al. 1997; Steck et al. 1997), the regulatory subunit p85 (*PIK3R1*) (Philp et al. 2001), and the catalytic subunit p110α (*PIK3CA*) (Samuels et al. 2004), and *PIK3R2* (Cheung et al. 2011). Almost 100 mutations have been found throughout the *PIK3CA* coding region. The Ras binding domain (RBD) appears to be spared from mutations and mutation "hot-spots" include the p85-binding domain, the helical domain, and the kinase domain (Vanhaesebroeck et al. 2010; Vogt et al. 2009). Many studies have documented the biochemical effects and transforming ability of *PTEN*-inactivation (Salmena et al. 2008) and various *PIK3CA* (Vogt et al. 2009) and *PIK3R1* mutations (Huang et al. 2007; Jaiswal et al. 2009; Philp et al. 2001; Sun et al. 2010; Wu et al. 2009). Mutations have not been found in genes encoding other PI3K catalytic subunits (*PIK3CB*, *PIK3CG*, *PIK3CD*). In contrast to p110α, however, which only shows transforming ability it its mutant form, overexpression of wild-type p110β, p110γ, and p110δ can transform chicken fibroblasts (Kang et al. 2006) and these PI3K family members may represent critical oncogenic units in certain genetic contexts (Berenjeno and Vanhaesebroeck 2009). In GBM, mutations in the PI(3)K-mTOR axis are most frequently found in the genes encoding the catalytic and regulatory subunit of PI(3)K (*PIK3CA* and *PIK3R1*, respectively) and in *PTEN* (Table 1 and Fig. 2).

4.1 Mutations in PIK3CA

The initial discovery of *PIK3CA* mutations in cancer reported a mutation prevalence of 26.7% (4/15) for GBM (Samuels et al. 2004). Subsequent studies in larger numbers of tumors suggest that these mutations occur less frequently in primary GBMs. Sequencing of exons 9 and 20 of *PIK3CA* in a diverse panel of primary brain tumors found mutations in 5/105 (5%) GBMs, 3/21 (14%) anaplastic oligodendrogliomas (WHO grade III), 1/31 (3%) anaplastic astrocytomas (WHO grade III), 0/24 (0%) WHO grade II astrocytomas, 4/78 (5%) medulloblastomas, and 0/26 (0%) ependymomas (Broderick et al. 2004). Other studies screened the entire *PIK3CA* coding region and reported mutations in 0/30 (0%) (Mueller et al. 2005) and 5/70 (7%) GBMs (Hartmann et al. 2005). Direct sequencing of a large part of the *PIK3CA* coding sequence (exons 1, 2, 4, 5, 7, 9, 12, 13, 18, 20) in 38 primary human GBMs identified mutations in 3/14 (21%) pediatric and 4/24 (17%) adult GBMs (Gallia et al. 2006). Another study focused on exons 9 and 20 of *PIK3CA* and reported mutations in 5/107 (5%) de novo GBMs and in 1/32 (3%) secondary GBMs (Kita et al. 2007). Differences between studies in the reported frequency of *PIK3CA* mutations are likely due to a combination of factors, including the sensitivity of the mutation detection assay (single strand conformational polymorphism versus direct bidirectional sequencing), gene coverage (mutation hot-spots versus entire coding sequence), glioma subtype, sample size, and inclusion of cell lines.

Amplification of the *PIK3CA* gene locus was first reported as oncogenic event in ovarian cancer (Shayesteh et al. 1999) and later in other cancers. No evidence for PIK3CA gene copy gain (>5-fold) or RNA overexpression was found in an analysis of 145 primary brain tumors (including 50 GBMs and 35 WHO grade III gliomas) (Broderick et al. 2004). Using a slighty less stringent cutoff for *PIK3CA* gene copy gain (>3-fold), Kita et al. reported *PIK3CA* amplifications in 14/107 (13%) de novo and 3/32 (9%) secondary GBMs (Kita et al. 2007).

4.2 Mutations in PIK3R1

A truncating mutation in *PIK3R1* was first reported in a GBM in 2004 (Mizoguchi et al. 2004). More recent studies reported mutations in *PIK3R1* in $\sim 10\%$ of GBMs (McLendon et al. 2008; Parsons et al. 2008). These mutations clustered in the N-terminal SH2-domain and the inter-SH2 domain of the PIK3R1 gene, regions that interact with the C2 and helical domains of p110α. Detailed characterization of selected p85 mutants showed that they were unable to negatively regulate p110α, p110β, and p110δ activity, despite retaining their ability to bind and stabilize them (Huang et al. 2007; Jaiswal et al. 2009; Wu et al. 2009). Peter Vogt's group expressed the full panel of GBM p85 mutants (G376R, E439del, KS459delN, D560Y, DKRMNS560del, N564K, R574fs, T576del, W583del) in chicken fibroblasts. All mutants induced a transformed phenotype, retained the ability to interact with p110α, stabilized the endogenous p110α protein, and stimulated phosphorylation of Akt and 4EBP-1. Efficiencies of transformation varied between mutants and did not clearly correlate with their biochemical effects on Akt and 4EBP1 (Sun et al. 2010).

4.3 Mutations in PTEN

Allelic loss of chromosome 10 has long been known to be common in high grade human glioma (James et al. 1988). After the identification of PTEN as tumor suppressor on chromosome 10 (Li et al. 1997; Steck et al. 1997), missense mutations in *PTEN* were reported in 17/63 (27%) of GBMs (Liu et al. 1997). Examination of the entire *PTEN* coding sequence in 331 gliomas reported *PTEN* missense mutations in 20/142 (14%) GBMs; homozygous *PTEN* deletions were observed in 7/142 (5%) GBMs (Duerr et al. 1998). Another study reported *PTEN* point mutations and homozygous deletions in 32/110 (29%) and 11/110 (10%) of GBMs (Smith et al. 2001). Later studies reported *PTEN* mutations in 14 (Hartmann et al. 2005) to 24% (Ohgaki et al. 2004). PTEN expression is silenced in additional GBMs through promoter methylation, micro-RNAs, and posttranslational modifications.

Genetically engineered mouse models (GEMMs) support a prominent tumor suppressor function of PTEN during glioma progression. Loss of PTEN in various cell types within the brain does not result in tumorigenesis (Fraser et al. 2004; Groszer et al. 2001; Kwon et al. 2001). Inactivation of *PTEN* in glioma-prone mice, in which oncogenic ^{V12}*H-Ras* is expressed from the GFAP promoter, greatly accelerated malignant glioma progression (Wei et al. 2006). In the *NF1/p53* astrocytoma model, haploinsufficiency of *PTEN* accelerated formation of WHO grade III astrocytomas, whereas loss of *PTEN* heterozygosity coincided with progression into WHO grade IV tumors (Kwon et al. 2008). Combined deletion of *PTEN* and *TP53* in neural stem cells of the subventricular zone is sufficient to induce glioma formation (Jacques et al. 2010; Zheng et al. 2008). Combined inactivation of PTEN and TP53 in mature astrocytes in the adult brain induced high grade gliomas that showed striking similarity to human GBMs in terms of secondary gene copy number alterations and genome wide RNA expression changes (Chow et al. 2011).

5 Experience with First-Generation RTK Inhibitors

The success with first-generation EGFR kinase inhibitors (gefitinib, erlotinib) in lung cancer and the high frequency of oncogenic *EGFR* alterations in GBM ($\sim$40%) raised expectations that these agents will show activity against GBM. This expectation has largely not been fulfilled. While most studies reported individual patients with tumor regressions in response to erlotinib or gefitinib, the frequency of these response is substantially lower (<5%) than the frequency of oncogenic EGFR alterations in GBM (Mellinghoff et al. 2011). The experience with imatinib, an ATP-site competitive inhibitor of the PDGFR, KIT and ABL-kinases has been similarly disappointing. A Phase II study of imatinib in 112 patients with recurrent gliomas reported a partial response for only 5 patients (Raymond et al. 2008). The radiographic response rates for the subgroup of GBM patients was 3/51 (6%) in this study. In a Phase I/II study of the North American Brain Tumor Consortium 3/57 (5%) GBM patients showed partial radiographic responses and no responses were observed for other histologic subgroups (Wen et al. 2006).

In contrast to the landmark clinical trials with imatinib in chronic myeloid leukemia (Druker et al. 2001) and with the HER2 antibody trastuzumab in breast cancer (Slamon et al. 2001), clinical trials with first-generation EGFR and PDGFR kinase inhibitors in GBM were not enriched for patients whose tumors harbored mutations in *EGFR* and *PDGFR-α*, respectively. This lack of molecular preselection likely contributed to the disappointing results in the clinic. Studies to identify determinants of EGFR kinase inhibitor response in GBM have associated tumor regressions with the presence of oncogenic EGFR alterations (*EGFR* gene amplification or EGFRvIII) and expression of the PTEN tumor suppressor protein or low p-AKT levels (Haas-Kogan et al. 2005; Mellinghoff et al. 2005). Other studies have questioned the relationship between oncogenic EGFR and EGFR kinase inhibitor response in GBM (van den Bent et al. 2009). This discrepancy may, at least in part, be attributable to differences in the determination of EGFRvIII status in tumor tissue.

Several lines of evidence support that PTEN inactivation mediates EGFR kinase inhibitor resistance: (1) PTEN restoration sensitizes *EGFR* amplified/*PTEN* deleted cancer cells to cell death induction by EGFR kinase inhibitors (Bianco et al. 2003); (2) PTEN knockdown is sufficient to render *EGFR* mutant cancer cells resistant to cell death induction by EGFR kinase inhibitors (Vivanco et al. 2010); and (3) PTEN emerged as most consistent resistance factor from a shRNA library screen performed in breast cancer cells to identify mechanisms of resistance to trastuzumab (which targets the EGFR co-receptor HER2) (Berns et al. 2007), and (4) GBMs with intact PTEN expression showed enhanced responsiveness to combination therapy of erlotinib plus temozolomide (Prados et al. 2009).

How does PTEN status influence EGFR kinase inhibitor response? By dephosphorylation the second messenger PIP3, PTEN plays an important role in signal termination downstream of many RTKs. Even if one RTK is effectively inhibited, PTEN loss may allow the accumulation of sufficient PIP3 to activate PIP3 effector molecules, such as the serine-threonine kinase Akt. In other words, PTEN deficient cells may be able to better compensate for single RTK inhibition than cells with intact PTEN. This concept of redundant RTK activation is supported by the biochemical evidence for RTK coactivation in primary GBM tumor samples and the experimental observation that inhibition of multiple RTK, but not a single RTK, induces cell death in certain GBM lines (Stommel et al. 2007). We recently made the surprising discovery that PTEN inactivation raises EGFR protein levels and EGFR kinase activity by interfering with the CBL-mediated downregulation of the activated EGF receptor. Of note, PTEN knockdown did not confer "absolute" EGFR kinase inhibitor resistance but instead right-shifted the cell-death response to EGFR kinase inhibition toward drug concentrations which are difficult to achieve in the central nervous system with currently available EGFR kinase inhibitors (Vivanco et al. 2010). Further studies are needed to determine whether more complete EGFR kinase inhibition, simultaneous inhibition of multiple RTKs, or both are required to overcome EGFR kinase inhibitor resistance in GBM.

In many ways, the current experience with EGFR and PDGFR inhibitors is reminiscent of the experience in melanoma where the disappointing clinical activity of RAF and MEK inhibitors questioned the role of mutant *BRAF* for the maintenance of these tumors (Smalley and Sondak 2010). The vast majority of clinical trials with RTK inhibitors in neurooncology did not include tumor biopsies during treatment and it is hence unknown to what extent a negative clinical trial result might be attributable to poor drug penetration into the brain tumor. The available data indeed suggests that first-generation RTK inhibitors, given at standard daily doses, result in only weak (if any) pathway inhibition in GBM. Fresh operative samples from three GBM patients who received erlotinib or gefitinib prior to surgery and for whom a frozen pretreatment sample was available showed inconsistent drug effects on phosphorylation of EGFR, Erk, and Akt (Lassman et al. 2005). A more extensive analysis of multiple candidate EGFR effector molecules (p-AKT, p-GSK-3α/β, p-NFκB p65, p-STAT3, p-ERK1/2, p-MEK1, p-p38MAPK, p-p90RSK, p-p70S6 Kinase, p-S6 ribosomal Protein, p-PDGFR-B, and p-SRC) in GBM patients treated with gefitinib similarly showed poor EGFR pathway inhibition (Hegi et al. 2011).

Conclusions regarding target inhibition in GBM have to be viewed as preliminary because tumors with the most informative genotype(s) and strong basal pathway activation were generally underpresented in these studies and because of difficulties to assemble a sufficiently large number of drug-naive "control" tumor samples. Genotype-enriched clinical trials with a surgical arm cohort (Cloughesy et al. 2008) could address this important issue and may be instrumental to "weed out" compounds that fail to achieve sufficient kinase inhibition in GBM tumor tissue and therefore do not warrant further clinical testing in GBM.

6 Clinical Experience with Rapalogs

The PI(3)K pathway represents a very active area of drug development in cancer. Strategies to target members of this pathway are of particular interest in GBM because the majority of these tumors harbor mutations in one or more genes that regulate this pathway (McLendon et al. 2008), including *EGFR, PDGFRA, MET, PTEN, NF1, PIK3CA* and *PIK3R1* (Fig. 1). Biochemical evidence for frequent PI(3)K pathway activation in GBM is provided by immunohistochemical studies which showed phosphorylation of the downstream pathway member S6 ribosomal protein in the majority of these tumors (Choe et al. 2003). The optimal strategy to target the PI(3)K pathway in glioma and other human cancers is currently unclear. Options include inhibitors of PI(3)K, the serine-threonine kinase Akt, the mammalian target of rapamycin (mTOR), and a combination thereof (Workman et al. 2010).

The first member of the PI(3)K pathway for which a clinical grade inhibitor became available was mTOR which exists as a member of two distinct protein complexes called complex I (mTORC1) and complex 2 (mTORC2). mTORC1 responds to a variety of stimuli (growth factors, changes in amino acid availability, energy status, oxygen levels, DNA damage) and promotes protein translation by phosphorylating p70 ribosomal S6 kinase (S6K) (Threonine 389) and eukaryotic initiation factor 4E-binding protein (4EBP) (Threonine 37/46). mTORC2 functions are incompletely understood and include phosphorylation of Akt (Serine 473), serum glucocorticoid-induced kinase (SGK), and specific Protein Kinase C isoforms (Mendoza et al. 2011; Sengupta et al. 2010). The natural product rapamycin inhibits mTORC1 functions allosterically by binding with high affinity to the immunophilin FK506-binding protein-12 (FKBP12).

The potent antiproliferative activity of rapamycin against PTEN-deficient tumor models (Neshat et al. 2001; Podsypanina et al. 2001) motivated a clinical trial with single-agent rapamycin for patients with PTEN-deficient, recurrent GBM. Screening for PTEN protein expression was performed by immunohistochemistry on the specimen from the initial tumor resection and rapamycin was given for 1–2 weeks prior to resection of recurrent tumor. Drug levels of rapamycin were measured in blood and tumor tissue and inhibition of mTOR was evaluated with phosphosite-specific antibodies against the S6K substrate S6 Ribosomal Protein and 40 kDa proline-rich AKT substrate (PRAS40). Inhibition of tumor cell proliferation by rapamycin correlated with mTOR pathway inhibition. About half the tumors showed increased phosphorylation of the Akt substrate PRAS40 during rapamycin treatment and PRAS40 hyperphosphorylation was associated with poor clinical outcome (Cloughesy et al. 2008). Akt activation during treatment with rapalogs has been observed in other cancers and has been attributed to de-inhibition of a negative feeback loop between the mTORC1 substrate S6K1 and adaptor protein insulin receptor substrate (IRS-1) (O'Reilly et al. 2006; Sun et al. 2005). Reactivation of the PI3-K pathway, and also the MAPK pathway (Carracedo et al. 2008), may contribute to the overall disappointing clinical activity of rapalogs in high grade glioma (Chang et al. 2005; Cloughesy et al. 2008; Galanis et al. 2005) and other human cancers (Dancey 2010).

Since PTEN-loss has been associated with EGFR kinase inhibitor resistance and mTOR represents an important effector protein downstream of PI(3)K, combined blockade of EGFR and mTOR might overcome this resistance. In GBM cell lines and other preclinical models, rapamycin indeed showed synergism with the EGFR kinase inhibitor erlotinib (Buck et al. 2006; Wang et al. 2006). However, the combination of rapalogs and first-generation EGFR kinase inhibitors in patients with recurrent GBM was complicated by toxicity requiring substantial dose reductions and failed to show compelling clinical activity (Kreisl et al. 2009b; Reardon et al. 2010).

7 New Approaches to Target the PI(3)K-mTOR Axis

The observed PI(3)K pathway activation in response to rapalogs suggests that inhibitors of PI(3)K (e.g., XL147, GDC-0941, GSK1059615, ZSTK474, PX866) or dual PI(3)K/mTOR inhibitors (e.g., XL765, SF1126, BEZ235, GSK1059615) might accomplish superior pathway blockade and biological activity. Many such inhibitors have been synthesized and have shown broad antiproliferative activity in preclinical GBM models (Fan et al. 2006; Guillard et al. 2009; Shuttleworth et al. 2011). The majority of first generation PI(3)K inhibitors entering the clinic block all members of the class I PI(3) K family and appear to be surprisingly well tolerated

(Shuttleworth et al. 2011) despite the central role of individual class I PI(3)Ks in glucose metabolism and immune function (Okkenhaug et al. 2002; Sasaki et al. 2000). Determination of their clinical activity in GBM is eagerly awaited.

Whether more selective inhibition of individual class I PI(3)Ks will widen the therapeutic window of these agents without compromising their activity (Foukas et al. 2010), is an open question. A screen of six GBM cell lines with a panel of chemotypically diverse and isoform-selective inhibitors of the PI(3)K family demonstrated that inhibitors of p110α or p110β were able to inhibit phosphorylation of Akt, but only p110α inhibitors induced proliferative arrest. The PI3K isoforms p110δ and p110γ were not expressed in these cells and inhibitors of p110β and p110δ had no effects on proliferation (Fan et al. 2006). More recent studies identified a critical role for p110β in certain PTEN-deficient malignancies (Jia et al. 2008; Wee et al. 2008). Further work is needed to determine which PI3K isoforms are most critical for tumor maintenance in GBM as many of these tumors harbor multiple lesions within the RTK/Ras/PI(3)-signaling axis (e.g., EGFR mutation and PTEN loss).

The only modest activity of rapalogs against many human cancers may, at least in part, be due to the fact that these drugs do not effectively block many functions of mTORC2 and mTORC1. This shortcoming could be overcome by a new class of *TOR* kinase domain inhibitors (also called TORKinibs). These "second-generation" mTOR inhibitors have shown compelling antiproliferative activity in a range of preclinical cancer models and have also advanced to clinical testing in GBM and other cancer types (Feldman and Shokat 2010; Liu et al. 2009a).

8 Leveraging the Cancer Genome Atlas for Clinical Drug Development

The clinical experience with kinase inhibitors as cancer therapeutics suggests that these drugs are most effective in patients whose tumors harbor gain-of-function mutations in the targeted kinase. Examples include *BCR-ABL* mutant leukemia, *KIT*- or *PDGFRA*-mutant sarcoma, *EGFR* or *ALK* mutant lung cancer, and *BRAF* or *KIT* mutant melanoma (Sawyers 2009). While the presence of an oncogenic mutation clearly does not guarantee response to the corresponding kinase inhibitor, the relationship between tumor genotype and drug response is compelling enough that mutational profiling is now routinely performed in the clinic for several human cancers (e.g., lung cancer, melanoma, colorectal cancer) and results incorporated into treatment decisions (Gerber and Minna 2010). A link between tumor genotype and drug response still remains to be proven for GBM, but many centers have begun to prospectively profile gliomas for the most commonly found alterations (e.g., *EGFR* gene amplification, *MGMT* methylation, *IDH1/2* mutations, *1p19q* deletion) (Jansen et al. 2010; Riemenschneider et al. 2010). The extent of profiling is currently driven by institutional expertise, assay cost, and tissue availability but is likely to increase in the near future as newer profiling platforms yield robust results from formalin-fixed and paraffin-embedded clinical specimen.

While the impact of tumor profiling on disease classification and treatment in GBM remains to be firmly established, currently its greatest utility may be for clinical drug development. A logistic obstacle toward genotype-focused clinical development in GBM is the low absolute number of patients with tumors of a particular tumor genotype. As discussed above, many presumed "driver" mutations in GBM (e.g., *PDGFRA, PIK3R1, PIK3CA, BRAF, MET*) occur in only a small subset of patients and a substantial number of these patients will be ineligible for clinical trial participation due to disease-related morbidity. By determining the distribution of mutations within a large number of patients with primary GBMs, TCGA (2005) has provided valuable information for clinical trial planning. For example, mutations in *EGFR* and *PDGFRA* are rarely found in the same tumor (Fig. 4) and one could envision using prospective genotyping information to assign patients to clinical trials targeting either of these lesions. Genotype-enriched trials for other presumed "driver" mutations, such as *MET* gene amplification, *PIK3CA* mutations, or *PIK3R1* mutations will require screening of a substantially larger number of patients as these mutations are even less common. Based on the distribution of mutations throughout the coding sequence of various pathway members (Fig. 2), perhaps a combination of phosphoproteomic "pathway activation" measurements (Solit and Mellinghoff 2010) and selected genotyping for mutation hotspots (Jansen et al. 2010) may represent the most cost-effective screening approach until predictive biomarkers have been properly validated.

9 Future Perspective

The clinical development of PI(3)K inhibitors for GBM would be greatly accelerated by enrichment of clinical trials for patients whose tumors that are more likely to respond. While several ATP-site competitive pan-class I PI(3)K inhibitors have shown antiproliferative activity against a broad panel of human GBM cell lines (Fan et al. 2006; Guillard et al. 2009; Koul et al. 2010; Liu et al. 2009b; Prasad et al. 2011), it is not clear whether any disease subgroup might exhibit a degree of PI(3)K pathway "addiction" associated with tumor cell death and tumor regressions in other cancers. In breast cancer, for example, such PI(3)K pathway addiction appears to exist for tumors with *PIK3CA* mutation and *HER2* gene amplification as evidenced by cell death induction in response to pan-class I PI(3)K inhibitors (Ihle et al. 2009; Junttila et al. 2009; Mallon et al. 2010; O'Brien et al. 2010; Serra et al. 2008), Akt inhibitors (She et al. 2008), and the emerging class of mTOR kinase domain inhibitors (Weigelt et al. 2011). Lung cancer cell lines harboring *EGFR* kinase mutations, on the other hand, do not appear to depend on PI(3)K signals for survival (Faber et al. 2009). More extensive testing of novel compounds in genetically faithful glioma models

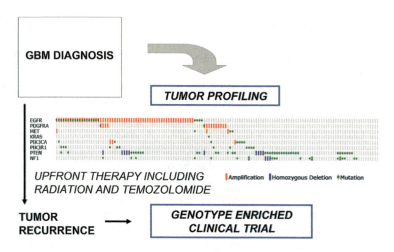

Fig. 4 Potential strategy for genotype-enriched clinical trials in GBM. Tumor tissue collected during the initial surgery ("GBM Diagnosis") is profiled to identify candidate "driver" mutations and clinical trial participation at the time of tumor recurrence (i.e., following standard "Upfront Therapy") is guided by the molecular profiling results. Shown is the distribution of mutations in 138 GBMs which were profiled by the TCGA (2005) and for whom complete Sanger Sequencing and Gene Copy Number data is available

(Hambardzumyan et al. 2011) and cell lines (Lee et al. 2006a) will provide the foundation to formulate hypotheses for genotype-enriched clinical trials.

Different dosing schedules (e.g., intermittent or "pulsatile" dosing) (Shah et al. 2008) and isoform-specific (e.g., PI3K) or mutant-specific (e.g., BRAF) compounds may increase the therapeutic window of individual kinase inhibitors. Ultimately, however, a combination of agents may be required to achieve clinically meaningful tumor regressions. Such therapies may include: (i) a combination of multiple selective RTK inhibitors, (ii) the simultaneous inhibition of multiple members within the same signaling pathway (e.g., PI3K and mTOR), (iii) a multi-pronged attack on key oncoproteins through distinct pharmacological approaches (e.g., RTK antibody plus RTK kinase inhibitor or HSP90 inhibitor plus RTK inhibitor), or (iv) a combination of agents based on synthetic lethal relationships between signaling pathways (Kaelin 2005). These strategies warrant rigorous testing in genetically faithful preclinical models.

One example for a rational combination therapy is the combination of autophagy inhibitors with PI(3)K-mTOR inhibitors. Autophagy is a process of "self-degradation" of cellular components which can provide substrates for energy production during periods of low extracellular nutrients. mTORC1 suppresses autophagy by blocking autophagosome initiation via phosphorylation of ATG13 and ULK1 (Zoncu et al. 2011). Conversely, inhibition of mTORC1 by rapamycin (Takeuchi et al. 2005) or dual pan-class I PI(3)K/mTOR inhibitors (Guillard et al. 2009; Liu et al. 2009b) induces autophagy in GBM cells. Induction of autophagy may represent an important survival mechanism during mTOR inhibitor therapy and explain why inhibitors of PI3K and mTOR induce growth arrest without cell death. Consistent with that model, recent studies show that inhibitors of autophagy can synergize with PI3K-mTOR inhibitors to induce apoptosis (Fan et al. 2010; Xu et al. 2011), representing an opportunity for mechanism-based combination therapy.

GBM has long been known as a disease with mutations in growth factor signaling pathways. The full extent of these alterations and their relationship to each other has emerged more clearly through The Cancer Genome Atlas. Despite discouraging clinical results with first-generation RTK inhibitors and rapalogs, there is considerable optimism that new RTK inhibitors, "second-generation" mTOR inhibitors, and compounds inhibiting class I PI(3)Ks will be better suited to effectively shut down critical signaling nodes in GBM. As the number of clinical grade inhibitors continues to grow, it will become increasingly important to develop an approach to clinical drug development which fully leverages our knowledge of the GBM cancer genome, lessons from kinase inhibitor therapy in other human cancers, and the ability to extract robust molecular information from small amounts of routinely collected human tumor tissue.

Acknowledgments We thank Ms. Farzeen Aslam for secretarial assistance. This work was supported through NIH U54 CA143798 and R21 CA137896 (IKM), NIH/NS 73831 (PSM), the Leon Levy Foundation (IKM), the Doris Duke Charitable Foundation (IKM), the Sontag Foundation (IKM), the James S. McDonnell Foundation (IKM), and an Advanced Clinical Research Award in Glioma from the American Society of Clinical Oncology (IKM). TFC acknowledges funding support by Art of the Brain, the Ziering Family Foundation in memory of Sigi Ziering, the Singleton Family Foundation, the Clarence Klein Fund for Neuro-Oncology, and the John W. Carson Foundation.

References

Alcantara Llaguno S, Chen J, Kwon CH, Jackson EL, Li Y, Burns DK, Alvarez-Buylla A, Parada LF (2009) Malignant astrocytomas originate from neural stem/progenitor cells in a somatic tumor suppressor mouse model. Cancer Cell 15:45–56. doi:S1535-6108(08)00409-[pii]10.1016/j.ccr.2008.12.006

Assanah M, Lochhead R, Ogden A, Bruce J, Goldman J, Canoll P (2006) Glial progenitors in adult white matter are driven to form malignant gliomas by platelet-derived growth factor-expressing retroviruses. J Neurosci 26:6781–6790. doi:26/25/6781[pii]10.1523/JNEUROSCI.0514-06.2006

Bachoo RM, Maher EA, Ligon KL, Sharpless NE, Chan SS, You MJ, Tang Y, DeFrances J, Stover E, Weissleder R, Rowitch DH, Louis DN, DePinho RA (2002) Epidermal growth factor receptor and Ink4a/Arf: convergent mechanisms governing terminal differentiation and transformation along the neural stem cell to astrocyte axis. Cancer Cell 1:269–277

Bajenaru ML, Hernandez MR, Perry A, Zhu Y, Parada LF, Garbow JR, Gutmann DH (2003) Optic nerve glioma in mice requires astrocyte Nf1 gene inactivation and Nf1 brain heterozygosity. Cancer Res 63:8573–8577

Bar EE, Lin A, Tihan T, Burger PC, Eberhart CG (2008) Frequent gains at chromosome 7q34 involving BRAF in pilocytic astrocytoma. J Neuropathol Exp Neurol 67:878–887. doi:10.1097/NEN.0b013e3181845622

Basto D, Trovisco V, Lopes JM, Martins A, Pardal F, Soares P, Reis RM (2005) Mutation analysis of B-RAF gene in human gliomas. Acta Neuropathol 109:207–210. doi:10.1007/s00401-004-0936-x

Batra SK, Castelino-Prabhu S, Wikstrand CJ, Zhu X, Humphrey PA, Friedman HS, Bigner DD (1995) Epidermal growth factor ligand-independent, unregulated, cell-transforming potential of a naturally occurring human mutant EGFRvIII gene. Cell Growth Differ 6:1251–1259

Bax DA, Mackay A, Little SE, Carvalho D, Viana-Pereira M, Tamber N, Grigoriadis AE, Ashworth A, Reis RM, Ellison DW, Al-Sarraj S, Hargrave D, Jones C (2010) A distinct spectrum of copy number aberrations in pediatric high-grade gliomas. Clin Cancer Res 16:3368–3377. doi:1078-0432.CCR-10-0438[pii]10.1158/1078-0432.CCR-10-0438

Berenjeno IM, Vanhaesebroeck B (2009) PI3K regulatory subunits lose control in cancer. Cancer Cell 16:449–450. doi:S1535-6108(09)00393-6[pii]10.1016/j.ccr.2009.11.017

Berns K, Horlings HM, Hennessy BT, Madiredjo M, Hijmans EM, Beelen K, Linn SC, Gonzalez-Angulo AM, Stemke-Hale K, Hauptmann M, Beijersbergen RL, Mills GB, van de Vijver MJ, Bernards R (2007) A functional genetic approach identifies the PI3K pathway as a major determinant of trastuzumab resistance in breast cancer. Cancer Cell 12:395–402. doi:S1535-6108(07)00262-0[pii]10.1016/j.ccr.2007.08.030

Beroukhim R, Getz G, Nghiemphu L, Barretina J, Hsueh T, Linhart D, Vivanco I, Lee JC, Huang JH, Alexander S, Du J, Kau T, Thomas RK, Shah K, Soto H, Perner S, Prensner J, Debiasi RM, Demichelis F, Hatton C, Rubin MA, Garraway LA, Nelson SF, Liau L, Mischel PS, Cloughesy TF, Meyerson M, Golub TA, Lander ES, Mellinghoff IK, Sellers WR (2007) Assessing the significance of chromosomal aberrations in cancer: methodology and application to glioma. Proc Natl Acad Sci U S A 104:20007–20012. doi:0710052104[pii]10.1073/pnas.0710052104

Beroukhim R, Getz G, Mellinghoff IK (2009) Genomic Identification of Significant Targets in Cancer (GISTIC): Methodology and Application to Glioma and Other Cancers. In: Van Meir E (ed) CNS Cancer. Models, Markers, Prognostic Factors, Targets, and Therapeutic Approaches. Springer, Berlin

Bianco R, Shin I, Ritter CA, Yakes FM, Basso A, Rosen N, Tsurutani J, Dennis PA, Mills GB, Arteaga CL (2003) Loss of PTEN/MMAC1/TEP in EGF receptor-expressing tumor cells counteracts the antitumor action of EGFR tyrosine kinase inhibitors. Oncogene 22:2812–2822

Blume-Jensen P, Hunter T (2001) Oncogenic kinase signalling. Nature 411:355–365

Broderick DK, Di C, Parrett TJ, Samuels YR, Cummins JM, McLendon RE, Fults DW, Velculescu VE, Bigner DD, Yan H (2004) Mutations of PIK3CA in anaplastic oligodendrogliomas, high-grade astrocytomas, and medulloblastomas. Cancer Res 64:5048–5050

Buck E, Eyzaguirre A, Brown E, Petti F, McCormack S, Haley JD, Iwata KK, Gibson NW, Griffin G (2006) Rapamycin synergizes with the epidermal growth factor receptor inhibitor erlotinib in non-small-cell lung, pancreatic, colon, and breast tumors. Mol Cancer Ther 5:2676–2684. doi:5/11/2676[pii]10.1158/1535-7163.MCT-06-0166

Buday L, Downward J (2008) Many faces of Ras activation. Biochim Biophys Acta. doi:S0304-419X(08)00024-3[pii]10.1016/j.bbcan.2008.05.001

Carracedo A, Ma L, Teruya-Feldstein J, Rojo F, Salmena L, Alimonti A, Egia A, Sasaki AT, Thomas G, Kozma SC, Papa A, Nardella C, Cantley LC, Baselga J, Pandolfi PP (2008) Inhibition of mTORC1 leads to MAPK pathway activation through a PI3K-dependent feedback loop in human cancer. J Clin Invest 118:3065–3074. doi:10.1172/JCI34739

Castellano E, Downward J (2011) RAS Interaction with PI3K: More Than Just Another Effector Pathway. Genes Cancer 2:261–274. doi:10.1177/1947601911408807910.1177_1947601911408079[pii]

Chang SM, Wen P, Cloughesy T, Greenberg H, Schiff D, Conrad C, Fink K, Robins HI, De Angelis L, Raizer J, Hess K, Aldape K, Lamborn KR, Kuhn J, Dancey J, Prados MD (2005) Phase II study of CCI-779 in patients with recurrent glioblastoma multiforme. Invest New Drugs 23:357–361

Chen WS, Lazar CS, Lund KA, Welsh JB, Chang CP, Walton GM, Der CJ, Wiley HS, Gill GN, Rosenfeld MG (1989) Functional independence of the epidermal growth factor receptor from a domain required for ligand-induced internalization and calcium regulation. Cell. 59(1):33–43. PMID: 2790960

Cheung LWT, Hennessy BT, Li J (2011) High Frequency of PIK3R1 and PIK3R2 Mutations in Endometrial Cancer Elucidates a Novel Mechansim for Regulation of PTEN Protein Stability. Cancer Discovery 1:170–185

Chi AS, Kwak EL, Clark JW, Wang DL, Louis DN, Iafrate AJ, Batchelor T (2011) Clinical improvement and rapid radiographic regression induced by a MET inhibitor in a patient with MET-amplified glioblastoma. J Clin Oncol 29: 2011 (suppl; abstr 2072)

Choe G, Horvath S, Cloughesy TF, Crosby K, Seligson D, Palotie A, Inge L, Smith BL, Sawyers CL, Mischel PS (2003) Analysis of the phosphatidylinositol 3'-kinase signaling pathway in glioblastoma patients in vivo. Cancer Res 63:2742–2746

Chow LM, Endersby R, Zhu X, Rankin S, Qu C, Zhang J, Broniscer A, Ellison DW, Baker SJ (2011) Cooperativity within and among Pten, p53, and Rb pathways induces high-grade astrocytoma in adult brain. Cancer Cell 19:305–316. doi:S1535-6108(11)00051-1[pii]10.1016/j.ccr.2011. 01.039

Cin H, Meyer C, Herr R, Janzarik WG, Lambert S, Jones DT, Jacob K, Benner A, Witt H, Remke M, Bender S, Falkenstein F, Van Anh TN, Olbrich H, von Deimling A, Pekrun A, Kulozik AE, Gnekow A, Scheurlen W, Witt O, Omran H, Jabado N, Collins VP, Brummer T, Marschalek R, Lichter P, Korshunov A, Pfister SM (2011) Oncogenic FAM131B-BRAF fusion resulting from 7q34 deletion comprises an alternative mechanism of MAPK pathway activation in pilocytic astrocytoma. Acta Neuropathol 121:763–774. doi:10.1007/s00401-011-0817-z

Clarke ID, Dirks PB (2003) A human brain tumor-derived PDGFR-alpha deletion mutant is transforming. Oncogene 22:722–733. doi:10.1038/sj.onc.12061601206160[pii]

Cloughesy TF, Yoshimoto K, Nghiemphu P, Brown K, Dang J, Zhu S, Hsueh T, Chen Y, Wang W, Youngkin D, Liau L, Martin N, Becker D, Bergsneider M, Lai A, Green R, Oglesby T, Koleto M, Trent J, Horvath S, Mischel PS, Mellinghoff IK, Sawyers CL (2008) Antitumor activity of rapamycin in a Phase I trial for patients with recurrent PTEN-deficient glioblastoma. PLoS Med 5:e8. doi:07-PLME-RA-0191[pii]10.1371/journal.pmed.0050008

Comoglio PM, Giordano S, Trusolino L (2008) Drug development of MET inhibitors: targeting oncogene addiction and expedience. Nat Rev Drug Discov 7:504–516. doi:nrd2530[pii]10.1038/ nrd2530

Dai C, Celestino JC, Okada Y, Louis DN, Fuller GN, Holland EC (2001) PDGF autocrine stimulation dedifferentiates cultured astrocytes and induces oligodendrogliomas and oligo-astrocytomas from neural progenitors and astrocytes in vivo. Genes Dev 15:1913–1925. doi:10.1101/gad.903001

Dancey J (2010) mTOR signaling and drug development in cancer. Nat Rev Clin Oncol 7:209–219. doi:nrclinonc.2010.21[pii]10.1038/nrclinonc.2010.21

de Vries NA, Bruggeman SW, Hulsman D, de Vries HI, Zevenhoven J, Buckle T, Hamans BC, Leenders WP, Beijnen JH, van Lohuizen M, Berns AJ, van Tellingen O (2010) Rapid and robust transgenic high-grade glioma mouse models for therapy intervention studies. Clin Cancer Res 16:3431–3441. doi:1078-0432.CCR-09-3414[pii]10.1158/1078-0432.CCR-09-3414

Decker SJ, Alexander C, Habib T (1992) Epidermal growth factor (EGF)-stimulated tyrosine phosphorylation and EGF receptor degradation in cells expressing EGF receptors truncated at residue 973. J Biol Chem 267:1104–1108

Deshmukh H, Yeh TH, Yu J, Sharma MK, Perry A, Leonard JR, Watson MA, Gutmann DH, Nagarajan R (2008) High-resolution, dual-platform aCGH analysis reveals frequent HIPK2 amplification and increased expression in pilocytic astrocytomas. Oncogene 27:4745–4751. doi:onc2008110[pii]10.1038/onc.2008.110

Di Fiore PP, Pierce JH, Fleming TP, Hazan R, Ullrich A, King CR, Schlessinger J, Aaronson SA (1987) Overexpression of the human EGF receptor confers an EGF-dependent transformed phenotype to NIH 3T3 cells. Cell 51:1063–1070

Ding H, Roncari L, Shannon P, Wu X, Lau N, Karaskova J, Gutmann DH, Squire JA, Nagy A, Guha A (2001) Astrocyte-specific expression of activated p21-ras results in malignant astrocytoma formation in a transgenic mouse model of human gliomas. Cancer Res 61: 3826–3836

Ding H, Shannon P, Lau N, Wu X, Roncari L, Baldwin RL, Takebayashi H, Nagy A, Gutmann DH, Guha A (2003) Oligodendrogliomas result from the expression of an activated mutant epidermal growth factor receptor in a RAS transgenic mouse astrocytoma model. Cancer Res 63:1106–1113

Dougherty MJ, Santi M, Brose MS, Ma C, Resnick AC, Sievert AJ, Storm PB, Biegel JA (2010) Activating mutations in BRAF characterize a spectrum of pediatric low-grade gliomas. Neuro Oncol. doi:noq007[pii]10.1093/neuonc/noq007

Druker BJ, Talpaz M, Resta DJ, Peng B, Buchdunger E, Ford JM, Lydon NB, Kantarjian H, Capdeville R, Ohno-Jones S, Sawyers CL (2001) Efficacy and safety of a specific inhibitor of the BCR-ABL tyrosine kinase in chronic myeloid leukemia. N Engl J Med 344:1031–1037

Duerr EM, Rollbrocker B, Hayashi Y, Peters N, Meyer-Puttlitz B, Louis DN, Schramm J, Wiestler OD, Parsons R, Eng C, von Deimling A (1998) PTEN mutations in gliomas and glioneuronal tumors. Oncogene 16:2259–2264. doi:10.1038/sj.onc.1201756

Eisenhardt AE, Olbrich H, Roring M, Janzarik W, Van Anh TN, Cin H, Remke M, Witt H, Korshunov A, Pfister SM, Omran H, Brummer T (2010) Functional characterization of a BRAF insertion mutant associated with pilocytic astrocytoma. Int J Cancer. doi:10.1002/ijc.25893

Ekstrand AJ, Sugawa N, James CD, Collins VP (1992) Amplified and rearranged epidermal growth factor receptor genes in human glioblastomas reveal deletions of sequences encoding portions of the N- and/or C-terminal tails. Proc Natl Acad Sci U S A 89:4309–4313

Ekstrand AJ, Longo N, Hamid ML, Olson JJ, Liu L, Collins VP, James CD (1994) Functional characterization of an EGF receptor with a truncated extracellular domain expressed in glioblastomas with EGFR gene amplification. Oncogene 9:2313–2320

Eley G, Frederick L, Wang XY, Smith DI, James CD (1998) 3' end structure and rearrangements of EGFR in glioblastomas. Genes Chromosomes Cancer 23:248–254. doi:10.1002/(SICI)1098-2264(199811)23:3<248:AID-GCC7>3.0.CO;2-1[pii]

El-Habr EA, Tsiorva P, Theodorou M, Levidou G, Korkolopoulou P, Vretakos G, Petraki L, Michalopoulos NV, Patsouris E, Saetta AA (2010) Analysis of PIK3CA and B-RAF gene mutations in human astrocytomas: association with activation of ERK and AKT. Clin Neuropathol 29:239–245. doi:7714[pii]

Eller JL, Longo SL, Hicklin DJ, Canute GW (2002) Activity of anti-epidermal growth factor receptor monoclonal antibody C225 against glioblastoma multiforme. Neurosurgery 51: 1005–1013 discussion 1013-4

Faber AC, Li D, Song Y, Liang MC, Yeap BY, Bronson RT, Lifshits E, Chen Z, Maira SM, Garcia-Echeverria C, Wong KK, Engelman JA (2009) Differential induction of apoptosis in HER2 and EGFR addicted cancers following PI3K inhibition. Proc Natl Acad Sci U S A 106:19503–19508. doi:0905056106[pii]10.1073/pnas.0905056106

Fan QW, Knight ZA, Goldenberg DD, Yu W, Mostov KE, Stokoe D, Shokat KM, Weiss WA (2006) A dual PI3 kinase/mTOR inhibitor reveals emergent efficacy in glioma. Cancer Cell 9:341–349

Fan QW, Cheng C, Hackett C, Feldman M, Houseman BT, Nicolaides T, Haas-Kogan D, James CD, Oakes SA, Debnath J, Shokat KM, Weiss WA (2010) Akt and autophagy cooperate to promote survival of drug-resistant glioma. Sci Signal 3: ra81. doi:3/147/ra81[pii]10.1126/scisignal.2001017

Feldman ME, Shokat KM (2010) New inhibitors of the PI3K-Akt-mTOR pathway: insights into mTOR signaling from a new generation of Tor Kinase Domain Inhibitors (TORKinibs). Curr Top Microbiol Immunol 347:241–262. doi:10.1007/82_2010_64

Fleming TP, Saxena A, Clark WC, Robertson JT, Oldfield EH, Aaronson SA, Ali IU (1992) Amplification and/or overexpression of platelet-derived growth factor receptors and epidermal growth factor receptor in human glial tumors. Cancer Res 52:4550–4553

Forshew T, Tatevossian RG, Lawson AR, Ma J, Neale G, Ogunkolade BW, Jones TA, Aarum J, Dalton J, Bailey S, Chaplin T, Carter RL, Gajjar A, Broniscer A, Young BD, Ellison DW,

Sheer D (2009) Activation of the ERK/MAPK pathway: a signature genetic defect in posterior fossa pilocytic astrocytomas. J Pathol 218:172–181. doi:10.1002/path.2558

Foukas LC, Berenjeno IM, Gray A, Khwaja A, Vanhaesebroeck B (2010) Activity of any class IA PI3K isoform can sustain cell proliferation and survival. Proc Natl Acad Sci U S A 107:11381–11386. doi:0906461107[pii]10.1073/pnas.0906461107

Fraser MM, Zhu X, Kwon CH, Uhlmann EJ, Gutmann DH, Baker SJ (2004) Pten loss causes hypertrophy and increased proliferation of astrocytes in vivo. Cancer Res 64:7773–7779. doi:64/21/7773[pii]10.1158/0008-5472.CAN-04-2487

Frederick L, Wang XY, Eley G, James CD (2000) Diversity and frequency of epidermal growth factor receptor mutations in human glioblastomas. Cancer Res 60:1383–1387

Friedman HS, Prados MD, Wen PY, Mikkelsen T, Schiff D, Abrey LE, Yung WK, Paleologos N, Nicholas MK, Jensen R, Vredenburgh J, Huang J, Zheng M, Cloughesy T (2009) Bevacizumab alone and in combination with irinotecan in recurrent glioblastoma. J Clin Oncol 27:4733–4740. doi:JCO.2008.19.8721[pii]10.1200/JCO.2008.19.8721

Galanis E, Buckner JC, Maurer MJ, Kreisberg JI, Ballman K, Boni J, Peralba JM, Jenkins RB, Dakhil SR, Morton RF, Jaeckle KA, Scheithauer BW, Dancey J, Hidalgo M, Walsh DJ (2005) Phase II trial of temsirolimus (CCI-779) in recurrent glioblastoma multiforme: a North Central Cancer Treatment Group Study. J Clin Oncol 23:5294–5304

Gallia GL, Rand V, Siu IM, Eberhart CG, James CD, Marie SK, Oba-Shinjo SM, Carlotti CG, Caballero OL, Simpson AJ, Brock MV, Massion PP, Carson BS Sr, Riggins GJ (2006) PIK3CA gene mutations in pediatric and adult glioblastoma multiforme. Mol Cancer Res 4:709–714. doi:4/10/709[pii]10.1158/1541-7786.MCR-06-0172

Gerber DE, Minna JD (2010) ALK inhibition for non-small cell lung cancer: from discovery to therapy in record time. Cancer Cell 18:548–551. doi:S1535-6108(10)00491-5[pii]10.1016/j.ccr.2010.11.033

Gronych J, Korshunov A, Bageritz J, Milde T, Jugold M, Hambardzumyan D, Remke M, Hartmann C, Witt H, Jones DT, Witt O, Heiland S, Bendszus M, Holland EC, Pfister S, Lichter P (2011) An activated mutant BRAF kinase domain is sufficient to induce pilocytic astrocytoma in mice. J Clin Invest 121:1344–1348. doi:44656[pii]10.1172/JCI44656

Groszer M, Erickson R, Scripture-Adams DD, Lesche R, Trumpp A, Zack JA, Kornblum HI, Liu X, Wu H (2001) Negative regulation of neural stem/progenitor cell proliferation by the Pten tumor suppressor gene in vivo. Science 294:2186–2189

Gschwind A, Fischer OM, Ullrich A (2004) The discovery of receptor tyrosine kinases: targets for cancer therapy. Nat Rev Cancer 4:361–370

Guillard S, Clarke PA, Te Poele R, Mohr Z, Bjerke L, Valenti M, Raynaud F, Eccles SA, Workman P (2009) Molecular pharmacology of phosphatidylinositol 3-kinase inhibition in human glioma. Cell Cycle 8:443–453. doi:7643[pii]

Gutmann DH, James CD, Poyhonen M, Louis DN, Ferner R, Guha A, Hariharan S, Viskochil D, Perry A (2003) Molecular analysis of astrocytomas presenting after age 10 in individuals with NF1. Neurology 61:1397–1400

Haas-Kogan DA, Prados MD, Tihan T, Eberhard DA, Jelluma N, Arvold ND, Baumber R, Lamborn KR, Kapadia A, Malec M, Berger MS, Stokoe D (2005) Epidermal growth factor receptor, protein kinase B/Akt, and glioma response to erlotinib. J Natl Cancer Inst 97:880–887

Hagemann C, Gloger J, Anacker J, Said HM, Gerngras S, Kuhnel S, Meyer C, Rapp UR, Kammerer U, Vordermark D, Flentje M, Roosen K, Vince GH (2009) RAF expression in human astrocytic tumors. Int J Mol Med 23:17–31

Haley JD, Hsuan JJ, Waterfield MD (1989) Analysis of mammalian fibroblast transformation by normal and mutated human EGF receptors. Oncogene 4:273–283

Hambardzumyan D, Parada LF, Holland EC, Charest A (2011) Genetic modeling of gliomas in mice: new tools to tackle old problems. Glia 59:1155–1168. doi:10.1002/glia.21142

Hartmann C, Bartels G, Gehlhaar C, Holtkamp N, von Deimling A (2005) PIK3CA mutations in glioblastoma multiforme. Acta Neuropathol 109:639–642. doi:10.1007/s00401-005-1000-1

Hegi ME, Diserens AC, Bady P, Kamoshima Y, Kouwenhoven MC, Delorenzi M, Lambiv WL, Hamou MF, Matter MS, Koch A, Heppner FL, Yonekawa Y, Merlo A, Frei K, Mariani L,

Hofer S (2011) Pathway Analysis of Glioblastoma Tissue after Preoperative Treatment with the EGFR Tyrosine Kinase Inhibitor Gefitinib–A Phase II Trial. Mol Cancer Ther 10:1102–1112. doi:1535-7163.MCT-11-0048[pii]10.1158/1535-7163.MCT-11-0048

Hermanson M, Funa K, Hartman M, Claesson-Welsh L, Heldin CH, Westermark B, Nister M (1992) Platelet-derived growth factor and its receptors in human glioma tissue: expression of messenger RNA and protein suggests the presence of autocrine and paracrine loops. Cancer Res 52:3213–3219

Hitoshi Y, Harris BT, Liu H, Popko B, Israel MA (2008) Spinal glioma: platelet-derived growth factor B-mediated oncogenesis in the spinal cord. Cancer Res 68:8507–8515. doi:68/20/8507[pii]10.1158/0008-5472.CAN-08-1063

Holland EC, Hively WP, DePinho RA, Varmus HE (1998) A constitutively active epidermal growth factor receptor cooperates with disruption of G1 cell-cycle arrest pathways to induce glioma-like lesions in mice. Genes Dev 12:3675–3685

Holland EC, Celestino J, Dai C, Schaefer L, Sawaya RE, Fuller GN (2000) Combined activation of Ras and Akt in neural progenitors induces glioblastoma formation in mice. Nat Genet 25:55–57

Holmen SL, Williams BO (2005) Essential role for Ras signaling in glioblastoma maintenance. Cancer Res 65:8250–8255. doi:65/18/8250[pii]10.1158/0008-5472.CAN-05-1173

Huang CH, Mandelker D, Schmidt-Kittler O, Samuels Y, Velculescu VE, Kinzler KW, Vogelstein B, Gabelli SB, Amzel LM (2007) The structure of a human p110alpha/p85alpha complex elucidates the effects of oncogenic PI3Kalpha mutations. Science 318:1744–1748. doi:318/5857/1744[pii]10.1126/science.1150799

Ihle NT, Lemos R Jr, Wipf P, Yacoub A, Mitchell C, Siwak D, Mills GB, Dent P, Kirkpatrick DL, Powis G (2009) Mutations in the phosphatidylinositol-3-kinase pathway predict for antitumor activity of the inhibitor PX-866 whereas oncogenic Ras is a dominant predictor for resistance. Cancer Res 69:143–150. doi:69/1/143[pii]10.1158/0008-5472.CAN-07-6656

Jacob K, Albrecht S, Sollier C, Faury D, Sader E, Montpetit A, Serre D, Hauser P, Garami M, Bognar L, Hanzely Z, Montes JL, Atkinson J, Farmer JP, Bouffet E, Hawkins C, Tabori U, Jabado N (2009) Duplication of 7q34 is specific to juvenile pilocytic astrocytomas and a hallmark of cerebellar and optic pathway tumours. Br J Cancer 101:722–733. doi:6605179[-pii]10.1038/sj.bjc.6605179

Jacques TS, Swales A, Brzozowski MJ, Henriquez NV, Linehan JM, Mirzadeh Z, OM C, Naumann H, Alvarez-Buylla A, Brandner S (2010) Combinations of genetic mutations in the adult neural stem cell compartment determine brain tumour phenotypes. EMBO J 29:222–235. doi:emboj2009327[pii]10.1038/emboj.2009.327

Jaiswal BS, Janakiraman V, Kljavin NM, Chaudhuri S, Stern HM, Wang W, Kan Z, Dbouk HA, Peters BA, Waring P, Dela Vega T, Kenski DM, Bowman KK, Lorenzo M, Li H, Wu J, Modrusan Z, Stinson J, Eby M, Yue P, Kaminker JS, de Sauvage FJ, Backer JM, Seshagiri S (2009) Somatic mutations in p85alpha promote tumorigenesis through class IA PI3K activation. Cancer Cell 16:463–474. doi:S1535-6108(09)00385-7[pii]10.1016/j.ccr.2009.10.016

James CD, Carlbom E, Dumanski JP, Hansen M, Nordenskjold M, Collins VP, Cavenee WK (1988) Clonal genomic alterations in glioma malignancy stages. Cancer Res 48:5546–5551

Jansen M, Yip S, Louis DN (2010) Molecular pathology in adult gliomas: diagnostic, prognostic, and predictive markers. Lancet Neurol 9:717–726. doi:S1474-4422(10)70105-8[pii]10.1016/S1474-4422(10)70105-8

Janzarik WG, Kratz CP, Loges NT, Olbrich H, Klein C, Schafer T, Scheurlen W, Roggendorf W, Weiller C, Niemeyer C, Korinthenberg R, Pfister S, Omran H (2007) Further evidence for a somatic KRAS mutation in a pilocytic astrocytoma. Neuropediatrics 38:61–63. doi:10.1055/s-2007-984451

Jeuken J, van den Broecke C, Gijsen S, Boots-Sprenger S, Wesseling P (2007) RAS/RAF pathway activation in gliomas: the result of copy number gains rather than activating mutations. Acta Neuropathol 114:121–133. doi:10.1007/s00401-007-0239-0

Jia S, Liu Z, Zhang S, Liu P, Zhang L, Lee SH, Zhang J, Signoretti S, Loda M, Roberts TM, Zhao JJ (2008) Essential roles of PI(3)K-p110beta in cell growth, metabolism and tumorigenesis. Nature 454:776–779. doi:nature07091[pii]10.1038/nature07091

Jones DT, Kocialkowski S, Liu L, Pearson DM, Backlund LM, Ichimura K, Collins VP (2008) Tandem duplication producing a novel oncogenic BRAF fusion gene defines the majority of pilocytic astrocytomas. Cancer Res 68:8673–8677. doi:68/21/8673[pii]10.1158/0008-5472.CAN-08-2097

Jones DT, Kocialkowski S, Liu L, Pearson DM, Ichimura K, Collins VP (2009) Oncogenic RAF1 rearrangement and a novel BRAF mutation as alternatives to KIAA1549:BRAF fusion in activating the MAPK pathway in pilocytic astrocytoma. Oncogene 28:2119–2123. doi:onc200973 [pii]10.1038/onc.2009.73

Junttila TT, Akita RW, Parsons K, Fields C, Lewis Phillips GD, Friedman LS, Sampath D, Sliwkowski MX (2009) Ligand-independent HER2/HER3/PI3K complex is disrupted by trastuzumab and is effectively inhibited by the PI3K inhibitor GDC-0941. Cancer Cell 15:429–440. doi:S1535-6108(09)00109-3[pii]10.1016/j.ccr.2009.03.020

Kaelin WG Jr (2005) The concept of synthetic lethality in the context of anticancer therapy. Nat Rev Cancer 5:689–698. doi:nrc1691[pii]10.1038/nrc1691

Kang S, Denley A, Vanhaesebroeck B, Vogt PK (2006) Oncogenic transformation induced by the p110beta, -gamma, and -delta isoforms of class I phosphoinositide 3-kinase. Proc Natl Acad Sci U S A 103:1289–1294. doi:0510772103[pii]10.1073/pnas.0510772103

Kita D, Yonekawa Y, Weller M, Ohgaki H (2007) PIK3CA alterations in primary (de novo) and secondary glioblastomas. Acta Neuropathol 113:295–302. doi:10.1007/s00401-006-0186-1

Knobbe CB, Reifenberger J, Reifenberger G (2004) Mutation analysis of the Ras pathway genes NRAS, HRAS, KRAS and BRAF in glioblastomas. Acta Neuropathol 108:467–470. doi:10.1007/s00401-004-0929-9

Koochekpour S, Jeffers M, Rulong S, Taylor G, Klineberg E, Hudson EA, Resau JH, Vande Woude GF (1997) Met and hepatocyte growth factor/scatter factor expression in human gliomas. Cancer Res 57:5391–5398

Kotliarov Y, Steed ME, Christopher N, Walling J, Su Q, Center A, Heiss J, Rosenblum M, Mikkelsen T, Zenklusen JC, Fine HA (2006) High-resolution global genomic survey of 178 gliomas reveals novel regions of copy number alteration and allelic imbalances. Cancer Res 66:9428–9436. doi:66/19/9428[pii]10.1158/0008-5472.CAN-06-1691

Koul D, Shen R, Kim YW, Kondo Y, Lu Y, Bankson J, Ronen SM, Kirkpatrick DL, Powis G, Yung WK (2010) Cellular and in vivo activity of a novel PI3K inhibitor, PX-866, against human glioblastoma. Neuro Oncol 12:559–569. doi:nop058[pii]10.1093/neuonc/nop058

Kreisl TN, Kim L, Moore K, Duic P, Royce C, Stroud I, Garren N, Mackey M, Butman JA, Camphausen K, Park J, Albert PS, Fine HA (2009a) Phase II trial of single-agent bevacizumab followed by bevacizumab plus irinotecan at tumor progression in recurrent glioblastoma. J Clin Oncol 27:740–745. doi:JCO.2008.16.3055[pii]10.1200/JCO.2008.16.3055

Kreisl TN, Lassman AB, Mischel PS, Rosen N, Scher HI, Teruya-Feldstein J, Shaffer D, Lis E, Abrey LE (2009b) A pilot study of everolimus and gefitinib in the treatment of recurrent glioblastoma (GBM). J Neurooncol 92:99–105. doi:10.1007/s11060-008-9741-z

Kumabe T, Sohma Y, Kayama T, Yoshimoto T, Yamamoto T (1992) Amplification of alpha-platelet-derived growth factor receptor gene lacking an exon coding for a portion of the extracellular region in a primary brain tumor of glial origin. Oncogene 7:627–633

Kwon CH, Zhu X, Zhang J, Knoop LL, Tharp R, Smeyne RJ, Eberhart CG, Burger PC, Baker SJ (2001) Pten regulates neuronal soma size: a mouse model of Lhermitte-Duclos disease. Nat Genet 29:404–411. doi:10.1038/ng781ng781[pii]

Kwon CH, Zhao D, Chen J, Alcantara S, Li Y, Burns DK, Mason RP, Lee EY, Wu H, Parada LF (2008) Pten haploinsufficiency accelerates formation of high-grade astrocytomas. Cancer Res 68:3286–3294. doi:68/9/3286[pii]10.1158/0008-5472.CAN-07-6867

Lai A, Kharbanda S, Pope WB et al (2011) Evidence for sequenced molecular evolution of IDH1 mutant glioblastoma from a distinct cell of origin. Journal of Clinical Oncology [in press]

Lassman AB, Rossi MR, Raizer JJ, Abrey LE, Lieberman FS, Grefe CN, Lamborn K, Pao W, Shih AH, Kuhn JG, Wilson R, Nowak NJ, Cowell JK, DeAngelis LM, Wen P, Gilbert MR, Chang S, Yung WA, Prados M, Holland EC (2005) Molecular study of malignant gliomas treated with epidermal growth factor receptor inhibitors: tissue analysis from North American Brain Tumor Consortium Trials 01–03 and 00–01. Clin Cancer Res 11:7841–7850. doi:11/21/7841[pii]10.1158/1078-0432.CCR-05-0421

Lee J, Kotliarova S, Kotliarov Y, Li A, Su Q, Donin NM, Pastorino S, Purow BW, Christopher N, Zhang W, Park JK, Fine HA (2006a) Tumor stem cells derived from glioblastomas cultured in bFGF and EGF more closely mirror the phenotype and genotype of primary tumors than do serum-cultured cell lines. Cancer Cell 9:391–403. doi:S1535-6108(06)00117-6[pii]10.1016/j.ccr.2006.03.030

Lee JC, Vivanco I, Beroukhim R, Huang JH, Feng WL, DeBiasi RM, Yoshimoto K, King JC, Nghiemphu P, Yuza Y, Xu Q, Greulich H, Thomas RK, Paez JG, Peck TC, Linhart DJ, Glatt KA, Getz G, Onofrio R, Ziaugra L, Levine RL, Gabriel S, Kawaguchi T, O'Neill K, Khan H, Liau LM, Nelson SF, Rao PN, Mischel P, Pieper RO, Cloughesy T, Leahy DJ, Sellers WR, Sawyers CL, Meyerson M, Mellinghoff IK (2006b) Epidermal growth factor receptor activation in glioblastoma through novel missense mutations in the extracellular domain. PLoS Med 3:e485. doi:06-PLME-RA-0223R2[pii]10.1371/journal.pmed.0030485

Lemmon MA, Schlessinger J (2010) Cell signaling by receptor tyrosine kinases. Cell 141:1117–1134. doi:S0092-8674(10)00665-3[pii]10.1016/j.cell.2010.06.011

Li Y, Bollag G, Clark R, Stevens J, Conroy L, Fults D, Ward K, Friedman E, Samowitz W, Robertson M et al (1992) Somatic mutations in the neurofibromatosis 1 gene in human tumors. Cell 69:275–281. doi:0092-8674(92)90408-5[pii]

Li J, Yen C, Liaw D, Podsypanina K, Bose S, Wang SI, Puc J, Miliaresis C, Rodgers L, McCombie R, Bigner SH, Giovanella BC, Ittmann M, Tycko B, Hibshoosh H, Wigler MH, Parsons R (1997) PTEN, a putative protein tyrosine phosphatase gene mutated in human brain, breast, and prostate cancer. Science 275:1943–1947

Libermann TA, Nusbaum HR, Razon N, Kris R, Lax I, Soreq H, Whittle N, Waterfield MD, Ullrich A, Schlessinger J (1985) Amplification, enhanced expression and possible rearrangement of EGF receptor gene in primary human brain tumours of glial origin. Nature 313:144–147

Listernick R, Charrow J, Gutmann DH (1999) Intracranial gliomas in neurofibromatosis type 1. Am J Med Genet 89:38–44. doi:10.1002/(SICI)1096-8628(19990326)89:1<38:AID-AJMG8>3.0. CO;2-M[pii]

Liu W, James CD, Frederick L, Alderete BE, Jenkins RB (1997) PTEN/MMAC1 mutations and EGFR amplification in glioblastomas. Cancer Res 57:5254–5257

Liu Q, Thoreen C, Wang J, Sabatini D, Gray NS (2009a) mTOR Mediated Anti-Cancer Drug Discovery. Drug Discov Today Ther Strateg 6:47–55. doi:10.1016/j.ddstr.2009.12.001

Liu TJ, Koul D, LaFortune T, Tiao N, Shen RJ, Maira SM, Garcia-Echevrria C, Yung WK (2009b) NVP-BEZ235, a novel dual phosphatidylinositol 3-kinase/mammalian target of rapamycin inhibitor, elicits multifaceted antitumor activities in human gliomas. Mol Cancer Ther 8:2204–2210. doi:1535-7163.MCT-09-0160[pii]10.1158/1535-7163.MCT-09-0160

Lokker NA, Sullivan CM, Hollenbach SJ, Israel MA, Giese NA (2002) Platelet-derived growth factor (PDGF) autocrine signaling regulates survival and mitogenic pathways in glioblastoma cells: evidence that the novel PDGF-C and PDGF-D ligands may play a role in the development of brain tumors. Cancer Res 62:3729–3735

Louis DN, Ohgaki H, Wiestler OD, Cavenee WK, Burger PC, Jouvet A, Scheithauer BW, Kleihues P (2007) The 2007 WHO classification of tumours of the central nervous system. Acta Neuropathol 114:97–109. doi:10.1007/s00401-007-0243-4

Lyustikman Y, Momota H, Pao W, Holland EC (2008) Constitutive activation of Raf-1 induces glioma formation in mice. Neoplasia 10:501–510

MacConaill LE, Campbell CD, Kehoe SM, Bass AJ, Hatton C, Niu L, Davis M, Yao K, Hanna M, Mondal C, Luongo L, Emery CM, Baker AC, Philips J, Goff DJ, Fiorentino M, Rubin MA, Polyak K, Chan J, Wang Y, Fletcher JA, Santagata S, Corso G, Roviello F, Shivdasani R, Kieran MW, Ligon KL, Stiles CD, Hahn WC, Meyerson ML, Garraway LA (2009) Profiling critical cancer gene mutations in clinical tumor samples. PLoS ONE 4:e7887. doi:10.1371/journal.pone.0007887

Malden LT, Novak U, Kaye AH, Burgess AW (1988) Selective amplification of the cytoplasmic domain of the epidermal growth factor receptor gene in glioblastoma multiforme. Cancer Res 48:2711–2714

Mallon R, Hollander I, Feldberg L, Lucas J, Soloveva V, Venkatesan A, Dehnhardt C, Delos Santos E, Chen Z, Dos Santos O, Ayral-Kaloustian S, Gibbons J (2010) Antitumor efficacy profile of PKI-402, a dual phosphatidylinositol 3-kinase/mammalian target of rapamycin inhibitor. Mol Cancer Ther 9:976–984. doi:1535-7163.MCT-09-0954[pii]10.1158/1535-7163.MCT-09-0954

Maltzman TH, Mueller BA, Schroeder J, Rutledge JC, Patterson K, Preston-Martin S, Faustman EM (1997) Ras oncogene mutations in childhood brain tumors. Cancer Epidemiol Biomarkers Prev 6:239–243

Martens T, Laabs Y, Gunther HS, Kemming D, Zhu Z, Witte L, Hagel C, Westphal M, Lamszus K (2008) Inhibition of glioblastoma growth in a highly invasive nude mouse model can be achieved by targeting epidermal growth factor receptor but not vascular endothelial growth factor receptor-2. Clin Cancer Res 14:5447–5458. doi:14/17/5447[pii]10.1158/1078-0432.CCR-08-0147

Marumoto T, Tashiro A, Friedmann-Morvinski D, Scadeng M, Soda Y, Gage FH, Verma IM (2009) Development of a novel mouse glioma model using lentiviral vectors. Nat Med 15:110–116. doi:nm.1863[pii]10.1038/nm.1863

Masui H, Wells A, Lazar CS, Rosenfeld MG, Gill GN (1991) Enhanced tumorigenesis of NR6 cells which express non-down-regulating epidermal growth factor receptors. Cancer Res. 51(22):6170–6175. PMID:1933876

McDermott U, Sharma SV, Dowell L, Greninger P, Montagut C, Lamb J, Archibald H, Raudales R, Tam A, Lee D, Rothenberg SM, Supko JG, Sordella R, Ulkus LE, Iafrate AJ, Maheswaran S, Njauw CN, Tsao H, Drew L, Hanke JH, Ma XJ, Erlander MG, Gray NS, Haber DA, Settleman J (2007) Identification of genotype-correlated sensitivity to selective kinase inhibitors by using high-throughput tumor cell line profiling. Proc Natl Acad Sci U S A 104:19936–19941. doi:0707498104[pii]10.1073/pnas.0707498104

McGillicuddy LT, Fromm JA, Hollstein PE, Kubek S, Beroukhim R, De Raedt T, Johnson BW, Williams SM, Nghiemphu P, Liau LM, Cloughesy TF, Mischel PS, Parret A, Seiler J, Moldenhauer G, Scheffzek K, Stemmer-Rachamimov AO, Sawyers CL, Brennan C, Messiaen L, Mellinghoff IK, Cichowski K (2009) Proteasomal and genetic inactivation of the NF1 tumor suppressor in gliomagenesis. Cancer Cell 16:44–54. doi:S1535-6108(09)00175-5[pii]10.1016/j.ccr.2009.05.009

McLendon R, Friedman A, Bigner D, Van Meir EG, Brat DJ, Mastrogianakis M, Olson JJ, Mikkelsen T, Lehman N, Aldape K, Alfred Yung WK, Bogler O, Vandenberg S, Berger M, Prados M, Muzny D, Morgan M, Scherer S, Sabo A, Nazareth L, Lewis L, Hall O, Zhu Y, Ren Y, Alvi O, Yao J, Hawes A, Jhangiani S, Fowler G, San Lucas A, Kovar C, Cree A, Dinh H, Santibanez J, Joshi V, Gonzalez-Garay ML, Miller CA, Milosavljevic A, Donehower L, Wheeler DA, Gibbs RA, Cibulskis K, Sougnez C, Fennell T, Mahan S, Wilkinson J, Ziaugra L, Onofrio R, Bloom T, Nicol R, Ardlie K, Baldwin J, Gabriel S, Lander ES, Ding L, Fulton RS, McLellan MD, Wallis J, Larson DE, Shi X, Abbott R, Fulton L, Chen K, Koboldt DC, Wendl MC, Meyer R, Tang Y, Lin L, Osborne JR, Dunford-Shore BH, Miner TL, Delehaunty K, Markovic C, Swift G, Courtney W, Pohl C, Abbott S, Hawkins A, Leong S, Haipek C, Schmidt H, Wiechert M, Vickery T, Scott S, Dooling DJ, Chinwalla A, Weinstock GM, Mardis ER, Wilson RK, Getz G, Winckler W, Verhaak RG, Lawrence MS, O'Kelly M, Robinson J, Alexe G, Beroukhim R, Carter S, Chiang D, Gould J et al (2008) Comprehensive genomic characterization defines human glioblastoma genes and core pathways. Nature 455:1061–1068

Mellinghoff IK, Wang MY, Vivanco I, Haas-Kogan DA, Zhu S, Dia EQ, Lu KV, Yoshimoto K, Huang JH, Chute DJ, Riggs BL, Horvath S, Liau LM, Cavenee WK, Rao PN, Beroukhim R, Peck TC, Lee JC, Sellers WR, Stokoe D, Prados M, Cloughesy TF, Sawyers CL, Mischel PS (2005) Molecular determinants of the response of glioblastomas to EGFR kinase inhibitors. N Engl J Med 353:2012–2024

Mellinghoff IK, Lassman AB, Wen PY (2011) Signal transduction inhibitors and antiangiogenic therapies for malignant glioma. Glia. doi: 10.1002/glia.21137

Mendoza MC, Er EE, Blenis J (2011) The Ras-ERK and PI3K-mTOR pathways: cross-talk and compensation. Trends Biochem Sci 36:320–328. doi:S0968-0004(11)00050-8[pii]10.1016/j.tibs.2011.03.006

Misra A, Pellarin M, Nigro J, Smirnov I, Moore D, Lamborn KR, Pinkel D, Albertson DG, Feuerstein BG (2005) Array comparative genomic hybridization identifies genetic subgroups in grade 4 human astrocytoma. Clin Cancer Res 11:2907–2918. doi:11/8/2907[pii]10.1158/1078-0432.CCR-04-0708

Mizoguchi M, Nutt CL, Mohapatra G, Louis DN (2004) Genetic alterations of phosphoinositide 3-kinase subunit genes in human glioblastomas. Brain Pathol 14:372–377

Mueller W, Mizoguchi M, Silen E, D'Amore K, Nutt CL, Louis DN (2005) Mutations of the PIK3CA gene are rare in human glioblastoma. Acta Neuropathol 109:654–655. doi:10.1007/s00401-005-1001-0

Neshat MS, Mellinghoff IK, Tran C, Stiles B, Thomas G, Petersen R, Frost P, Gibbons JJ, Wu H, Sawyers CL (2001) Enhanced sensitivity of PTEN-deficient tumors to inhibition of FRAP/mTOR. Proc Natl Acad Sci U S A 98:10314–10319. doi:10.1073/pnas.171076798171076798[pii]

Nishikawa R, Ji XD, Harmon RC, Lazar CS, Gill GN, Cavenee WK, Huang HJ (1994) A mutant epidermal growth factor receptor common in human glioma confers enhanced tumorigenicity. Proc Natl Acad Sci U S A 91:7727–7731

O'Brien C, Wallin JJ, Sampath D, GuhaThakurta D, Savage H, Punnoose EA, Guan J, Berry L, Prior WW, Amler LC, Belvin M, Friedman LS, Lackner MR (2010) Predictive biomarkers of sensitivity to the phosphatidylinositol 3' kinase inhibitor GDC-0941 in breast cancer preclinical models. Clin Cancer Res 16:3670–3683. doi:1078-0432.CCR-09-2828[pii]10.1158/1078-0432.CCR-09-2828

Ohgaki H, Kleihues P (2007) Genetic pathways to primary and secondary glioblastoma. Am J Pathol 170:1445–1453. doi:S0002-9440(10)61358-2[pii]10.2353/ajpath.2007.070011

Ohgaki H, Dessen P, Jourde B, Horstmann S, Nishikawa T, Di Patre PL, Burkhard C, Schuler D, Probst-Hensch NM, Maiorka PC, Baeza N, Pisani P, Yonekawa Y, Yasargil MG, Lutolf UM, Kleihues P (2004) Genetic pathways to glioblastoma: a population-based study. Cancer Res 64:6892–6899. doi:64/19/6892[pii]10.1158/0008-5472.CAN-04-1337

Okkenhaug K, Bilancio A, Farjot G, Priddle H, Sancho S, Peskett E, Pearce W, Meek SE, Salpekar A, Waterfield MD, Smith AJ, Vanhaesebroeck B (2002) Impaired B and T cell antigen receptor signaling in p110delta PI 3-kinase mutant mice. Science 297:1031–1034. doi:10.1126/science.10735601073560[pii]

O'Reilly KE, Rojo F, She QB, Solit D, Mills GB, Smith D, Lane H, Hofmann F, Hicklin DJ, Ludwig DL, Baselga J, Rosen N (2006) mTOR inhibition induces upstream receptor tyrosine kinase signaling and activates Akt. Cancer Res 66:1500–1508

Ostman A, Heldin CH (2007) PDGF receptors as targets in tumor treatment. Adv Cancer Res 97:247–274. doi:S0065-230X(06)97011-0[pii]10.1016/S0065-230X(06)97011-0

Ozawa T, Brennan CW, Wang L, Squatrito M, Sasayama T, Nakada M, Huse JT, Pedraza A, Utsuki S, Yasui Y, Tandon A, Fomchenko EI, Oka H, Levine RL, Fujii K, Ladanyi M, Holland EC (2010) PDGFRA gene rearrangements are frequent genetic events in PDGFRA-amplified glioblastomas. Genes Dev 24:2205–2218. doi:24/19/2205[pii]10.1101/gad.1972310

Parsons DW, Jones S, Zhang X, Lin JC, Leary RJ, Angenendt P, Mankoo P, Carter H, Siu IM, Gallia GL, Olivi A, McLendon R, Rasheed BA, Keir S, Nikolskaya T, Nikolsky Y, Busam DA, Tekleab H, Diaz LA Jr, Hartigan J, Smith DR, Strausberg RL, Marie SK, Shinjo SM, Yan H, Riggins GJ, Bigner DD, Karchin R, Papadopoulos N, Parmigiani G, Vogelstein B, Velculescu VE, Kinzler KW (2008) An integrated genomic analysis of human glioblastoma multiforme. Science 321:1807–1812. doi:1164382[pii]10.1126/science.1164382

Paugh BS, Qu C, Jones C, Liu Z, Adamowicz-Brice M, Zhang J, Bax DA, Coyle B, Barrow J, Hargrave D, Lowe J, Gajjar A, Zhao W, Broniscer A, Ellison DW, Grundy RG, Baker SJ (2010) Integrated molecular genetic profiling of pediatric high-grade gliomas reveals key differences with the adult disease. J Clin Oncol 28:3061–3068. doi:JCO.2009.26.7252[-pii]10.1200/JCO.2009.26.7252

Pfister S, Janzarik WG, Remke M, Ernst A, Werft W, Becker N, Toedt G, Wittmann A, Kratz C, Olbrich H, Ahmadi R, Thieme B, Joos S, Radlwimmer B, Kulozik A, Pietsch T, Herold-Mende C, Gnekow A, Reifenberger G, Korshunov A, Scheurlen W, Omran H, Lichter P (2008) BRAF gene duplication constitutes a mechanism of MAPK pathway activation in low-grade astrocytomas. J Clin Invest 118:1739–1749. doi:10.1172/JCI33656

Phillips HS, Kharbanda S, Chen R, Forrest WF, Soriano RH, Wu TD, Misra A, Nigro JM, Colman H, Soroceanu L, Williams PM, Modrusan Z, Feuerstein BG, Aldape K (2006) Molecular subclasses of high-grade glioma predict prognosis, delineate a pattern of disease progression, and resemble stages in neurogenesis. Cancer Cell 9:157–173. doi:S1535-6108(06)00056-0[pii]10.1016/j.ccr.2006.02.019

Philp AJ, Campbell IG, Leet C, Vincan E, Rockman SP, Whitehead RH, Thomas RJ, Phillips WA (2001) The phosphatidylinositol 3'-kinase p85alpha gene is an oncogene in human ovarian and colon tumors. Cancer Res 61:7426–7429

Podsypanina K, Lee RT, Politis C, Hennessy I, Crane A, Puc J, Neshat M, Wang H, Yang L, Gibbons J, Frost P, Dreisbach V, Blenis J, Gaciong Z, Fisher P, Sawyers C, Hedrick-Ellenson L, Parsons R (2001) An inhibitor of mTOR reduces neoplasia and normalizes p70/S6 kinase activity in Pten ± mice. Proc Natl Acad Sci U S A 98:10320–10325

Prados MD, Chang SM, Butowski N, DeBoer R, Parvataneni R, Carliner H, Kabuubi P, Ayers-Ringler J, Rabbitt J, Page M, Fedoroff A, Sneed PK, Berger MS, McDermott MW, Parsa AT, Vandenberg S, James CD, Lamborn KR, Stokoe D, Haas-Kogan DA (2009) Phase II study of erlotinib plus temozolomide during and after radiation therapy in patients with newly diagnosed glioblastoma multiforme or gliosarcoma. J Clin Oncol 27:579–584. doi:JCO.2008.18.9639[pii]10.1200/JCO.2008.18.9639

Prasad G, Sottero T, Yang X, Mueller S, James CD, Weiss WA, Polley MY, Ozawa T, Berger MS, Aftab DT, Prados MD, Haas-Kogan DA (2011) Inhibition of PI3K/mTOR pathways in glioblastoma and implications for combination therapy with temozolomide. Neuro Oncol 13:384–392. doi:noq193[pii]10.1093/neuonc/noq193

Rand V, Huang J, Stockwell T, Ferriera S, Buzko O, Levy S, Busam D, Li K, Edwards JB, Eberhart C, Murphy KM, Tsiamouri A, Beeson K, Simpson AJ, Venter JC, Riggins GJ, Strausberg RL (2005) Sequence survey of receptor tyrosine kinases reveals mutations in glioblastomas. Proc Natl Acad Sci U S A 102:14344–14349. doi:0507200102[pii]10.1073/pnas.0507200102

Raymond E, Brandes AA, Dittrich C, Fumoleau P, Coudert B, Clement PM, Frenay M, Rampling R, Stupp R, Kros JM, Heinrich MC, Gorlia T, Lacombe D, van den Bent MJ (2008) Phase II study of imatinib in patients with recurrent gliomas of various histologies: a European Organisation for Research and Treatment of Cancer Brain Tumor Group Study. J Clin Oncol 26:4659–4665. doi:26/28/4659[pii]10.1200/JCO.2008.16.9235

Reardon DA, Desjardins A, Vredenburgh JJ, Gururangan S, Friedman AH, Herndon JE 2nd, Marcello J, Norfleet JA, McLendon RE, Sampson JH, Friedman HS (2010) Phase 2 trial of erlotinib plus sirolimus in adults with recurrent glioblastoma. J Neurooncol 96:219–230. doi:10.1007/s11060-009-9950-0

Reilly KM, Loisel DA, Bronson RT, McLaughlin ME, Jacks T (2000) Nf1;Trp53 mutant mice develop glioblastoma with evidence of strain-specific effects. Nat Genet 26:109–113. doi:10.1038/79075

Richardson WD, Pringle N, Mosley MJ, Westermark B, Dubois-Dalcq M (1988) A role for platelet-derived growth factor in normal gliogenesis in the central nervous system. Cell 53:309–319. doi:0092-8674(88)90392-3[pii]

Riemenschneider MJ, Jeuken JW, Wesseling P, Reifenberger G (2010) Molecular diagnostics of gliomas: state of the art. Acta Neuropathol 120:567–584. doi:10.1007/s00401-010-0736-4

Robinson JP, VanBrocklin MW, Guilbeault AR, Signorelli DL, Brandner S, Holmen SL (2010) Activated BRAF induces gliomas in mice when combined with Ink4a/Arf loss or Akt activation. Oncogene 29:335–344. doi:onc2009333[pii]10.1038/onc.2009.333

Robinson JP, Vanbrocklin MW, Lastwika KJ, McKinney AJ, Brandner S, Holmen SL (2011) Activated MEK cooperates with Ink4a/Arf loss or Akt activation to induce gliomas in vivo. Oncogene 30:1341–1350. doi:onc2010513[pii]10.1038/onc.2010.513

Rodriguez FJ, Perry A, Gutmann DH, O'Neill BP, Leonard J, Bryant S, Giannini C (2008) Gliomas in neurofibromatosis type 1: a clinicopathologic study of 100 patients. J Neuropathol Exp Neurol 67:240–249. doi:10.1097/NEN.0b013e318165eb7500005072-200803000-00007[pii]

Salmena L, Carracedo A, Pandolfi PP (2008) Tenets of PTEN tumor suppression. Cell 133:403–414. doi:S0092-8674(08)00504-7[pii]10.1016/j.cell.2008.04.013

Samuels Y, Wang Z, Bardelli A, Silliman N, Ptak J, Szabo S, Yan H, Gazdar A, Powell SM, Riggins GJ, Willson JK, Markowitz S, Kinzler KW, Vogelstein B, Velculescu VE (2004) High frequency of mutations of the PIK3CA gene in human cancers. Science 304:554

Sarkaria JN, Yang L, Grogan PT, Kitange GJ, Carlson BL, Schroeder MA, Galanis E, Giannini C, Wu W, Dinca EB, James CD (2007) Identification of molecular characteristics correlated with glioblastoma sensitivity to EGFR kinase inhibition through use of an intracranial xenograft test panel. Mol Cancer Ther 6:1167–1174. doi:6/3/1167[pii]10.1158/1535-7163.MCT-06-0691

Sasaki T, Irie-Sasaki J, Jones RG, Oliveira-dos-Santos AJ, Stanford WL, Bolon B, Wakeham A, Itie A, Bouchard D, Kozieradzki I, Joza N, Mak TW, Ohashi PS, Suzuki A, Penninger JM (2000) Function of PI3Kgamma in thymocyte development, T cell activation, and neutrophil migration. Science 287:1040–1046. doi:8264[pii]

Sawyers CL (2009) Shifting paradigms: the seeds of oncogene addiction. Nat Med 15:1158–1161. doi:nm1009-1158[pii]10.1038/nm1009-1158

Schatzman RC, Evan GI, Privalsky ML, Bishop JM (1986) Orientation of the v-erb-B gene product in the plasma membrane. Mol Cell Biol 6:1329–1333

Schiffman JD, Hodgson JG, VandenBerg SR, Flaherty P, Polley MY, Yu M, Fisher PG, Rowitch DH, Ford JM, Berger MS, Ji H, Gutmann DH, James CD (2010) Oncogenic BRAF mutation with CDKN2A inactivation is characteristic of a subset of pediatric malignant astrocytomas. Cancer Res 70:512–519. doi:0008-5472.CAN-09-1851[pii]10.1158/0008-5472.CAN-09-1851

Schindler G, Capper D, Meyer J, Janzarik W, Omran H, Herold-Mende C, Schmieder K, Wesseling P, Mawrin C, Hasselblatt M, Louis DN, Korshunov A, Pfister S, Hartmann C, Paulus W, Reifenberger G, von Deimling A (2011) Analysis of BRAF V600E mutation in 1, 320 nervous system tumors reveals high mutation frequencies in pleomorphic xanthoastrocytoma, ganglioglioma and extra-cerebellar pilocytic astrocytoma. Acta Neuropathol 121:397–405. doi:10.1007/s00401-011-0802-6

Sengupta S, Peterson TR, Sabatini DM (2010) Regulation of the mTOR complex 1 pathway by nutrients, growth factors, and stress. Mol Cell 40:310–322. doi:S1097-2765(10)00754-9[pii]10.1016/j.molcel.2010.09.026

Serra V, Markman B, Scaltriti M, Eichhorn PJ, Valero V, Guzman M, Botero ML, Llonch E, Atzori F, Di Cosimo S, Maira M, Garcia-Echeverria C, Parra JL, Arribas J, Baselga J (2008) NVP-BEZ235, a dual PI3K/mTOR inhibitor, prevents PI3K signaling and inhibits the growth of cancer cells with activating PI3K mutations. Cancer Res 68:8022–8030. doi:68/19/8022[pii]10.1158/0008-5472.CAN-08-1385

Shah NP, Kasap C, Weier C, Balbas M, Nicoll JM, Bleickardt E, Nicaise C, Sawyers CL (2008) Transient potent BCR-ABL inhibition is sufficient to commit chronic myeloid leukemia cells irreversibly to apoptosis. Cancer Cell 14:485–493. doi:S1535-6108(08)00368-1[pii]10.1016/j.ccr.2008.11.001

Sharma MK, Zehnbauer BA, Watson MA, Gutmann DH (2005) RAS pathway activation and an oncogenic RAS mutation in sporadic pilocytic astrocytoma. Neurology 65:1335–1336. doi:65/8/1335[pii]10.1212/01.wnl.0000180409.78098.d7

Shaw RJ, Cantley LC (2006) Ras, PI(3)K and mTOR signalling controls tumour cell growth. Nature 441:424–430

Shayesteh L, Lu Y, Kuo WL, Baldocchi R, Godfrey T, Collins C, Pinkel D, Powell B, Mills GB, Gray JW (1999) PIK3CA is implicated as an oncogene in ovarian cancer. Nat Genet 21:99–102. doi:10.1038/5042

She QB, Chandarlapaty S, Ye Q, Lobo J, Haskell KM, Leander KR, DeFeo-Jones D, Huber HE, Rosen N (2008) Breast tumor cells with PI3K mutation or HER2 amplification are selectively addicted to Akt signaling. PLoS ONE 3:e3065. doi:10.1371/journal.pone.0003065

Shuttleworth SJ, Silva FA, Cecil AR, Tomassi CD, Hill TJ, Raynaud FI, Clarke PA, Workman P (2011) Progress in the Preclinical Discovery and Clinical Development of Class I and Dual Class I/IV Phosphoinositide 3-Kinase (PI3K) Inhibitors. Curr Med Chem 18:2686–2714. doi:BSP/CMC/E-Pub/2011/181[pii]

Sievert AJ, Jackson EM, Gai X, Hakonarson H, Judkins AR, Resnick AC, Sutton LN, Storm PB, Shaikh TH, Biegel JA (2009) Duplication of 7q34 in pediatric low-grade astrocytomas detected by high-density single-nucleotide polymorphism-based genotype arrays results in a novel BRAF fusion gene. Brain Pathol 19:449–458. doi:BPA225[pii]10.1111/j.1750-3639.2008.00225.x

Slamon DJ, Leyland-Jones B, Shak S, Fuchs H, Paton V, Bajamonde A, Fleming T, Eiermann W, Wolter J, Pegram M, Baselga J, Norton L (2001) Use of chemotherapy plus a monoclonal antibody against HER2 for metastatic breast cancer that overexpresses HER2. N Engl J Med 344:783–792

Smalley KS, Sondak VK (2010) Melanoma–an unlikely poster child for personalized cancer therapy. N Engl J Med 363:876–878. doi:10.1056/NEJMe1005370

Smith JS, Tachibana I, Passe SM, Huntley BK, Borell TJ, Iturria N, O'Fallon JR, Schaefer PL, Scheithauer BW, James CD, Buckner JC, Jenkins RB (2001) PTEN mutation, EGFR amplification, and outcome in patients with anaplastic astrocytoma and glioblastoma multiforme. J Natl Cancer Inst 93:1246–1256

Solit DB, Mellinghoff IK (2010) Tracing cancer networks with phosphoproteomics. Nat Biotechnol 28:1028–1029. doi:nbt1010-1028[pii]10.1038/nbt1010-1028

Steck PA, Pershouse MA, Jasser SA, Yung WK, Lin H, Ligon AH, Langford LA, Baumgard ML, Hattier T, Davis T, Frye C, Hu R, Swedlund B, Teng DH, Tavtigian SV (1997) Identification of a candidate tumour suppressor gene, MMAC1, at chromosome 10q23.3 that is mutated in multiple advanced cancers. Nat Genet 15:356–362

Stommel JM, Kimmelman AC, Ying H, Nabioullin R, Ponugoti AH, Wiedemeyer R, Stegh AH, Bradner JE, Ligon KL, Brennan C, Chin L, DePinho RA (2007) Coactivation of receptor tyrosine kinases affects the response of tumor cells to targeted therapies. Science 318:287–290. doi:1142946[pii]10.1126/science.1142946

Stupp R, Mason WP, van den Bent MJ, Weller M, Fisher B, Taphoorn MJ, Belanger K, Brandes AA, Marosi C, Bogdahn U, Curschmann J, Janzer RC, Ludwin SK, Gorlia T, Allgeier A, Lacombe D, Cairncross JG, Eisenhauer E, Mirimanoff RO (2005) Radiotherapy plus concomitant and adjuvant temozolomide for glioblastoma. N Engl J Med 352:987–996

Sugawa N, Ekstrand AJ, James CD, Collins VP (1990) Identical splicing of aberrant epidermal growth factor receptor transcripts from amplified rearranged genes in human glioblastomas. Proc Natl Acad Sci U S A 87:8602–8606

Sun SY, Rosenberg LM, Wang X, Zhou Z, Yue P, Fu H, Khuri FR (2005) Activation of Akt and eIF4E survival pathways by rapamycin-mediated mammalian target of rapamycin inhibition. Cancer Res 65:7052–7058

Sun M, Hillmann P, Hofmann BT, Hart JR, Vogt PK (2010) Cancer-derived mutations in the regulatory subunit p85alpha of phosphoinositide 3-kinase function through the catalytic subunit p110alpha. Proc Natl Acad Sci U S A 107:15547–15552. doi:1009652107[-pii]10.1073/pnas.1009652107

Takeuchi H, Kondo Y, Fujiwara K, Kanzawa T, Aoki H, Mills GB, Kondo S (2005) Synergistic augmentation of rapamycin-induced autophagy in malignant glioma cells by phosphatidyl-inositol 3-kinase/protein kinase B inhibitors. Cancer Res 65:3336–3346. doi:65/8/3336[pii]10.1158/0008-5472.CAN-04-3640

The Cancer Genome Atlas Research Network (TCGA) (2005)

Thiel G, Marczinek K, Neumann R, Witkowski R, Marchuk DA, Nurnberg P (1995) Somatic mutations in the neurofibromatosis 1 gene in gliomas and primitive neuroectodermal tumours. Anticancer Res 15:2495–2499

Uhrbom L, Hesselager G, Nister M, Westermark B (1998) Induction of brain tumors in mice using a recombinant platelet-derived growth factor B-chain retrovirus. Cancer Res 58: 5275–5279

Uhrbom L, Dai C, Celestino JC, Rosenblum MK, Fuller GN, Holland EC (2002) Ink4a-Arf loss cooperates with KRas activation in astrocytes and neural progenitors to generate glioblastomas of various morphologies depending on activated Akt. Cancer Res 62:5551–5558

van den Bent MJ, Brandes AA, Rampling R, Kouwenhoven MC, Kros JM, Carpentier AF, Clement PM, Frenay M, Campone M, Baurain JF, Armand JP, Taphoorn MJ, Tosoni A, Kletzl H, Klughammer B, Lacombe D, Gorlia T (2009) Randomized phase II trial of erlotinib versus temozolomide or carmustine in recurrent glioblastoma: EORTC brain tumor group study 26034. J Clin Oncol 27:1268–1274. doi:JCO.2008.17.5984[pii]10.1200/JCO.2008.17.5984

Vanhaesebroeck B, Guillermet-Guibert J, Graupera M, Bilanges B (2010) The emerging mechanisms of isoform-specific PI3K signalling. Nat Rev Mol Cell Biol 11:329–341. doi:nrm2882[pii]10.1038/nrm2882

Verhaak RG, Hoadley KA, Purdom E, Wang V, Qi Y, Wilkerson MD, Miller CR, Ding L, Golub T, Mesirov JP, Alexe G, Lawrence M, O'Kelly M, Tamayo P, Weir BA, Gabriel S, Winckler W, Gupta S, Jakkula L, Feiler HS, Hodgson JG, James CD, Sarkaria JN, Brennan C, Kahn A, Spellman PT, Wilson RK, Speed TP, Gray JW, Meyerson M, Getz G, Perou CM, Hayes DN (2010) Integrated genomic analysis identifies clinically relevant subtypes of glioblastoma characterized by abnormalities in PDGFRA, IDH1, EGFR, and NF1. Cancer Cell 17:98–110. doi:S1535-6108(09)00432-2[pii]10.1016/j.ccr.2009.12.020

Vivanco I, Rohle D, Versele M, Iwanami A, Kuga D, Oldrini B, Tanaka K, Dang J, Kubek S, Palaskas N, Hsueh T, Evans M, Mulholland D, Wolle D, Rajasekaran S, Rajasekaran A, Liau LM, Cloughesy TF, Dikic I, Brennan C, Wu H, Mischel PS, Perera T, Mellinghoff IK (2010) The phosphatase and tensin homolog regulates epidermal growth factor receptor (EGFR) inhibitor response by targeting EGFR for degradation. Proc Natl Acad Sci U S A 107:6459–6464. doi:0911188107[pii]10.1073/pnas.0911188107

Vogt PK, Gymnopoulos M, Hart JR (2009) PI 3-kinase and cancer: changing accents. Curr Opin Genet Dev 19:12–17. doi:S0959-437X(08)00188-3[pii]10.1016/j.gde.2008.11.011

Wang MY, Lu KV, Zhu S, Dia EQ, Vivanco I, Shackleford GM, Cavenee WK, Mellinghoff IK, Cloughesy TF, Sawyers CL, Mischel PS (2006) Mammalian target of rapamycin inhibition promotes response to epidermal growth factor receptor kinase inhibitors in PTEN-deficient and PTEN-intact glioblastoma cells. Cancer Res 66:7864–7869. doi:66/16/7864[pii]10.1158/0008-5472.CAN-04-4392

Wee S, Wiederschain D, Maira SM, Loo A, Miller C, deBeaumont R, Stegmeier F, Yao YM, Lengauer C (2008) PTEN-deficient cancers depend on PIK3CB. Proc Natl Acad Sci U S A 105:13057–13062. doi:0802655105[pii]10.1073/pnas.0802655105

Wei Q, Clarke L, Scheidenhelm DK, Qian B, Tong A, Sabha N, Karim Z, Bock NA, Reti R, Swoboda R, Purev E, Lavoie JF, Bajenaru ML, Shannon P, Herlyn D, Kaplan D, Henkelman RM, Gutmann DH, Guha A (2006) High-grade glioma formation results from postnatal pten loss or mutant epidermal growth factor receptor expression in a transgenic mouse glioma model. Cancer Res 66:7429–7437. doi:66/15/7429[pii]10.1158/0008-5472.CAN-06-0712

Weigelt B, Warne PH, Downward J (2011) PIK3CA mutation, but not PTEN loss of function, determines the sensitivity of breast cancer cells to mTOR inhibitory drugs. Oncogene 30:3222–3233. doi:onc201142[pii]10.1038/onc.2011.42

Weiss WA, Burns MJ, Hackett C, Aldape K, Hill JR, Kuriyama H, Kuriyama N, Milshteyn N, Roberts T, Wendland MF, DePinho R, Israel MA (2003) Genetic determinants of malignancy in a mouse model for oligodendroglioma. Cancer Res 63:1589–1595

Wells A, Welsh JB, Lazar CS, Wiley HS, Gill GN, Rosenfeld MG (1990) Ligand-induced transformation by a noninternalizing epidermal growth factor receptor. Science. 247(4945): 962–964. PMID:2305263

Wen PY, Yung WK, Lamborn KR, Dahia PL, Wang Y, Peng B, Abrey LE, Raizer J, Cloughesy TF, Fink K, Gilbert M, Chang S, Junck L, Schiff D, Lieberman F, Fine HA, Mehta M, Robins HI, DeAngelis LM, Groves MD, Puduvalli VK, Levin V, Conrad C,

Maher EA, Aldape K, Hayes M, Letvak L, Egorin MJ, Capdeville R, Kaplan R, Murgo AJ, Stiles C, Prados MD (2006) Phase I/II study of imatinib mesylate for recurrent malignant gliomas: North American Brain Tumor Consortium Study 99–08. Clin Cancer Res 12:4899–4907. doi:12/16/4899[pii]10.1158/1078-0432.CCR-06-0773

Wong AJ, Bigner SH, Bigner DD, Kinzler KW, Hamilton SR, Vogelstein B (1987) Increased expression of the epidermal growth factor receptor gene in malignant gliomas is invariably associated with gene amplification. Proc Natl Acad Sci U S A 84:6899–6903

Workman P, Clarke PA, Raynaud FI, van Montfort RL (2010) Drugging the PI3 kinome: from chemical tools to drugs in the clinic. Cancer Res 70:2146–2157. doi:0008-5472.CAN-09-4355[pii]10.1158/0008-5472.CAN-09-4355

Wu H, Shekar SC, Flinn RJ, El-Sibai M, Jaiswal BS, Sen KI, Janakiraman V, Seshagiri S, Gerfen GJ, Girvin ME, Backer JM (2009) Regulation of Class IA PI 3-kinases: C2 domain-iSH2 domain contacts inhibit p85/p110alpha and are disrupted in oncogenic p85 mutants. Proc Natl Acad Sci U S A 106:20258–20263. doi:0902369106[pii]10.1073/pnas.0902369106

Xu CX, Zhao L, Yue P, Fang G, Tao H, Owonikoko TK, Ramalingam SS, Khuri FR, Sun SY (2011) Augmentation of NVP-BEZ235's anticancer activity against human lung cancer cells by blockage of autophagy. Cancer Biol Ther 12. doi:16397 [pii]

Yamazaki H, Fukui Y, Ueyama Y, Tamaoki N, Kawamoto T, Taniguchi S, Shibuya M (1988) Amplification of the structurally and functionally altered epidermal growth factor receptor gene (c-erbB) in human brain tumors. Mol Cell Biol 8:1816–1820

Yu J, Deshmukh H, Gutmann RJ, Emnett RJ, Rodriguez FJ, Watson MA, Nagarajan R, Gutmann DH (2009) Alterations of BRAF and HIPK2 loci predominate in sporadic pilocytic astrocytoma. Neurology 73:1526–1531. doi:WNL.0b013e3181c0664a[pii]10.1212/WNL.0b013e3181c0664a

Zheng H, Ying H, Yan H, Kimmelman AC, Hiller DJ, Chen AJ, Perry SR, Tonon G, Chu GC, Ding Z, Stommel JM, Dunn KL, Wiedemeyer R, You MJ, Brennan C, Wang YA, Ligon KL, Wong WH, Chin L, DePinho RA (2008) p53 and Pten control neural and glioma stem/progenitor cell renewal and differentiation. Nature 455:1129–1133. doi:nature07443[-pii]10.1038/nature07443

Zhu Y, Guignard F, Zhao D, Liu L, Burns DK, Mason RP, Messing A, Parada LF (2005a) Early inactivation of p53 tumor suppressor gene cooperating with NF1 loss induces malignant astrocytoma. Cancer Cell 8:119–130. doi:S1535-6108(05)00228-X[pii]10.1016/j.ccr.2005.07.004

Zhu Y, Harada T, Liu L, Lush ME, Guignard F, Harada C, Burns DK, Bajenaru ML, Gutmann DH, Parada LF (2005b) Inactivation of NF1 in CNS causes increased glial progenitor proliferation and optic glioma formation. Development 132:5577–5588. doi:132/24/5577[pii]10.1242/dev.02162

Zhu H, Acquaviva J, Ramachandran P, Boskovitz A, Woolfenden S, Pfannl R, Bronson RT, Chen JW, Weissleder R, Housman DE, Charest A (2009) Oncogenic EGFR signaling cooperates with loss of tumor suppressor gene functions in gliomagenesis. Proc Natl Acad Sci U S A 106:2712–2716. doi:0813314106[pii]10.1073/pnas.0813314106

Zoncu R, Efeyan A, Sabatini DM (2011) mTOR: from growth signal integration to cancer, diabetes and ageing. Nat Rev Mol Cell Biol 12:21–35. doi:nrm3025[pii]10.1038/nrm3025

Part III
Perspectives

Predictive Genomic Biomarkers

Rakesh Kumar and Rafael G. Amado

Abstract Advances in the biological characterization of tumors has led to the design and development of anticancer agents targeting specific molecular alterations. The majority of these agents are designed to silence phosphorylation signals that are required for the development and maintenance of the cancer phenotype in specific tumor types. Prospective identification of cancer subsets containing particular target alterations is a requirement for these development programs, which in theory, should include smaller trials and result in larger therapeutic benefits. In this review, we will examine relevant examples of selection markers effectively utilized in oncology, and discuss important considerations pertaining to the codevelopment of drugs and diagnostics, including current regulatory paths, the incorporation of selection markers emerging late in development, and future directions in the area of personalized oncology.

Keywords Biomarker · Mutation · EGFR · KRAS · ErbB-2 · Bcr-Abl

Contents

1 Introduction	174
2 Examples for Positive and Negative Selection Markers	175
3 Co-Development of Biomarkers and Therapeutics: Regulatory Considerations	182
4 Future Directions	184
References	185

R. Kumar · R. G. Amado (✉)
Oncology Research and Development, GlaxoSmithKline,
Collegeville, PA 19426, USA
e-mail: rafael.g.amado@gsk.com

Current Topics in Microbiology and Immunology (2012) 355: 173–188
DOI: 10.1007/82_2011_164
© Springer-Verlag Berlin Heidelberg 2011
Published Online: 30 August 2011

1 Introduction

Historically, medical anti-cancer treatments have been based on broad-spectrum chemotherapy, which indiscriminately target cell proliferation or DNA metabolism, resulting, with few exceptions, in modest efficacy and high toxicity. These agents have traditionally been developed empirically in multiple tumor types without patient selection, and have formed the basis for established combination regimens in oncology indications. Subsequent additions of agents to these regimens sometimes resulted in multi-agent combinations with higher efficacy but narrower therapeutic windows than the parental regimens. Consequently, treatments have become cumbersome, and the associated small efficacy gains and added toxicities are increasingly being deemed unacceptable by patients, physicians, regulators, and payers.

Advancements in the molecular understanding of the origin of various cancers have led to the development of precise treatment approaches that match designer molecules to targets identified through biological characterization of tumors. These agents are simplifying existing treatments, and are delivering significantly greater therapeutic benefits in specific indications. Focused development programs that employ patient selection are improving the therapeutic windows of new drugs by limiting indications to selected patient populations. Patient selection is based on either positive predictive markers that select populations sensitive to the therapeutic or negative selection markers that enrich for sensitive populations by excluding non-responders. While an early example of targeted therapy can be found in the use of antiestrogens and aromatase inhibitors for patients with hormone receptor positive breast cancer, these advances in precision medicine have generally followed more recent discoveries in cancer genetics and signal transduction.

Driver oncogenes can be classified in a number of protein classes, e.g., kinases, transcription factors, GTPases, nuclear receptors, cell surface receptors, and other enzyme classes. To date, clinical success in oncology using targeted therapeutics is largely due to blockade of oncogenic kinases, either by small molecule inhibitors or by antibodies targeting cell surface receptor tyrosine kinases. Kinases are enzymes that phosphorylate proteins or lipids leading to change in their functional activity. Of the 518 identified human kinases, a small proportion has been shown to be activated in different tumors by mutation, amplification, translocation, overexpression, or dysregulation of upstream events. Positive predictive biomarkers generally measure the various activated states of the drug target, and usually form the basis for development of therapeutics from the inception of the development programs. Negative predictors, on the other hand, can include activation of other components of the signal pathway being targeted, or of alternative pathways, and as such, are more diverse and challenging to identify early on in the drug development process. In this review, we will describe the relevant examples illustrating the use of both positive and negative predictive markers for development of small molecules and biologic agents targeting oncogenic kinases. We will also review regulatory considerations important to attain this goal of precision medicine in oncology.

2 Examples for Positive and Negative Selection Markers

1. *ErbB-2 (Her2/neu)-directed therapy*: Interdiction of the ErbB-2 oncogene is regarded as the first example of precision medicine in oncology. ErbB-2 amplification and overexpression have been reported in a number of human tumors including approximately 25% of human breast cancers as well as in subsets of patients with ovarian cancers, gastric carcinoma, and salivary gland tumors (Baselga and Swain 2009; Slamon et al. 1987). In breast cancer patients, ErbB-2 overexpression correlates with an aggressive phenotype and poor prognosis. Trastuzumab, a humanized monoclonal antibody directed against the extracellular domain of the ErbB-2 receptor, is highly active against ErbB-2 overexpressing breast cancer. From the inception of the development program, trastuzumab was developed as a targeted therapeutic coupled to a diagnostic test, namely immunohistochemistry. The efficacy and safety of trastuzumab was evaluated in a Phase III randomized trial of 469 women with ErbB-2 overexpressed metastatic breast cancer (Slamon et al. 2001). Patients were randomized to receive standard chemotherapy with trastuzumab ($N = 235$) or standard chemotherapy alone ($N = 234$). Both time to progression (TTP) and overall survival (OS) were longer in the trastuzumab arm (median TTP was 7.4 vs. 4.6 months; $P < 0.001$, and median OS was 25.1 vs. 20.3 months; $P = 0.046$, for trastuzumab and control respective). FDA approved Trastuzumab in 1998 for the treatment of Her2/neu overexpressing metastatic breast cancer. In 2006, the label was expanded to include adjuvant treatment after several trials showed reductions in the rate of relapse of approximately 50% and improvement in OS of 33% when trastuzumab is delivered concurrently or sequentially with chemotherapy in women with node-positive or high-risk node-negative ErbB-2 positive breast cancer (Joensuu et al. 2006; Piccart-Gebhart et al. 2005; Romond et al. 2005). Lapatinib, a small molecule tyrosine kinase inhibitor of both epidermal growth factor receptor (EGFR) and ErbB-2 has also shown prolongation of TTP when given in combination with capecitabine to patients with ErbB-2 positive, trastuzumab-refractory breast cancer (Geyer et al. 2006).

By all accounts, trastuzumab has been a true example of personalized medicine drug development (see also "Adjuvant Trials of Targeted Agents: The Newest Battleground in the War on Cancer"), where a therapeutic was coupled with a diagnostic aimed to detect a particular molecular alteration from the inception of the program. The initial approval of trastuzumab in 1998 occurred together with the approval of an immunohistochemistry (IHC) test (HercepTest[TM]) for the detection of ErbB-2 overexpression. Overexpression was defined as 2+ or 3+ staining. Accrual of ErbB-2 positive patients to the pivotal trastuzumab trials drastically shortened the time needed to demonstrate drug effect in ErbB-2 positive patients. However, since marker negative patients were not studied, the original trial did not establish the lack of effect of trastuzumab in ErbB-2 negative patients. Subsequent studies showed lack of activity of trastuzumab in patients with 0 or 1+, non-amplified ErbB-2 status (Seidman et al. 2004).

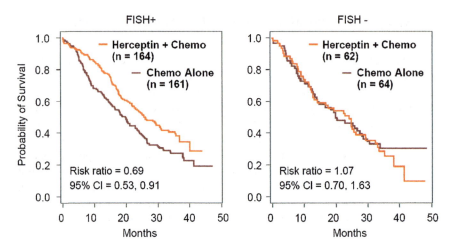

Fig. 1 Retrospective analyses of overall survival outcomes by treatment arm (chemotherapy vs. chemotherapy plus trastuzumab) of patients with metastatic breast cancer selected for Her2–Neu expression in the trastuzumab pivotal trial H0648g (Slamon et al. 1987). Results are displayed by FISH score (*top panel*, FISH positive subgroup, *bottom panel*, FISH negative subgroup) (from Mass et al. 2005)

Presently, several commercial assays are FDA approved for the selection of patients eligible for treatment with trastuzumab. These include two IHC assays (HercepTest™ and Pathway® HER-2/neu) and two HER2 FISH assays (PathVysion® and pharmDx™). Approval of FISH assays by FDA in 2002 relied on retrospective bridging studies to ascertain concordance with the IHC Hercep-Test™. These analyses suggested no benefit for trastuzumab in patients with IHC positive, FISH negative tumors (Fig. 1) (Mass et al. 2005). FISH positivity is now thought to be required for activity of ErbB-2-directed therapy in IHC 2+ tumors. The American Society of Clinical Oncology together with the College of American Pathologists issued guidelines to standardize clinical testing of ErbB-2 using both IHC and FISH (Wolff et al. 2007).

Despite the success of trastuzumab and lapatinib, breast cancer in some patients with ErbB-2 amplification does not respond to these therapies, and those who respond eventually develop resistance. Understanding the mechanism of both primary and secondary resistance to ErbB-2 targeted therapies is being pursued both in laboratories and in translational clinical studies. For instance, a truncated form of ErbB-2 receptor is postulated to mediate resistance to trastuzumab in a fraction of ErbB-2 positive tumors (Arribas et al. 2011). A number of a novel ErbB-2 targeted agents, including antibodies, antibody–drug conjugates, vaccines, and small molecule kinase inhibitors, are in various stages of clinical development (Bedard et al. 2009; Browne et al. 2009). Understanding the biological mechanism of resistance to ErbB2-directed therapy may result in the advent of targeted secondary therapies which will likely involve novel diagnostic biomarkers.

2. *Anti-EGFR antibodies in colorectal cancer*: While trastuzumab is widely recognized to be an example of personalized therapy, where an effective biomarker existed in the program since its inception, the story of anti-EGFR antibodies in colorectal cancer (CRC) reflects the evolution of science during the development programs of a therapeutic, resulting in the adaptation of ongoing clinical research to incorporate scientific discoveries.

EGFR is overexpressed in many human tumors of different histologies. Two different monoclonal antibodies directed against EGFR, cetuximab, and panitumumab, are now approved for metastatic colorectal cancer and have shown improved response rate, TTP, or progression-free survival (PFS), and in the case of cetuximab, OS (Cunningham et al. 2004; Jonker et al. 2007; Van Cutsem et al. 2007). Like trastuzumab, these agents were developed in CRC with EGFR IHC as a selection biomarker. Subsequent studies found that expression of EGFR is not a reliable predictor of clinical outcome (Chung et al. 2005). While it is acknowledged that the presence of the target must be a requirement for anti-tumor activity, this lack of ability to predict response based on EGFR status highlights the limitations of testing therapeutics in biomarker positive populations only, when the role of the target is not sufficiently characterized. There are a number of possible explanations for the demonstrated lack of relationship between clinical outcomes in patients treated with EGFR-inhibiting antibodies and EGFR expression measured by IHC, including variability in staining with different tissue fixation techniques, interobserver variability with regard to scoring, tissue sample storage time, and site of tissue collection (primary tumor vs. metastatic) (Atkins et al. 2004).

As anti-EGFR antibodies were approved in the broad EGFR-expressing CRC population, mutations in the downstream signaling components of the EGFR pathway were being investigated as alternative predictive biomarkers of activity. Initially validated in retrospective analysis, the mutational status of the KRAS oncogene is now recognized as a reliable negative predictive marker of activity for these agents. KRAS is a member of the RAS family of small G-proteins involved in intracellular signaling. When receptor tyrosine kinases such as EGFR bind ligands (such as EGF, TGF-α, epiregulin, or amphiregulin), the receptor dimerizes and undergoes a conformational change that results in phosphorylation of tyrosine residues within the intracellular domain, which in turn leads to activation of protein kinase signaling cascades including the Ras-Raf-MAP kinase pathway (Malumbres and Barbacid 2003). Activation of KRAS kinase activity occurs upon binding of GTP. Deactivation of the kinase activity in normal cells occurs when GTP is hydrolyzed; however, oncogenic mutations in KRAS have been described in which GTP signaling is constitutive (Bos 1989). Constitutive activation of the Ras-Raf-MAP Kinase pathway as a result of KRAS mutation results was postulated to result in resistance to inhibition of upstream elements of the pathway, such as EGFR. Activating KRAS mutations are among the most commonly found oncogenic mutations (Bos 1989).

The first evidence of the utility of KRAS genotyping arose from single-arm clinical trial retrospective series where responses were largely confined to subjects whose tumors harbored wild-type KRAS (Benvenuti et al. 2007;

De Roock et al. 2008; Di Fiore et al. 2007; Lievre et al. 2006). The first demonstration of KRAS mutational status as a predictive biomarker of resistance to an anti-EGFR antibody arose from the retrospective analysis of a randomized controlled trial of panitumumab in patients with chemotherapy refractory metastatic CRC. The study randomized patients to panitumumab monotherapy or best supportive care (BSC), and allowed patients progressing on BSC to receive panitumumab in an open label single-arm study. In the primary analysis, a statistically significant improvement in PFS was observed for the panitumumab arm (HR $= 0.542$, 95% CI: 0.443, 0.663; $P < 0.0001$). Response rate was 10% in the panitumumab versus 0 in the BSC arm. No differences in OS were observed likely due to panitumumab treatment upon progression in the majority of patients randomized to the BSC arm.

Based on phase II data, a hypothesis was postulated that the treatment effect on PFS in this study would be larger among patients with wild-type versus mutant-KRAS status. Blinded to KRAS status, a statistical analysis plan was designed to confirm the KRAS hypothesis. In this study, pre-treatment tumor biopsy samples were available for all patients due to the central laboratory determination of EGFR by IHC for study eligibility. The primary objective of the KRAS analysis was to assess whether the effect of panitumumab on PFS was significantly greater among subjects with wild-type versus mutant-KRAS status. The secondary objective was to assess whether panitumumab plus BSC improve PFS and response rate compared with BSC alone for subjects having tumors with wild-type KRAS. Analysis of KRAS mutation status was performed with an assay that utilizes allele-specific PCR amplification using amplification refractory mutation system technology (ARMS^{TM}) by means of real-time PCR (Newton et al. 1989; Thelwell et al. 2000). KRAS status was determined in 92% of subjects. PFS was statistically significantly prolonged with panitumumab treatment in the wild-type versus mutant-KRAS stratum (quantitative interaction test $P < 0.0001$) (Fig. 2). The hazard ratio (95% CI) in the wild-type stratum was 0.45 (0.34–0.59), versus 0.99 (0.73–1.36) in the mutant stratum. All responses were in the wild-type KRAS strata (17 vs. 0%). Likely due to the rapid high rate of crossover, the difference in OS within the wild-type KRAS stratum was not statistically significant [HR $= 0.99$ (95% CI: 0.75–1.29); $P = 0.139$] (Amado et al. 2008).

Similar results were obtained with the antibody cetuximab. NCIC CO.17/BMS-025 was a randomized Phase III study of cetuximab and best BSC versus BSC in subjects with chemotherapy pretreated EGFR-positive metastatic CRC. Crossover to cetuximab from BSC was not allowed in this trial. Addition of cetuximab prolonged survival in the overall study population; the median survival was 6.1 months in cetuximab plus BSC arm versus 4.6 months in BSC alone arm [HR $= 0.77$ (95% CI: 0.64–0.92); $P = 0.0046$] (Jonker et al. 2007). A retrospective analysis of efficacy by KRAS status was conducted (Karapetis et al. 2008). Of the overall study population, 69% of tumor samples were evaluable for KRAS analyses. Cetuximab provided significant improvement in OS in subjects with KRAS wild-type tumors (median OS 9.5 months vs. 4.8 months in BSC alone, HR $= 0.55$; 95% CI, 0.41–0.74; $P < 0.001$). As was observed with

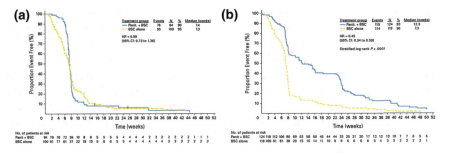

Fig. 2 Progression-free survival (PFS) by randomized treatment in (**a**) mutant, and (**b**) wild-type KRAS groups treatment in patients with colorectal cancer treated with either panitumumab or best supportive care (BSC). PFS Hazard ratios (HR) are shown for panitumumab (panit.) versus BSC adjusted for randomization factors (Eastern Cooperative Oncology Group score, geographic region) (from Amado et al. 2008)

panitumumab, subjects with KRAS mutations did not derive benefit from the addition of cetuximab to BSC. Moreover, the results showed that KRAS is not a prognostic factor in CRC, but a strong predictor for cetuximab activity.

Similar results have been obtained in the setting of combination chemotherapy with both antibodies. The data with cetuximab in this setting are retrospective. In untreated patients, a modest improvement in PFS was observed when cetuximab was added to FOLFIRI (median PFS in cetuximab + FOLFIRI arm was 8.9 months vs. 8.0 months with FOLFIRI alone; HR = 0.85; 95% CI, 0.72–0.99; $P = 0.048$). KRAS analyses in a subset of patients with sample availability showed that the benefit of adding cetuximab to FOLFIRI was confined to subjects with KRAS wild-type (Van Cutsem et al. 2009). A phase III study of irinotecan with or without cetuximab in second line also showed results in a retrospective analysis that segregated by KRAS status (Sobrero et al. 2008). A recent study of panitumumab established the role of this biomarker prospectively in the combination setting. This study compared the efficacy of panitumumab in combination with FOLFIRI chemotherapy to FOLFIRI alone, in patients with previously treated metastatic CRC. A total of 1,186 subjects were randomized; KRAS ascertainment was 91%. PFS was superior in the treatment arm with a median of 5.9 months versus 3.9 months (HR = 0.73, 95% CI: 0.59–0.90; $P = 0.004$). No differences in OS were observed, and there were no significant differences in PFS or OS between arms in the KRAS mutant group (Peeters et al. 2010).

The accrual of biomarker negative (mutant KRAS) patients in panitumumab and cetuximab trials allowed us to establish its predictive value, and has led to a finding with important clinical consequences, namely that subjects with mutant KRAS tumors treated with oxaliplatin-based chemotherapy and either anti-EGFR antibodies, experience worse outcomes compared to chemotherapy alone. This finding was first suggested by a phase II studies of FOLFOX with or without cetuximab (Bokemeyer et al. 2009), and was recently prospectively confirmed in a phase III randomized trial of FOLFOX with or without panitumumab (Douillard et al. 2010). This phenomenon appears to be specific for the use of FOLFOX chemotherapy in combination with these antibodies; the reasons for these findings are unknown and may include excess toxicity compromising chemotherapy delivery or induction of resistance to oxaliplatin by EGFR inhibitors.

3. *Anti-EGFR small molecules in non-small cell lung cancer*: Small molecule inhibitors of EGFR tyrosine kinase have been developed in non-small cell lung cancer (NSCLC) as second and third line therapies in the metastatic setting, with one of the agents, namely erlotinib, demonstrating a survival benefit compared to BSC (Shepherd et al. 2005) (see also EGFR Mutant Lung Cancer). When used in combination with chemotherapy, no clinical benefit was demonstrated. Early in development it was identified that the benefit was realized at the expense of about 10% of patients who had rapid and impressive responses to treatment. Clinical characteristics that defined this responsive population included non-smoker women with adenocarcinoma, and patients of Asian descent. Subsequent work identified that specific somatic mutations in the tyrosine kinase domain of EGFR resulting in ligand-independent receptor activation were present at higher frequency in patients with these characteristics (Lynch et al. 2004; Paez et al. 2004), specifically, base pair deletions at exon19 (del 746–750) and point mutations at exon 21 (L858R). Although the initial studies with EGFR kinase inhibitors in NSCLC did not select patients with activated EGFR, retrospective analysis and subsequent studies clearly demonstrate the role of somatic mutations in EGFR gene. These alterations are found in 5–20% of Caucasians and 20–40% of Asian patients with NSCLC. The presence of activating mutations has been associated with a high response rate of up to 80%, compared with <10% in patients with wild-type EGFR (John et al. 2009). A secondary mutation in codon 790 (T790 M) in the EGFR gene has been associated with approximately 50% of cases with acquired resistance (Pao et al. 2005), and overexpression of the MET gene has also been implicated in resistance to anti-EGFR agents (Engelman et al. 2007).

The discovery of EGFR mutations rendering tumors highly sensitive to small molecule EGFR inhibitors represents another example of biological findings evolving after therapeutics are developed and drugs are already in the market. Two studies have established the role of EGFR mutations as selection markers for anti-EGFR therapy in NSCLC. One study performed in East Asia enriched for patients with EGFR mutations by selecting for clinical characteristics such as adenocarcinoma histology and non-or former light smokers (Mok et al. 2009). Patients were randomized to receive gefitinib ($N = 609$) or carboplatin and pac-litaxel ($N = 608$). PFS was superior in the gefitinib arm (HR = 0.74; 95% CI: 0.65–0.85; $P < 0.001$), with a more pronounced effect observed in the subgroup of patients ($N = 261$) who were positive for EGFR mutations (HR = 0.48; 95% CI, 0.36–0.64; $P < 0.001$). Interestingly, an inferior outcome was observed with gefitinib in the subgroup of patients ($N = 176$) without EGFR mutations, (HR = 2.85; 95% CI, 2.05–3.98; $P < 0.001$) highlighting the importance of genotyping over clinical selection. Another study screened 2,105 patients with adenocarcinoma of the lung for EGFR mutations. Mutations were identified in 350 of 2,105 patients (16.6%). PFS and OS for those patients with mutations who received erlotinib were 14 months and 27 months, respectively (Rosell et al. 2009). After a decade of research of anti-EGFR small molecules in NSCLC, these studies determined that EGFR mutant NSCLC is a distinct clinical entity that should be treated with anti-EGFR small molecules regardless of line of therapy, and firmly established the role of EGFR genotyping in NSCLC.

4. *Bcr-Abl-directed therapies*: A prime example of targeted therapy in oncology associated with a predictive marker is chronic myelogenous leukemia (CML) (Will Kinase Inhibitors Make it as GlioBlastoma Drugs?). This entity is defined by the Bcr-Abl translocation. Imatinib, a small molecule kinase inhibitor of Abl kinase, is currently the first line therapy for CML owing to high activity in patients with all stages of the disease (Druker et al. 2001). The development of imatinib in CML resulting in its commercial availability spurred research into other clinical entities defined by alterations also addressed by imatinib, such as platelet derived growth factor (PDGF) rearrangements in myelodysplastic and hypereosinophilic syndromes, and c-Kit and PDGFR alterations in gastrointestinal stromal tumors (GIST) (see below). Despite the impressive activity of imatinib in CML, acquired resistance has been observed. Dose escalation with imatinib is used in some patients who do not respond to the standard dose of 400 mg. Imatinib resistance is generally associated with point mutations in the Abl kinase domain of Bcr-Abl, leading to reactivation of Bcr-Abl signaling. Although many mutations have been reported, amino acid substitutions at 13 residues may account for approximately 90% of all resistance-associated mutations (Hughes et al. 2006; O'Hare et al. 2005; Soverini et al. 2006).

Two second generation Abl kinase inhibitors with activity against imatinib-resistant Bcr-Abl mutants, nilotinib, and dasatinib, are now approved. Nilotinib is a more potent analog of imatinib, with in vitro evidence suggesting activity against all imatinib-resistant Bcr-Abl mutations except T315I, and with diminished activity against P-loop mutations and other imatinib-resistant mutations, including F359C 47 (O'Hare et al. 2005; Weisberg et al. 2005). In clinical studies, nilotinib showed activity in patients with many imatinib-resistant Bcr-Abl mutations (except T315I) (Cortes et al. 2007; Kantarjian et al. 2007).

Dasatinib, is a multi-targeted kinase inhibitor with activity against Src family kinases, c-kit, and Abl kinases (Shah et al. 2004). Differences in the binding mode to Abl kinase, may explain why dasatinib is active against the majority of imatinib-resistant mutations, except T315I. Clinical studies have validated preclinical data as patients with imatinib-resistant Bcr-Abl mutations have responded to dasatinib (Talpaz et al. 2006). Although nilotinib and dasatinib provide options to patients with imatinib-resistant mutations, secondary resistance to these agents has already been observed at the expense of additional mutations rather than additional genetic alterations (Cortes et al. 2007; O'Hare et al. 2008). In general, dasatinib may be more effective in patients with P-loop or F359C mutations; nilotinib may be more effective in those with F317L mutations. Recently, dasatinib has been proven superior to imatinib as first line agent in CML (Kantarjian et al. 2010). Quantitative RT-PCR for Bcr-Abl rearrangement, is routinely used to monitor response to therapy with these agents.

5. *Kit and PDGFRα-directed therapies*: GIST carry c-Kit mutations in approximately 80% of cases, with another 6% harboring PDGFRα mutations. IHC for CD117 (c-Kit) is used in the diagnosis of this clinical entity. Most of the c-Kit

mutations are located in the juxtamembrane region (exon 11; 68%) or the extra-cellular region (exon 9; 10%), whereas mutations in the kinase I (exon 13) and kinase II (exon 17) domains occur in 1% each (Corless and Heinrich 2008). Responsiveness to imatinib is related to the type of c-Kit mutation, with 71% response rate in patients with exon 11 mutations compared to 38 and 28% in patients with exon 9 mutation or wild-type c-Kit respectively. PFS and overall survival are also significantly superior for imatinib-treated patients with c-Kit exon 11 mutations than for those with c-Kit exon 9 mutations, or wild-type c-Kit tumors (Corless and Heinrich 2008; Nilsson et al. 2009). Although several of the PDGFRα mutations observed in GIST are sensitive to imatinib, D842 V is imatinib-resistant (Heinrich et al. 2006a). In one-half to two-third of patients who initially respond to imatinib, acquired resistance is observed due to secondary mutations in c-Kit. Although the acquired mutations are present in exons 13, 14, and 17, the most common secondary mutation is the V654A, mainly in GIST harboring an exon 11 primary mutation (Maleddu et al. 2009).

Sunitinib is a multi-targeted small molecule kinase inhibitor with high affinity for c-Kit, PDGFRα and β, VEGFR1-3, RET, FLT-3, and a number of other kinases (Grimaldi et al. 2007). Sunitinib has shown an improvement in both the TTP and OS in imatinib-resistant GIST patients. The best responses were seen in patients with primary KIT exon 9 mutations or wt tumors; also patients with acquired KIT exon 13 or PDGFRA exon 14 mutations (kinase I regions) had benefit of such treatment (Demetri et al. 2006; Heinrich et al. 2006b). The inhibitory effect of sunitinib on c-Kit kinase activity was not substantially affected by secondary mutations in TK1. However, GIST with TK2 secondary mutations was resistant to sunitinib treatment (Heinrich et al. 2007). As with CML, extensive characterization of the alterations of the oncogenic targets, and the availability of several therapies with diverse molecular specificity, underscore the need for customized therapy in these diseases guided by validated companion diagnostics.

3 Co-Development of Biomarkers and Therapeutics: Regulatory Considerations

Diagnostics are central to personalized medicine. The standard for approval by FDA of in vitro diagnostic devices (IVD) are, as with drugs, safety, and efficacy. Because IVDs are used to drive clinical decisions, the risk for the test is equivalent to the risk for the drug whose use is guided by the test result. In the United States, companion diagnostics follow two development paths. FDA review class II and III tests through processes termed pre-marketing notification and pre-marketing application. These reviews involve elements of analytical performance (accuracy, precision, specificity, limit of detection), and clinical validity, and are limited to IVDs and not laboratory-developed tests (LDT). LTDs are generally developed by laboratory and pathology practices and evolve with the practice of medicine. They are regulated under the 1988 Clinical Laboratory Improvement Amendments (CLIA), which involves Centers for Medicare and Medicaid Services (CMS) oversight and certification of clinical laboratory quality, including physician office laboratories. CLIA-certification is required for Medicare and Medicaid reimbursement. These pathways are not in conflict. Indeed, as new discoveries elicit new understandings of disease, tests are first developed by laboratory and pathology experts in academic institutions and eventually offered in CLIA-certified laboratories. Overtime, tests are optimized, standardized, and developed in the form of IVD kits that are eventually cleared by FDA. For instance, while HercepTest[TM] and PathVysion[®] are FDA approved IVDs, current tests measuring KRAS for use with anti-EGFR antibodies, EGFR mutations for small molecule anti-EGFR therapy in NSCLC, and mutational analysis tests to guide CML and GIST therapy are LTDs performed in CLIA laboratories. Although these paths can be seen as complementary, it is worth noting that FDA approval of IVDs generally require clinical validation in the context of lengthy and costly research programs, whereas LTDs are generally cleared based on analytical performance and generally do not undergo FDA review.

While ideally biomarkers should be validated prospectively in clinical trials, retrospective validation may be adequate under certain circumstances, and should arguably be sufficient to gain regulatory approval when analyses meet certain conditions. These include (a) the hypothesis that a given biomarker may have clinical applicability should arise independently from the sample that will be used for retrospective validation, (b) to avoid multiple testing error, only one biomarker should be tested in the validation samples, (c) the analyses need to be sufficiently powered and prespecified before knowledge of test results, (d) the test should be analytically validated and, ideally, testing should be performed by an independent laboratory without patient-level knowledge of clinical outcomes and (e) ascertainment of marker status should be available in the large majority of subjects. Examples of biomarkers identified via retrospective analyses include FISH selection for trastuzumab (performed using bridging studies), KRAS for EGFR-inhibiting antibodies, EGFR mutations for small molecule EGFR inhibitors, and OncotypeDx for chemotherapy in ER positive/node negative breast cancer. An advantage of retrospective validation is that it allows for the assessment of the predictive potential of the biomarker in both biomarker positive and negative patients. Indeed, biomarkers used for patient selection upfront where subjects without biomarker positive are not randomized cannot be characterized for sensitivity, specificity, or negative predictive value, as no reliable information about outcomes in biomarker negative patients is generally available. This practice should only be employed in situations where there is sufficient information to ensure that the therapeutic being tested would not be effective in biomarker negative patients, and where the biomarker is sufficiently well characterized on its ability to reliably segregate patients into positive and negative groups. Indeed the broad applicability of a practice of studying biomarker negative patients would negate an obvious advantage of the use of selection markers, namely the ability to conduct smaller trials that lead to effective patient allocation and resource utilization. However, such an approach is not optimal for markers not well characterized preclinically and in Phase II trials in non-selected populations (as was the case for EGFR IHC in the case of anti-EGFR antibodies in CRC), or for tests not validated to read in binary format.

4 Future Directions

Kinase inhibitors have proven successful in the treatment of patients with certain tumors containing activation of the target kinase. Additional examples of effective interdiction of kinase targets resulting in clinical benefit, such as BRAF inhibitors in melanoma ("Targeting Oncogenic Braf in Human Cancer"), and JAK-2 inhibitors in myelofibrosis (JAK-Muatant Myeloproliferative Neoplasms) continue to emerge (Flaherty et al. 2010; Verstovsek et al. 2010). There are however, a large number of tumors in which kinase inhibitors may not be effective. Kinases represent a small fraction of the human proteome and thus other protein classes will need to be exploited in drug discovery. Transcription factors compose one such class of targets; these are often dysregulated in various cancers, e.g., ETS, HIF-1a, β-catenin, Myc, etc. Developing small molecule inhibitors against transcription factors has historically been challenging as it involves interfering with protein–protein or protein–DNA interactions; however, there is emerging data suggesting potential opportunities with this target class (Berg 2008). Similarly, there are active efforts to target epigenetic changes (acetylation, methylation), proteosomal pathway (ubiquitylation), metabolism, and stem cells.

Secondary resistance will occur with most targeted agents, as is evident from Bcr-Abl, Kit, EGFR, and other kinase inhibitor experiences, thus necessitating the next generation of agents either against the same or other targets or pathways. Combinations of targeted agents with the hope of circumventing resistance, a concept borrowed from the infectious disease field, is being evaluated in the clinic with several agents, driven by encouraging preclinical data, e.g., PI3K and MAPK pathway inhibitors.

The field of oncology is evolving from a setting where multiple, non-specific anti-proliferative agents existed against tumors characterized morphologically and by location, to a setting where diagnosis is made on the basis of cell of origin and molecular characteristics, and where drugs are often defining the biology of the disease through retrospective discoveries that elucidate the correct alteration addressed by already existing targeted agents (e.g., KRAS and anti-EGFR antibodies in CRC, EGFR mutations, and anti-EGFR small molecules in NSCLC). Ideally, future development programs will co-develop therapeutics with effective molecular diagnostics from the inception of the development programs, leading to smaller trials, lower attrition in phase III, and larger therapeutic benefit in clinically important endpoints, including potentially cures. While other targets are emerging, kinases such as FLT3, BRAF, ALK, c-MET, JAK2, PI3K, AKT, and RET continue to be exploited with custom-designed therapies coupled with companion diagnostics. The success obtained with kinase inhibitors, as therapeutic

Predictive Genomic Biomarkers

tools at the forefront of this paradigm change in oncology care, illustrates that the goal of personalized medicine in oncology is attainable, and while for the majority of cancer patients this goal is not yet met, the field provides researchers, drug developers, and physicians with important challenges and opportunities.

References

Amado RG, Wolf M, Peeters M, Van Cutsem E, Siena S, Freeman DJ, Juan T, Sikorski R, Suggs S, Radinsky R (2008) Wild-type KRAS is required for panitumumab efficacy in patients with metastatic colorectal cancer. J Clin Oncol 26:1626–1634

Arribas J, Baselga J, Pedersen K, Parra-Palau JL (2011) p95HER2 and breast cancer. Cancer Res 71:1515–1519

Atkins D, Reiffen KA, Tegtmeier CL, Winther H, Bonato MS, Störkel S (2004) Immunohistochemical detection of EGFR in paraffin-embedded tumor tissues. J Histochem Cytochem 52:893–901

Baselga J, Swain SM (2009) Novel anticancer targets: revisiting ERBB2 and discovering ERBB3. Nat Rev Cancer 9:463–475

Bedard PL, de Azambuja E, Cardoso F (2009) Beyond trastuzumab: overcoming resistance to targeted HER-2 therapy in breast cancer. Curr Cancer Drug Targets 9:148–162

Benvenuti S, Sartore-Bianchi A, Di Nicolantonio F, Zanon C, Moroni M, Veronese S, Siena S, Bardelli A (2007) Oncogenic activation of the RAS/RAF signaling pathway impairs the response of metastatic colorectal cancers to anti-epidermal growth factor receptor antibody therapies. Cancer Res 67:2643–2648

Berg T (2008) Inhibition of transcription factors with small organic molecules. Curr Opin Chem Biol 12:464–471

Bokemeyer C, Bondarenko I, Makhson A, Hartmann JT, Aparicio J, de Braud F, Donea S, Ludwig H, Schuch G, Stroh C (2009) Fluorouracil, leucovorin, and oxaliplatin with and without cetuximab in the first-line treatment of metastatic colorectal cancer. J Clin Oncol 27:663–671

Bos JL (1989) Ras oncogenes in human cancer: a review. Cancer Res 49:4682–4689

Browne BC, OBrien N, Duffy MJ, Crown J, ODonovan N (2009) HER-2 signaling and inhibition in breast cancer. Curr Cancer Drug Targets 9:419–438

Chung KY, Shia J, Kemeny NE, Shah M, Schwartz GK, Tse A, Hamilton A, Pan D, Schrag D, Schwartz L (2005) Cetuximab shows activity in colorectal cancer patients with tumors that do not express the epidermal growth factor receptor by immunohistochemistry. J Clin Oncol 23:1803–1810

Corless CL, Heinrich MC (2008) Molecular pathobiology of gastrointestinal stromal sarcomas. Annu Rev Pathol 3:557–586

Cortes J, Jabbour E, Kantarjian H, Yin CC, Shan J, O'Brien S, Garcia-Manero G, Giles F, Breeden M, Reeves N (2007) Dynamics of BCR-ABL kinase domain mutations in chronic myeloid leukemia after sequential treatment with multiple tyrosine kinase inhibitors. Blood 110:4005–4011

Cunningham D, Humblet Y, Siena S, Khayat D, Bleiberg H, Santoro A, Bets D, Mueser M, Harstrick A, Verslype C (2004) Cetuximab monotherapy and cetuximab plus irinotecan in irinotecan-refractory metastatic colorectal cancer. New Engl J Med 351:337–345

De Roock W, Piessevaux H, De Schutter J, Janssens M, De Hertogh G, Personeni N, Biesmans B, Van Laethem JL, Peeters M, Humblet Y (2008) KRAS wild-type state predicts survival and is associated to early radiological response in metastatic colorectal cancer treated with cetuximab. Ann Oncol 19:508–515

Demetri GD, van Oosterom AT, Garrett CR, Blackstein ME, Shah MH, Verweij J, McArthur G, Judson IR, Heinrich MC, Morgan JA (2006) Efficacy and safety of sunitinib in patients with advanced gastrointestinal stromal tumour after failure of imatinib: a randomised controlled trial. Lancet 368:1329–1338

Di Fiore F, Blanchard F, Charbonnier F, Le Pessot F, Lamy A, Galais MP, Bastit L, Killian A, Sesboüé R, Tuech JJ (2007) Clinical relevance of KRAS mutation detection in metastatic colorectal cancer treated by cetuximab plus chemotherapy. Br J Cancer 96:1166–1169

Douillard JY, Siena S, Cassidy J, Tabernero J, Burkes R, Barugel M, Humblet Y, Bodoky G, Cunningham D, Jassem J (2010) Randomized, phase III trial of panitumumab with infusional fluorouracil, leucovorin, and oxaliplatin (FOLFOX4) versus FOLFOX4 alone as first-line treatment in patients with previously untreated metastatic colorectal cancer: the PRIME study. J Clin Oncol 28:4697–4705

Druker BJ, Talpaz M, Resta DJ, Peng B, Buchdunger E, Ford JM, Lydon NB, Kantarjian H, Capdeville R, Ohno-Jones S (2001) Efficacy and safety of a specific inhibitor of the BCR-ABL tyrosine kinase in chronic myeloid leukemia. New Engl J Med 344:1031–1037

Engelman JA, Zejnullahu K, Mitsudomi T, Song Y, Hyland C, Park JO, Lindeman N, Gale CM, Zhao X, Christensen J (2007) MET amplification leads to gefitinib resistance in lung cancer by activating ERBB3 signaling. Science 316:1039–1043

Flaherty KT, Puzanov I, Kim KB, Ribas A, McArthur GA, Sosman JA, O'Dwyer PJ, Lee RJ, Grippo JF, Nolop K (2010) Inhibition of mutated, activated BRAF in metastatic melanoma. New Engl J Med 363:809–819

Geyer CE, Forster J, Lindquist D, Chan S, Romieu CG, Pienkowski T, Jagiello-Gruszfeld A, Crown J, Chan A, Kaufman B (2006) Lapatinib plus capecitabine for HER2-positive advanced breast cancer. New Engl J Med 355:2733–2743

Grimaldi AM, Guida T, D'Attino R, Perrotta E, Otero M, Masala A, Cartení G (2007) Sunitinib: bridging present and future cancer treatment. Ann Oncol 18:31–34

Heinrich MC, Corless CL, Blanke CD, Demetri GD, Joensuu H, Roberts PJ, Eisenberg BL, von Mehren M, Fletcher CDM, Sandau K (2006a) Molecular correlates of imatinib resistance in gastrointestinal stromal tumors. J Clin Oncol 24:4764–4774

Heinrich MC, Maki RG, Corless CL, Antonescu CR, Fletcher JA, Fletcher CD, Huang X, Baum CM, Demetri GD (2006b) Sunitinib (SU) response in imatinib-resistant (IM-R) GIST correlates with KIT and PDGFRA mutation status. J Clin Oncol 24:9502

Heinrich MC, Corless CL, Liegl B, Fletcher CD, Raut CP, Donsky R, Bertagnolli MM, Harlow A, Demetri GD, Fletcher JA (2007) Mechanisms of sunitinib malate (SU) resistance in gastrointestinal stromal tumors (GISTs). J Clin Oncol 25:10006

Hughes T, Deininger M, Hochhaus A, Branford S, Radich J, Kaeda J, Baccarani M, Cortes J, Cross NCP, Druker BJ (2006) Monitoring CML patients responding to treatment with tyrosine kinase inhibitors: review and recommendations for harmonizing current methodology for detecting BCR-ABL transcripts and kinase domain mutations and for expressing results. Blood 108:28–37

Joensuu H, Kellokumpu-Lehtinen PL, Bono P, Alanko T, Kataja V, Asola R, Utriainen T, Kokko R, Hemminki A, Tarkkanen M (2006) Adjuvant docetaxel or vinorelbine with or without trastuzumab for breast cancer. New Engl J Med 354:809–820

John T, Liu G, Tsao MS (2009) Overview of molecular testing in non-small-cell lung cancer: mutational analysis, gene copy number, protein expression and other biomarkers of EGFR for the prediction of response to tyrosine kinase inhibitors. Oncogene 28:S14–S23

Jonker DJ, O'Callaghan CJ, Karapetis CS, Zalcberg JR, Tu D, Au HJ, Berry SR, Krahn M, Price T, Simes RJ (2007) Cetuximab for the treatment of colorectal cancer. New Engl J Med 357:2040–2048

Kantarjian HM, Giles F, Gattermann N, Bhalla K, Alimena G, Palandri F, Ossenkoppele GJ, Nicolini FE, O'Brien SG, Litzow M (2007) Nilotinib (formerly AMN107), a highly selective BCR-ABL tyrosine kinase inhibitor, is effective in patients with Philadelphia chromosome-positive chronic myelogenous leukemia in chronic phase following imatinib resistance and intolerance. Blood 110:3540–3546

Kantarjian H, Shah NP, Hochhaus A, Cortes J, Shah S, Ayala M, Moiraghi B, Shen Z, Mayer J, Pasquini R (2010) Dasatinib versus imatinib in newly diagnosed chronic-phase chronic myeloid leukemia. New Engl J Med 362:2260–2270

Karapetis CS, Khambata-Ford S, Jonker DJ, O'Callaghan CJ, Tu D, Tebbutt NC, Simes RJ, Chalchal H, Shapiro JD, Robitaille S (2008) K-ras mutations and benefit from cetuximab in advanced colorectal cancer. New Engl J Med 359:1757–1765

Lievre A, Bachet JB, Le Corre D, Boige V, Landi B, Emile JF, Côté JF, Tomasic G, Penna C, Ducreux M (2006) KRAS mutation status is predictive of response to cetuximab therapy in colorectal cancer. Cancer Res 66:3992–3995

Lynch TJ, Bell DW, Sordella R, Gurubhagavatula S, Okimoto RA, Brannigan BW, Harris PL, Haserlat SM, Supko JG, Haluska FG (2004) Activating mutations in the epidermal growth factor receptor underlying responsiveness of non-small-cell lung cancer to gefitinib. New Engl J Med 350:2129–2139

Maleddu A, Pantaleo MA, Nannini M, Di Battista M, Saponara M, Lolli C, Biasco G (2009) Mechanisms of secondary resistance to tyrosine kinase inhibitors in gastrointestinal stromal tumours (Review). Oncol Rep 21:1359–1366

Malumbres M, Barbacid M (2003) RAS oncogenes: the first 30 years. Nat Rev Cancer 3:459–465

Mass RD, Press MF, Anderson S, Cobleigh MA, Vogel CL, Dybdal N, Leiberman G, Slamon DJ (2005) Evaluation of clinical outcomes according to HER2 detection by fluorescence in situ hybridization in women with metastatic breast cancer treated with trastuzumab. Clin Breast Cancer 6:240–246

Mok TS, Wu YL, Thongprasert S, Yang CH, Chu DT, Saijo N, Sunpaweravong P, Han B, Margono B, Ichinose Y (2009) Gefitinib or carboplatin-paclitaxel in pulmonary adenocarcinoma. New Engl J Med 361:947–957

Newton CR, Graham A, Heptinstall LE, Powell SJ, Summers C, Kalsheker N, Smith JC, Markham AF (1989) Analysis of any point mutation in DNA. The amplification refractory mutation system (ARMS). Nucleic Acids Res 17:2503–2516

Nilsson B, Nilsson O, Ahlman H (2009) Treatment of gastrointestinal stromal tumours: imatinib, sunitinib-and then? Expert Opin Investig Drugs 18:457–468

O'Hare T, Walters DK, Stoffregen EP, Jia T, Manley PW, Mestan J, Cowan-Jacob SW, Lee FY, Heinrich MC, Deininger MWN (2005) In vitro activity of Bcr-Abl inhibitors AMN107 and BMS-354825 against clinically relevant imatinib-resistant Abl kinase domain mutants. Cancer Res 65:4500–4505

O'Hare T, Eide CA, Deininger MW (2008) New Bcr-Abl inhibitors in chronic myeloid leukemia: keeping resistance in check. Expert Opin Investig Drugs 17:865–878

Paez JG, Jänne PA, Lee JC, Tracy S, Greulich H, Gabriel S, Herman P, Kaye FJ, Lindeman N, Boggon TJ (2004) EGFR mutations in lung cancer: correlation with clinical response to gefitinib therapy. Science 304:1497–1500

Pao W, Miller VA, Politi KA, Ricly GJ, Somwar R, Zakowski MF, Kris MG, Varmus H (2005) Acquired resistance of lung adenocarcinomas to gefitinib or erlotinib is associated with a second mutation in the EGFR kinase domain. PLoS Med 2:e73

Peeters M, Price TJ, Cervantes A, Sobrero AF, Ducreux M, Hotko Y, André T, Chan E, Lordick F, Punt CJA (2010) Randomized phase III study of panitumumab with fluorouracil, leucovorin, and irinotecan (FOLFIRI) compared with FOLFIRI alone as second-line treatment in patients with metastatic colorectal cancer. J Clin Oncol 28:4706–4713

Piccart-Gebhart MJ, Procter M, Leyland-Jones B, Goldhirsch A, Untch M, Smith I, Gianni L, Baselga J, Bell R, Jackisch C (2005) Trastuzumab after adjuvant chemotherapy in HER2-positive breast cancer. New Engl J Med 353:1659–1672

Romond EH, Perez EA, Bryant J, Suman VJ, Geyer CE Jr, Davidson NE, Tan-Chiu E, Martino S, Paik S, Kaufman PA (2005) Trastuzumab plus adjuvant chemotherapy for operable HER2-positive breast cancer. New Engl J Med 353:1673–1684

Rosell R, Moran T, Queralt C, Porta R, Cardenal F, Camps C, Majem M, Lopez-Vivanco G, Isla D, Provencio M (2009) Screening for epidermal growth factor receptor mutations in lung cancer. New Engl J Med 361:958–967

Seidman AD, Berry D, Cirrincione C, Harris L, Dressler L, Muss H, Norton L, Winer E, Hudis C (2004) CALGB 9840: Phase III study of weekly (W) paclitaxel (P) via 1-hour (h) infusion versus standard (S) 3 h infusion every third week in the treatment of metastatic breast cancer

(MBC), with trastuzumab (T) for HER2 positive MBC and randomized for T in HER2 normal MBC. J Clin Oncol 22:6s (Abs 512)

Shah NP, Tran C, Lee FY, Chen P, Norris D, Sawyers CL (2004) Overriding imatinib resistance with a novel ABL kinase inhibitor. Science 305:399–401

Shepherd FA, Rodrigues Pereira J, Ciuleanu T, Tan EH, Hirsh V, Thongprasert S, Campos D, Maoleekoonpiroj S, Smylie M, Martins R (2005) Erlotinib in previously treated non-small-cell lung cancer. New Engl J Med 353:123–132

Slamon DJ, Clark GM, Wong SG, Levin WJ, Ullrich A, McGuire WL (1987) Human breast cancer: correlation of relapse and survival with amplification of the HER-2/neu oncogene. Science 235:177–182

Slamon DJ, Leyland-Jones B, Shak S, Fuchs H, Paton V, Bajamonde A, Fleming T, Eiermann W, Wolter J, Pegram M (2001) Use of chemotherapy plus a monoclonal antibody against HER2 for metastatic breast cancer that overexpresses HER2. New Engl J Med 344:783–792

Sobrero AF, Maurel J, Fehrenbacher L, Scheithauer W, Abubakr YA, Lutz MP, Vega-Villegas ME, Eng C, Steinhauer EU, Prausova J (2008) EPIC: phase III trial of cetuximab plus irinotecan after fluoropyrimidine and oxaliplatin failure in patients with metastatic colorectal cancer. J Clin Oncol 26:2311–2319

Soverini S, Colarossi S, Gnani A, Rosti G, Castagnetti F, Poerio A, Iacobucci I, Amabile M, Abruzzese E, Orlandi E (2006) Contribution of ABL kinase domain mutations to imatinib resistance in different subsets of Philadelphia-positive patients: by the GIMEMA working party on chronic myeloid leukemia. Clin Cancer Res 12:7374–7379

Talpaz M, Shah NP, Kantarjian H, Donato N, Nicoll J, Paquette R, Cortes J, O'Brien S, Nicaise C, Bleickardt E (2006) Dasatinib in imatinib-resistant Philadelphia chromosome-positive leukemias. New Engl J Med 354:2531–2541

Thelwell N, Millington S, Solinas A, Booth J, Brown T (2000) Mode of action and application of Scorpion primers to mutation detection. Nucleic Acids Res 28:3752–3756

Van Cutsem E, Peeters M, Siena S, Humblet Y, Hendlisz A, Neyns B, Canon JL, Van Laethem JL, Maurel J, Richardson G (2007) Open-label phase III trial of panitumumab plus best supportive care compared with best supportive care alone in patients with chemotherapy-refractory metastatic colorectal cancer. J Clin Oncol 25:1658–1664

Van Cutsem E, Köhne CH, Hitre E, Zaluski J, Chang Chien CR, Makhson A, D'Haens G, Pintér T, Lim R, Bodoky G (2009) Cetuximab and chemotherapy as initial treatment for metastatic colorectal cancer. New Engl J Med 360:1408–1417

Verstovsek S, Kantarjian H, Mesa RA, Pardanani AD, Cortes-Franco J, Thomas DA, Estrov Z, Fridman JS, Bradley EC, Erickson-Viitanen S (2010) Safety and efficacy of INCB018424, a JAK1 and JAK2 inhibitor, in myelofibrosis. New Engl J Med 363:1117–1127

Weisberg E, Manley PW, Breitenstein W, Bruggen J, Cowan-Jacob SW, Ray A, Huntly B, Fabbro D, Fendrich G, Hall-Meyers E (2005) Characterization of AMN107, a selective inhibitor of native and mutant Bcr-Abl. Cancer cell 7:129–141

Wolff AC, Hammond MEH, Schwartz JN, Hagerty KL, Allred DC, Cote RJ, Dowsett M, Fitzgibbons PL, Hanna WM, Langer A (2007) American society of clinical oncology/college of American pathologists guideline recommendations for human epidermal growth factor receptor 2 testing in breast cancer. Arch Pathol Lab Med 131:18–43

Epigenetic Biomarkers

Timothy A. Chan and Stephen B. Baylin

Abstract Profound changes in the epigenetic landscape of cancer cells underlie the development of human malignancies. These changes include large-scale DNA methylation changes throughout the genome as well as alterations in the compendium of post-translational chromatin modifications. Epigenetic aberrations impact multiple steps during tumorigenesis, ultimately promoting the selection of neoplastic cells with increasing pathogenicity. Identification of these alterations for use as predictive and prognostic biomarkers has been a highly sought after goal. Recent advances in the field have not only greatly expanded our knowledge of the epigenetic changes driving neoplasia but also demonstrated their significant clinical utility as cancer biomarkers. These biomarkers have proved to be useful for identifying patients whose malignancies are sensitive to specific cytotoxic chemotherapies and may hold promise for predicting which patients will benefit from newer targeted agents directed at oncogenes. The recent application of global analysis strategies has further accelerated our understanding of the epigenome and promises to enhance the identification of epigenomic programs underlying cancer progression and treatment response.

T. A. Chan (✉)
Memorial Sloan Kettering Cancer Center,
New York, NY 10065, USA
e-mail: chant@mskcc.org

S. B. Baylin
Johns Hopkins School of Medicine,
Sidney Kimmel Comprehensive Cancer Center,
Baltimore, MD 21231, USA

Contents

1	Introduction	190
2	Changes in DNA Methylation	190
3	Changes in the Histone Code	194
4	Suitability of Epigenetic Alterations as Biomarkers	195
5	Examples of Prognostic Epigenetic Biomarkers	196
6	Epigenetic Determinants of Treatment Response	203
7	Oncogenes, Epigenetics, and Targeted Therapies	205
8	Future Perspectives	208
References		208

1 Introduction

Epigenetic alterations are heritable changes in the structure and function of the genome that occur without changes in DNA sequence. In mammalian cells, these epigenetic marks consist primarily of DNA methylation and post-translational histone modifications. Both types of modifications have been shown to play critical roles in normal growth, development, and differentiation in a multitude of organisms (Jaenisch and Young 2008; Reik et al. 2001; Wolf and Migeon 1982). From embryogenesis to the late stages of terminal differentiation, complex programs of DNA methylation alterations and chromatin state changes act to properly activate and repress appropriate transcriptional programs during development. These programs are fundamentally important for ontogeny and cell fate determination.

Epigenetic modifications involve heritable changes that provide additional layers of control that regulate how chromatin is organized and how genes are expressed. These marks confer a structural adaptation of genes and entire chromosomal regions that can register, signal, or perpetuate functional states. Such instructions ensure proper patterns of gene expression and genomic integrity. Overwhelming evidence now shows that many of these same processes are markedly distorted in cancer cells, contributing to oncogenesis and tumor progression. Recently, excellent reviews have summarized our understanding of epigenetic mechanisms underlying cancer development. Here, we highlight key concepts in cancer epigenetics and then specifically focus on describing our state of knowledge of epigenetic cancer biomarkers and their use in clinical decision-making (Herman and Baylin 2003; Jones and Baylin 2007; Jones and Laird 1999).

2 Changes in DNA Methylation

DNA methylation plays a central role in the epigenetic control of genomic programs in both normal and cancer cells. In mammalian genomic DNA, methylation takes place on the $5'$ position of cytosine bases that are part of CpG dinucleotides (m^5C). CpG dinucleotides have been progressively depleted from the eukaryotic genome

Epigenetic Biomarkers 191

over the course of evolution (Ng and Bird 1999). The remaining CpG dinucleotides in the mammalian genome are often methylated. m^5C constitutes approximately 1–2% of total DNA bases and thus affects about 70% of all CpG dinucleotides in the genome (Ehrlich et al. 1982). This methylation is thought to play an important role in the coordination of chromosomal structure and integrity, facilitating the functional segregation of active and silent chromatin. Repetitive sequences such as Alu repeats and transposons are frequently very heavily methylated, and this state may serve to maintain a transcriptionally repressed state in these regions (Bestor and Tycko 1996; Szpakowski et al. 2009).

Maintenance of DNA methylation is important for preventing chromosomal instability, translocations, and disruption of gene function by reactivation of endo-parasitic elements in the genome (Walsh et al. 1998; Yoder et al. 1997). Loss of DNA methylation has been proposed to lead to widespread genomic instability and tumor formation (Gaudet et al. 2003). CpG dinucleotides are not uniformly distributed throughout the human genome. Rather, they are concentrated in specific regions—termed CpG islands—which are located in the 5' ends (promoter, exon 1, etc.) of many genes and at other regions as well. Computational analyses estimate that, in humans, approximately 60% of all genes possess CpG islands of which the majority are unmethylated in all tissue types and throughout development (Antequera and Bird 1993, 1999). It is estimated that there are 28,000–29,000 CpG islands in the human genome (Antequera and Bird 1994). Methylation of these CpG islands is a primary method by which stable, heritable gene silencing is achieved.

In normal physiology, DNA methylation plays an integral role in the epigenetic control of germ-line, developmental, and tissue-specific transcriptional programs. For example, normal germ-line-specific expression of members of the melanoma-associated antigen (*MAGE*) gene family and the nuclear RNA export factor 2 (*NXF2*) requires DNA CpG island methylation (Bodey et al. 2002; Loriot et al. 2003). Similarly, DNA methylation constitutes a primary mechanistic basis of genomic imprinting. During imprinting, one of two parental alleles of a gene undergoes hypermethylation. This leads to the preferential expression of the unmethylated allele. Disruption of this imprinting process can lead to developmental abnormalities. Examples of monogenic epigenetic diseases involving aberrant methylation are Beckwith–Wiedemann syndrome, which involves disrupted imprinting in sub-domains of chromosome 11p15 (includes *H19/IGF2* and *p57KIP2*); and the Prader–Willi and Angelman syndromes, which involve adjacent reciprocally imprinted genes (*SNRPN* and *UBE3A*) (Diaz-Meyer et al. 2005; Horsthemke and Buiting 2006; Ohlsson et al. 1993; Weksberg et al. 1993). DNA methylation is critical for genomic imprinting as deletion of the DNA methylation catalyzing enzyme, *DNMT1*, leads to disruption of monoallelic expression of imprinted genes (Li et al. 1993). Like imprinting, X inactivation also selectively silences one allele, leaving the other copy unaffected. Multiple layers of epigenetic control are required for proper X chromosome inactivation in females, including expression of the *Xist* non-coding chromosomal RNA and DNA methylation (Reik and Lewis 2005). During this process, expression of the *Xist* RNA leads to stable silencing of genomic regions in *cis*. This is followed by wide-spread methylation of CpG islands and repression of the targeted region of the genome. As such, acquisition of DNA methylation at CpG islands is thought to establish stable transcriptional silencing of genes, essentially "locking in" the inactive state.

In human cancers, many significant changes in DNA methylation patterns occur during oncogenesis and tumor progression. These changes can be either broad-based changes that involve large regions of DNA or locus-specific changes that control the transcription of specific genes. One of the first epigenetic alterations noted in tumors was global hypomethylation. Hypomethylation occurs broadly throughout the DNA of cancer cells, affecting repetitive sequences, intergenic areas, and promoter CpG islands associated with genes (Feinberg and Vogelstein 1983). While much remains to be elucidated about the functional significance of this global genomic hypomethylation in cancer cells, it is clear that this change may help to increase genomic instability and can drive the tumorigenic process by enabling chromosomal breaks, translocations, and aneuploidy to occur (Hoffmann and Schulz 2005; Howard et al. 2008). Hypomethylation can also occur at the CpG islands of specific genes, resulting in aberrant overexpression of oncogenes. Examples of genes activated by hypomethylation include *HRAS*, *CCND2*, and *SERPINB5* in gastric cancer, *CA9* in renal cell cancer, and *PAX2* in endometrial cancer (Oshimo et al. 2003; Wilson et al. 2007; Wu et al. 2005). In cancer, abnormal decreases of DNA methylation in the promoters of such genes contribute to a growth advantage during tumorigenesis. The hypomethylation events may cooperate with mutational activation of oncogenes to drive cancer cell growth.

The most studied abnormality of DNA methylation in cancer is an abnormal gain of DNA methylation—hypermethylation—which is now established as a very common event in cancer cells which often involves normally unmethylated gene promoter CpG islands (Herman and Baylin 2003). This promoter change can be associated with transcriptional silencing, and thus loss of function, of tumor suppressor genes and may be a key event contributing to the oncogenic process (Jones and Baylin 2007; Laird 1997; Wajed et al. 2001). Aberrant hypermethylation can be passed on to daughter cells and forms the basis for an epigenetic "cellular memory." Specific methylation events can impart a survival advantage and as such, serve as a basis for clonal selection during tumorigenesis. This method of tumor suppressor inactivation is one of the most prevalent modes in cancer and is found in nearly every type of human malignancy (Esteller 2008; Jones and Baylin 2007). The tumor suppressors that are inactivated by hypermethylation can affect DNA repair, programmed cell death, angiogenesis, cell cycle regulation, and tumor cell invasion. For example, the mismatch repair gene *hMLH1* is frequently silenced by methylation and results in mismatch repair deficiency in cancers of the colon, stomach, and endometrium (Gu et al. 2009; Herman et al. 1996; Jacinto and Esteller 2007; Kane et al. 1997). Other well-known examples of genes silenced by hypermethylation include the *VHL* tumor suppressor in renal cell carcinoma (Herman et al. 1994), the *BRCA1* tumor suppressor (Esteller et al. 2000b), the cyclin-dependent kinase inhibitor *CDKN2A* (p16) (Merlo et al. 1995), and the retinoblastoma susceptibility gene *RB1* (Greger et al. 1989). In any given tumor, current estimates place the number of genes

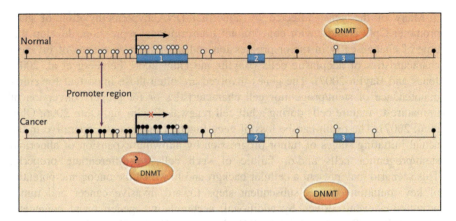

Fig. 1 Differences in methylation patterns between normal and cancer cells. *Circles* represent individual CpG islands, with *closed circles* representing methylated CpGs and *open circles* representing unmethylated CpGs. In contrast to normal cells, cancers tend to have local hypermethylation at promoter CpG islands in a setting of global hypomethylation. The *arrow* represents the transcriptional start site. DNMT, DNA methyltransferase. Diagram from Herman and Baylin (2003)

abnormally silenced by methylation in any given tumor at several hundred (Chan et al. 2008; Hoque et al. 2008; Schuebel et al. 2007). Figure 1 illustrates the concept of DNA hypermethylation in cancer cells.

How does promoter hypermethylation result in transcriptional silencing? Currently, there are thought to be two primary methods by which this occurs. First, in a number of experimental systems, it appears that DNA methylation results in the recruitment of specific chromatin-binding proteins which mediate gene silencing (Esteller 2008; Jones and Baylin 2007). Once a promoter CpG island is methylated by DNA methyltransferases (DNMTs), the methylated CpGs become bound to methyl-CpG binding proteins (MeCP) (Bird and Wolffe 1999). A family of 5 such proteins has been characterized, each containing a region highly homologous to the methyl-CpG binding domain of MeCP2 (Cross et al. 1997; Nan et al. 1993, 1998). These proteins have been shown to play a critical role in mediating methylation-dependent transcriptional repression (Jones et al. 1998). The methyl-cytosine binding proteins associate with histone deacetylases (HDAC) which help effect transcriptional silencing by regulating the transcriptional permissiveness of chromatin (Bird and Wolffe 1999). Alternatively, methylated DNA may interfere with the binding of proteins required for active transcription. Numerous DNA binding factors are known to bind CpG-containing sequences, and CpG methylation prevents some from binding. For example, the CTCF protein, a factor that is important for the proper imprinting of the *H19/IGF2* locus, can bind to a specific sequence between the promoter and a downstream enhancer (Bell and Felsenfeld 2000; Hark et al. 2000). This binding occurs in the maternal copy of the gene and is critical for maintaining silencing of the allele. At the paternal locus, CpG methylation of the sequence prevents binding of CTCF and allows the downstream enhancer to activate the gene.

Many of the genes affected by abnormal DNA hypermethylation of gene promoter CpG islands, with concomitant transcriptional repression, develop this type of change early in tumor progression and prior to the presence of invasive characteristics of neoplastic cells (Baylin and Ohm 2006; Feinberg et al. 2006; Jones and Baylin 2007). The genes involved are often those important for either maintenance of stem/progenitor cell characteristics or for proper conversion of immature to mature cells during adult cell renewal (Baylin and Ohm 2006; Ohm et al. 2007). The result can be loss of gene function that may be operative in the actual initiating stages of tumor progression by allowing expansion of abnormal stem/progenitor cells and/or failure of such cells to differentiate properly. This scenario may present a cellular background in which the oncogenic potential of key mutations propel subsequent steps toward invasive cancer and tumor progression events driven by additional, accumulating, genetic, and epigenetic abnormalities (Baylin and Ohm 2006; Jones and Baylin 2007). Recognition of these potential roles for epigenetic abnormalities in tumorigenesis emphasizes how a compilation of the genes involved can provide potential biomarkers for key stages of tumor progression and behavior.

3 Changes in the Histone Code

In cancer cells, abnormal DNA methylation occurs alongside a number of other types of epigenetic aberrations. Of these alterations, post-translational histone modifications are of paramount importance. Chromatin is composed of DNA, histones, and various other proteins. The amino-terminal tails of some histones project out of the nucleosome core and are subject to a number of post-translational modifications—or marks–including acetylation, phosphorylation, ubiquitination, and methylation (Esteller 2008). Acetylation and methylation of histones are the alterations that have been the most intensely studied thus far. These two types of modifications can remodel chromatin, and the nature of the resultant functional change depends on the histone modified and the location of the modification along the histone polypeptide. As such, they can control the functional state of chromatin and, thereby, dictate whether genes in the domain affected are activated or repressed.

Recently, there has been a flurry of activity in this field and an increasing number of histone marks have been identified. Some of these marks are implicated in activation of transcription. Examples include acetylation of H3K4 (histone 3 lysine 4) and methylation of H3K4, H3K36, and H3K79 (Bannister et al. 2005; Liang et al. 2004; Ng et al. 2003; Singer et al. 1998). In contrast, other marks result in an inactive chromatin state and transcriptional repression. The primary examples of these types of modifications include methylation of H3K9, H3K27, and H4K20 (Peters et al. 2002, 2003; Sims et al. 2006). Acetylation of histones is controlled by three main families of acetyltransferases—GNAT, MYST, and CBP/p300—and deacetylation is carried out by members of three classes of histone deacetylases—classes 1–3 (Kouzarides 2007; Sterner and Berger 2000). Histone methylation is carried out by any number of histone lysine methyltransferases such as those in the polycomb complex; and demethylation is carried out by a number of demethylases such as LSD1 and the Jumonji-C domain containing proteins (Shi et al. 2004; Wissmann et al. 2007; Yamane et al. 2006). Systematic changes of these and other histone marks have been found to be present in a wide range of malignancies, suggesting that abnormalities in chromatic state may be present in cancer cells.

Using global profiling, abnormal histone marks have been found to affect a large number of genes in both cancer cell lines and primary tumors (Fraga et al. 2005). In this particular study, tumor cells were shown to possess decreased monoacetylated and trimethylated histone H4, which at times are associated with promoter hypermethylation. Particularly interesting was the finding that these alterations occurred early in oncogenesis and accumulated as tumors continued to grow. Changes in histone marks such as these disrupt a wide range of normal cellular processes that eventually leads to tumor development. As with DNA methylation, histone modifications in cancer are being increasingly recognized as biomarkers that can predict cancer prognosis.

4 Suitability of Epigenetic Alterations as Biomarkers

Cancer-specific hypermethylation of CpG islands comprise one of the most prevalent molecular changes in cancer cells, and detection of abnormal methylation has proven to be of great use in the clinic. This is due to several inherent advantages in strategies for the detection of hypermethylation. First, DNA is a relatively stable substance and can be obtained from a wide range of sources. It can be stored for long periods after collection from patients. Compared to mRNA, DNA samples require fewer precautions to prevent sample degradation. Second, DNA methylation is a widespread alteration throughout the cancer genome. This allows for the possibility of using assays to query many points in the genome and combining their use in highly predictive models. Third, highly sensitive and specific technologies now exist that can query the methylation state of specific DNA locations using minimal amounts of nucleic acid that can be obtained from a wide array of clinical specimens. These techniques include methylation-specific PCR (MSP), high-performance liquid chromatography (HPLC), mass spectrometry-based methylation detection (EpiTYPER), Methy-Light, and pyrosequencing (Eads et al. 2000; Ehrich et al. 2005; Fraga and Esteller 2002; Herman et al. 1996; Uhlmann et al. 2002). Assays like MSP and EpiTYPER are able to detect DNA methylation from even minute amounts of material such as urine and saliva, and capable of utilizing DNA from both frozen and paraffin-embedded archived tissue. These advantages have enabled investigators to evaluate the diagnostic and prognostic utility of methylation of a large number of genes in a many tumor types (reviewed in Esteller (2007)).

The need to identify the entire spectrum of epigenetic alterations is spurring many approaches to perform genome-wide analyses of cancer DNA for abnormal DNA methylation marks and chromatin alterations. Currently used techniques include treating cells with drugs which induce re-expression of abnormally silenced genes and detection of their transcripts on expression microarrays (Chan et al. 2008; Schuebel et al. 2007; Suzuki et al. 2002), immunoprecipitation of methylcytosine residues and use of genomic arrays to identify associated genes (Keshet et al. 2006; Weber et al. 2005), hybridization array strategies for detecting methylated DNA such as the Infinium platform by Illumina (TCGA 2008), and deep genomic sequencing strategies for identifying DNA methylation sites (Lister et al. 2009). These approaches have led to identification of some of the gene promoter DNA methylation markers, such as the Secreted frizzled-related proteins (SFRPs) (Suzuki et al. 2004), which will be discussed below.

A current example of the use of genome screening for DNA methylation changes in cancer is the use of the Infinium platform in the Cancer Genome Atlas project (TCGA), to detect gene promoter alterations. By matching DNA modifications to DNA sequencing and expression changes, important discoveries were made regarding epigenetic silencing of *MGMT* (TCGA 2008). A sharp increase in the total number of gene mutations was seen in GBM DNA taken from patients with DNA hypermethylation and silencing of this gene who had received previous treatment with radiation and alkylating agent therapy (TCGA 2008). The mechanism appears to involve a selection of tumor cells for mutations in mismatch repair genes in such individuals. While initial loss of MGMT function, as discussed earlier, makes glioblastoma cells sensitive to killing by alkylating agents, the mechanism of cell death involves a futile attempt at DNA repair of the resultant guanosine adducts by the mismatch repair enzymes (Hirose et al. 2003; Kaina et al. 2007). Thus, cells are subsequently vulnerable to selection of mutations in the mismatch repair enzymes which then, in turn, promotes cell survival with accruing gene mutations due to loss of function of these enzymes. No doubt, such cancer genome screening endeavors for epigenetic changes, especially coupled with simultaneous screens for genetic abnormalities, will produce many more valuable associations. In turn, we will continue to unravel the contribution of epigenetic abnormalities to cancer pathobiology and acquire more valuable biomarkers for cancer risk assessment, early detection, monitoring of prognosis, and monitoring of therapeutic outcomes.

5 Examples of Prognostic Epigenetic Biomarkers

One of the most compelling studies performed to date was reported by Brock et al. (2008). This nested, case control study examined the utility of using a panel of methylated genes to predict disease recurrence after curative resection in patients with Stage I lung cancer. Most patients with Stage I lung cancer are cured after surgical resection (65–75%), but a significant subset develop recurrence of their

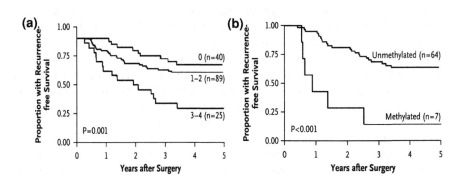

Fig. 2 Kaplan–Meier estimates of recurrence-free survival among patients with Stage I non-small-cell lung cancer according to the status of methylated genes. a Recurrence-free survival of patients according to the number of methylated genes (*CDKN2A*, *RASSF1A*, *CDH13*, and *APC*) in the primary tumor. Number of patients are shown in each cohort. b Recurrence-free survival according to methylation status of *CDKN2A* and *CDH13* in primary tumor and mediastinal nodes. Number of patients in each cohort is shown. Figure is derived from Brock et al. (2008)

disease, which usually leads to death. Currently, no diagnostic test exists that can identify the patients that are at risk for failure. In their study, Brock et al. showed that promoter hypermethylation of just four genes—*CDH13*, *RASSF1A*, *APC*, and *CDKN2A* (*p16*)—was able to predict tumor recurrence, identifying Stage I patients who essentially behaved like Stage 3 patients. Methylation of the promoters of two genes, *CDKN2A* and *CDH13*, provided most of the predictive power. When both genes were methylated in the primary tumor and mediastinal nodes, the odds ratio for recurrence was an impressive 15.5. Figure 2 shows the association of gene methylation with lung cancer recurrence as reported by Brock et al. (2008). Several points can be concluded from this study. First, it is clear that the epigenetic status of tumors can strongly influence a given tumor's clinical behavior and aggressiveness. Second, molecular examination of the epigenetic status of lung cancers may improve upon histologic criteria and anatomic staging for the purposes of providing prognostic information. And third, epigenetic staging appears to be an efficient strategy for the molecular staging of cancer, utilizing fewer genes than expression signature-based approaches. Independent prospective validation of the Brock study is currently underway and will be necessary before the widespread application of this biomarker panel in the clinic.

Disruption of the WNT pathway is well established as an important contributor to cancer development and progression (Kinzler and Vogelstein 1996). Mutation of *APC* and *CTNNB1*, two genes encoding protein products that function in WNT signaling, leads to the development of colorectal cancers (Kinzler and Vogelstein 1997; Morin et al. 1997). WNT signaling dysfunction extends beyond colorectal cancers and has been observed in a wide range of human cancers. SFRPs, inhibitors of WNT receptor binding, have been found to be frequently silenced by hypermethylation in a number of malignancies, including cancers of the colon, cervix, and breast (Lin et al. 2009; Suzuki et al. 2004, 2008). SFRPs are antagonists of the growth and survival promoting WNT signaling cascade, and they function as tumor suppressors. Interestingly, SFRP silencing is significantly associated with a reduced overall survival and is an independent predictor of prognosis in malignancies such as breast and renal cell carcinoma (Urakami et al. 2006; Veeck et al. 2008). Perhaps methylation and silencing of these genes results in constitutively active WNT signaling, promoting cancer cell growth, and tumor progression.

Aberrant silencing of the death-associated protein kinase (DAPK) is another common cancer-associated epigenetic lesion that has been linked to clinical outcomes. DAPK is a 16kD Ca+/calmodulin-regulated serine threonine kinase with a conserved death domain that functions as a positive mediator of diverse apoptotic systems (Deiss et al. 1995; Inbal et al. 2000). The *DAPK* gene has an extensive promoter CpG island and is subject to silencing by hypermethylation in a number of human cancers, including those of the colon, breast, ovary, lung, head and neck, and leukemia (Esteller et al. 2001; Steinmann et al. 2009). Silencing of DAPK has been found to predict tumor progression and poor outcome in a number of cancer types. For example, Iliopoulos and colleagues have found that methylation of DAPK increased during cervical cancer progression and was associated with high-risk pathological features (Iliopoulos et al. 2009). In bladder cancer, Jarmalaite et al. observed that hypermethylation of *DAPK* significantly increased the risk of relapse after therapy. Silencing of DAPK disrupts the normal apoptotic machinery. Such a disruption may impart resistance to programmed cell death, enabling affected cells to acquire additional lesions that impart increasing pathogenicity during clonal selection (Jarmalaite et al. 2008).

Aside from the Brock study, a number of reports have evaluated the prognostic value of methylation of a combination of genes in human tumors. Many gene sets appear to be very promising. In breast cancer, methylation of *BRCA1*, *RB1*, *ERalpha*, *GSTP1*, *RASSF1A*, *CDKN2A*, and *RARbeta2* heralded poor prognosis, with a hazard ratio of 14.58 (Sharma et al. 2009). Interestingly, concurrent methylation of multiple genes in the set was a frequent event and likely reflects a more aggressive tumor biology. Aggerholm et al. examined the clinical impact of methylation of *CDKN2B* (*p*15), *HIC1*, *CDH1*, and *ER* (Aggerholm et al. 2006). Concurrent methylation of three or more of these genes was associated with leukemic transformation of patients with early-stage myelodysplastic syndrome (MDS). Patients with hypermethylation had a median survival of 17 months compared to 67 months for those without hypermethylation. These data suggest that epigenetic modification of *CDKN2B* (*p*15), *HIC1*, *CDH1*, and *ER* may contribute to the development and outcome of MDS.

The finding of high frequencies of concurrent CpG island methylation of multiple genes in some tumors and lack of methylation in others has given rise to the hypothesis that certain tumors display a distinct "hypermethylator phenotype." This CpG island methylator phenotype (CIMP) is perhaps best described for colon cancer (Toyota et al. 1999). In CIMP+ tumors, concomitant methylation of a number of genes occurs, leading to the inactivation of multiple tumor suppressors. Genes that are affected include *MLH1*, *CDKN2A*, *THBS1*, and others (Toyota et al. 2000). Peter Laird and colleagues systematically examined 295 primary human colorectal tumors, analyzing 195 CpG islands using MethyLight technology, and showed that CIMP+ tumors convincingly represented a distinct subset of colon tumors (Weisenberger et al. 2006). Furthermore, they found that CIMP+ tumors encompassed nearly all cases of tumors with BRAF mutation (odds ratio = 203). In addition, sporadic cases of mismatch repair deficiency (MSI) occurred almost exclusively as a consequence of CIMP-associated methylation of *MLH1*. These findings are consistent with observations from a number of other investigators, who together, have validated CIMP tumors as a molecular subgroup of colon cancer (Oue et al. 2002; van Rijnsoever et al. 2002). Additional analyses showed that the CIMP phenotype, in combination with specific genetic lesions, can be used to further classify colon cancer into three molecular subclasses, each arising from a different pathway. These pathways expand on the classic model of colon cancer evolution ("the Vogelgram") and have important clinical consequences. One pathway is characterized by the CIMP phenotype. These tumors have concomitant mutations of BRAF and are associated with serrated adenomas (Park et al. 2003). They are characterized by inactivation of *MLH1* by epigenetic silencing and the development of MSI. Compared to tumors with chromosomal instability, which demonstrate genetic instability at the level of whole or large sections of chromosomes, these tumors tend to occur in the proximal colon and in older patients. Patients with CIMP+, MSI+ tumors constitute 10–20% of all patients and tended to have excellent prognosis (Ogino et al. 2009; Thibodeau et al. 1993). CIMP+, MSI−tumors, on the other hand, are associated with poor prognosis and a poor responsiveness to 5-fluorouracil and cetuximab (Karapetis et al. 2008; Ogino et al. 2007). This subset is associated with *KRAS* and *APC* mutation and commonly arises from villous adenomas (Kakar et al. 2008; Rashid et al. 2001). Patients with this type of tumor constitute 10–30% of all cases of colon cancer (Shen et al. 2007). The third group of tumors are those characterized by chromosomal instability (CIN). These tumors do not display the CIMP phenotype and are associated with *APC* and *p*53 mutations. They arise from tubular adenomas and typically are located in the distal colon. Patients with these types of tumors constitute 50–70% of all cases and their prognosis is intermediate between the two classes mentioned above (Goel et al. 2007; Issa 2008). Figure 3 shows the three molecular subgroups of colon cancers.

The clinical implications of multiple pathways for colon cancer initiation impact both diagnosis and treatment. The finding of distinct subgroups of colon cancer associated with vastly different prognoses—in a large part differentiated by the CIMP phenotype—suggests that the use of epigenetic biomarkers to detect CIMP, integrated with information on specific genetic loci such as *APC* and *KRAS*, may be useful for providing valuable prognostic information for patients. Such biomarkers may also have a important impact on therapy decisions. Current clinical practice is only now beginning to progress from a uniformity in treating colon cancer to a more personalized approach. Already, there is increased recognition of the different responsiveness of MSI+ (both CIMP+ and −) to 5-FU.

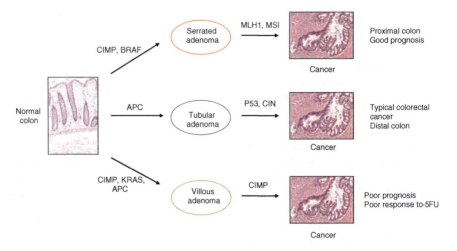

Fig. 3 Molecular subtypes of colon cancer. Multiple pathways can lead to colon cancer, each with distinct clinical implications. *CIMP* CpG island methylator phenotype, *CIN* chromosomal instability. Modified from Issa (2008)

As such, methylation markers will have an increasing role in dictating therapeutic options. Indeed, it has been hypothesized that patients who are MSI+/CIMP+ may not need extensive adjuvant therapy after surgical resection. Ongoing and future prospective trials are needed to test the clinical effectiveness of treating these patients differently.

Aside from colon cancer, CIMP has been shown to be present in several types of human malignancies. The Cancer Genome Atlas (TCGA) has described the presence of CIMP in malignant gliomas. In glioblastomas (GBM), glioma CIMP, or G-CIMP, defines a distinct subgroup of tumors marked by high-coordinate hypermethylation at a large number of CpG islands (Noushmehr et al. 2010; TCGA 2008). G-CIMP+ GBMs are associated with mutations in the *IDH1* or *IDH2* genes and the proneural subgroup of gliomas, and impart significantly better prognosis than G-CIMP−GBMs. Interestingly, while the G-CIMP+ tumors possess a high degree of epigenetic dysfunction, these tumors possess relatively few alterations in chromosome number and structure. CIMP has also recently been described in breast cancer. As with colon cancer and GBM, CIMP in breast cancer (B-CIMP) is associated with high-coordinate hypermethylation at many loci and is a strong predictor of good prognosis. Interestingly, B-CIMP modulates the expression of many metastasis-associated genes and was found to be a root cause of much of the transcriptional diversity underlying prognostic signatures for metastatic risk (Fang et al. 2011).

Genes coding for protein products that regulate DNA methylation have been found to have altered expression or be mutated in cancer. For example, recently, several groups have found that *TET2* is mutated in a number of myeloid malignancies, including acute myeloid leukemia, myeloproliferative disorders, and myelodysplastic syndromes (Abdel-Wahab et al. 2009; Delhommeau et al. 2009; Langemeijer et al. 2009). The frequency of tumors harboring *TET2* mutations ranges from 1–2% to approximately 25%, depending of the type of myeloid malignancy examined. Interestingly, the TET family proteins have been shown to catalyze the conversion of 5-methylcytosine to 5-hydroxymethylcytosine. As such, the TET proteins may have important roles in epigenetic regulation and, when mutated, a disruption in this normal function may contribute to the development of cancers. Mutation in *TET2* seems to predict a worse overall survival in patients with acute myeloid leukemia (Abdel-Wahab et al. 2009). A number of investigators also observe elevated levels of DNMTs and methyl-CpG binding proteins (MBDs) in human tumors (Ahluwalia et al. 2001; Girault et al. 2003; Lopez-Serra et al. 2006). Ley et al. (2010) has recently reported mutations in the *DNMT3A* gene in these hematopoietic malignancies. *DNMT3A* mutations were found to be strongly associated with poor prognosis. Mutations in other DNMTs and MBDs are rare in most cancers. However, crossing cancer-prone murine strains with mice carrying genetic defects in these two classes of proteins alters the timing and risk of tumorigenesis, suggesting that they have the potential to promote tumor progression (Mager and Bartolomei 2005).

Aberrant histone modifications, working together with or independently of DNA methylation changes, can also contribute to the development and progression of cancers. These alterations involve key histone marks that are critical for the regulation of genes that govern cell fate, growth, and survival. Among the most compelling evidence implicating the histone code in carcinogenesis is the finding that a significant number of proteins that regulate histone modifications are themselves the target of genetic alteration in tumors. Chinnaiyan and colleagues have identified the polycomb group protein Enhancer of Zeste 2 (EZH2) as a critical player in prostate cancer carcinogenesis (Varambally et al. 2002). EZH2 is a component of the polycomb repressive complex 2 (PRC2) which is required for establishing transcriptionally silent chromatin by methylating histone H3 on lysine 27 (H3K27me3). EZH2 was shown to be overexpressed in hormone-refractory, metastatic prostate cancer. Clinically localized prostate tumors that expressed higher concentrations of EZH2 were associated with a higher distant failure rate and poorer prognosis. In addition to prostate cancer, EZH2 overexpression is associated with poor clinical outcomes in breast cancer, esophageal cancer, and head and neck cancers (Kidani et al. 2009; Kleer et al. 2003). High levels of EZH2 results in the aberrant silencing of a number of genes, which promotes neoplastic transformation and tumor cell aggressiveness. Supporting this hypothesis is the observation that tumors demonstrating repression of genes targeted by the polycomb proteins (the polycomb repression signature) are associated with significantly worse survival (Yu et al. 2007). Interestingly, EZH2 has been found to be mutated in nearly 22% of germinal center–derived diffuse large B cell lymphomas (Morin et al. 2010). Surprisingly, these mutations appear to decrease the enzymatic activity of the gene product, suggesting that EZH2 may function as a tumor suppressor in some lymphomas. Together, these studies show that the polycomb proteins and their histone targets are important elements dictating the behavior of malignancies.

Another histone modifying protein found to play a significant role in cancer aggressiveness is the lysine-specific demethylase 1 (LSD1). LSD1 is an anime oxidase that catalyzes histone demethylation. It regulates histone configuration by removing the mono- and di-methyl groups from H3K4. By removing these methyl groups, LSD1 functions as a transcriptional repressor. This histone demethylase is an integral component of several corepressor complexes that play roles in regulating gene activity, including CoREST and NuRD. Recently, Wang et al. showed that LSD1 can modulate the genetic programs that lead to metastasis in breast cancer (Wang et al. 2009). Using a chromatin immunoprecipitation approach coupled with microarray analysis, they showed that the LSD1/NuRD complex targets a number of genes implicated in epithelial-to-mesenchymal transition and metastasis, including *TGFB1*, *EGFR*, *COL6A* (collagen VI), *RHOA*, and *EDN1* (endothelin-1). LSD1 is frequently downregulated in primary breast carcinomas, and functional studies show that LDS1 suppresses breast cancer cell invasiveness in vitro and metastatic potential in vivo. This effect was found to be partly due to the ability of LSD1 to suppress the expression of TGFB1 expression (Wang et al. 2009). Together, the data show that LSD1 inactivation may promote breast cancer aggressiveness and distant failures.

However, there is, paradoxical to the above findings, another facet of LSD1 transcriptional repression that indicates a tumor suppressive effect, in the setting of epigenetic gene silencing and inhibition of this enzyme. This protein has been localized to the promoters of several genes silenced in cancer cells in association with DNA hypermethylation of their promoters (Huang et al. 2007). Inhibition of the demethylase activity of LSD1 here can lead to reactivation of the silenced genes (Huang et al. 2009). Moreover, synergy has been observed for such inhibition with inhibition of DNA methyltransferases by 5-aza-cytidine (Huang et al. 2009). Most recently, synergy for both inhibitors has been seen for anti-tumor effects on human colon cancer cells grown as xenografts in immunocompromised mice (Huang et al. 2009). These effects may reflect the fact that restoration of the H3K4me2 modification with inhibition of LSD1 would favor prevention of recruitment of DNA methyltransferases to gene promoter regions. This type of synergy demonstrated by drugs with epigenetic effects highlights the promise for construction of future anti-cancer therapies built upon such concepts.

Other histone modifying factors that are disrupted in cancer include the histone acetyltransferases *p300*, *CBP*, *pCAF*, *MOZ*, and *MORF*; the histone deacetylase *HDAC1* and *HDAC2*; the histone methyltrasferases *MLL1-3*, *NSD1*, and *RIZ1*; *and* the histone demethylases *UTX* and *GASC1* (Esteller 2007; van Haaften et al. 2009). Ongoing characterization of cancer genomes will likely reveal the full extent of mutational alteration of the histone code regulating machinery in human cancers. A significant future challenge will be to decipher the prognostic and predictive significance of these changes in human cancers.

6 Epigenetic Determinants of Treatment Response

From the discussion above, it is clear that some epigenetic alterations in cancer possess clinically significant prognostic value. Specific epigenetic markers, however, also possess very significant predictive value for cancer therapy. Why would epigenetic alterations arise during clonal selection and tumorigenesis impart a better response to specific anti-cancer treatments? Several hypotheses have been suggested that may explain this phenomenon. First, it is possible that epigenetic inactivation of specific genes, such as those encoding DNA repair enzymes, may lead to a mutator phenotype and promote the acquisition of mutations in tumor suppressor genes during tumor development. Inactivation of these same genes may lead to an inability to repair DNA damage from treatment with cytotoxic agents, leading to an increased sensitivity and greater response of the tumor cells to these drugs. Secondly, it is possible that under conditions in which tumor cells are treated with chemotherapy, specific epigenetic alterations may bring about a synthetic lethal phenotype that is accentuated in the setting of genotoxic stress. Third, it is possible that some predictive epigenetic markers are simply passenger events, tightly linked to another genetic or epigenetic alteration that provides clonal selection but are themselves not drivers of tumorigenesis. Such biomarkers may be predictive of response to specific therapies but not be functionally related to the direct biological response to those therapies.

Perhaps the most compelling example of the utility of epigenetic markers for prediction of treatment response is the use of *MGMT* (O^6-methylguanine-DNA methyltransferase) promoter methylation to determine response to alkylating agents among patients with glioblastoma. Alkylating agents such as BCNU (1,3-bis(2-chloroethyl)-1-nitrosourea), temozolomide, and procarbazine are commonly used chemotherapeutics that generate a variety of adducts on DNA, which leads to tumor cell death. The ability of alkylating agents to exert their effects on cells can be diminished by the presence of MGMT, which is a DNA repair enzyme that reverses the DNA adducts at the O^6 position of guanine formed by the drugs. The efficiency of DNA repair in the cancer cell is an important determinant of therapeutic resistance and the inactivation of MGMT can cause cells to become more sensitive to alkylating agents. This is in fact what is observed in the clinic. Herman and colleagues identified *MGMT* methylation as a significant independent predictor of response to BCNU (Esteller et al. 2000a). *MGMT* methylation was associated with regression of tumors and a prolonged overall and disease-free survival. It was a stronger prognostic factor than age, stage, tumor grade, or performance status. The results of this retrospective study were confirmed by a large study conducted by the European Organization for Research and Treatment of Cancer (EORTC) and the National Cancer Institute of Canada (NCIC) randomizing GBM patients following surgical resection to treatment with radiation versus radiation and temozolomide (Stupp et al. 2005). This trial showed that patients treated with adjuvant treatment with radiation and temozolomide had superior overall survival compared to those treated with radiation alone. The design of the

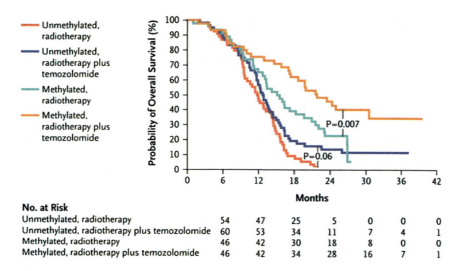

Fig. 4 Glioblastoma patients with *MGMT* methylation have improved survival following treatment adjuvant radiotherapy and temozolomide. Kaplan-Meier curves are shown for each cohort labeled. Number of patients in each cohort is shown below the graph. *P*-value is calculated by the log-rank method. Figure is derived from Hegi et al. (2005)

study included the collection of tumor tissue from the randomized patients and analysis of *MGMT* promoter methylation. Analysis of the tissue indicated that *MGMT* methylation strongly predicted for improved survival following treatment with radiation and temozolomide (Hegi et al. 2005). *MGMT* was methylated in 45% of the patients analyzed. Among patients whose tumor contained a methylated *MGMT* promoter, patients treated with temozolomide and radiotherapy had a median survival of 21.7 months, as compared with 15.3 months among those who were assigned to only radiotherapy ($p = 0.007$ by the log-rank test). Figure 4 shows the survival results of *MGMT* methylated and unmethylated patients on the EORTC/NCIC trial. Since these data were reported, some investigators have raised the possibility that MGMT methylation is prognostic for outcome but not predictive for treatment response. It may be that patients with *MGMT* methylation do better irrespective of treatment with an alkylating agent. Furthermore, in trials of other anaplastic gliomas, *MGMT* methylation appeared to be prognostic but not predictive for alkylator therapy (van den Bent et al. 2009). However, given the significantly different survival outcomes of *MGMT* methylated patients treated with temozolomide and those who were not, *MGMT* methylation is likely to be, at least in part, predictive of treatment response. In fact, follow-up studies have confirmed that the survival advantage of patients with tumors having methylated MGMT seems to be dependent on the use of alkylating agents as part of adjuvant therapy (Criniere et al. 2007). It is important to note that these are not mutually exclusive qualities, and that *MGMT* methylation may possess both predictive and prognostic value, as in the case of estrogen receptor status (ER) in breast cancer patients.

In addition to *MGMT* methylation, other epigenetic alterations are beginning to show promise for predicting response to chemotherapy. One such marker is *BRCA1* hypermethylation. Inactivation of *BRCA1* by hypermethylation is common in sporadic tumors in malignancies such as breast and ovarian cancer (Esteller et al. 2000b; Rice et al. 2000). Chaudhry et al. investigated the clinical utility of *BRCA1* promoter methylation in predicting response of epithelial ovarian cancer to platinum-based chemotherapeutics (Chaudhry et al. 2009). They observe that *BRCA1* methylation predicts chemosensitivity and clinical response to cisplatin. Similarly, methylation of *GSTP1* and *MLH1* has been shown to predict response to systemic therapies for several cancer types. Confirmation of the clinical utility of markers such as those prior to widespread clinical use requires a long and arduous but necessary process. All of these promising candidate biomarkers will need to be independently validated in a prospective manner prior to their use in clinical decision-making.

7 Oncogenes, Epigenetics, and Targeted Therapies

It is now well established that aberrant activation of oncogenes plays a crucial role in the development of the nearly every type of human malignancy. In normal cells, these genes usually function to regulate cell growth and death. In cancers, however, oncogenes inappropriately activate growth promoting and pro-survival programs, which ultimately lead to unchecked cell proliferation and defective apoptosis. Aberrant activation of oncogenic activity usually results from somatic mutations within an oncogene itself, which leads to a constitutively active protein product, or mutations in a tumor suppressor which normally shuts down growth promoting pathways. Examples of oncogenes linked to human cancers include *KRAS, HRAS, NRAS, EGFR, PIK3CA, MYC, JAK2, HER2*, and *BCR-ABL*.

The signaling cascades that are activated by oncogenes such as Ras have been intensively studied and are reasonably well worked out. Upon binding to their ligands, growth factor receptors and their adapter proteins can activate Ras. Activated Ras binds GTP and activates Raf kinase. Raf, in turn, phosphorylates and activates MEK, which activates ERK. This signaling cascade subsequently leads to a number of changes in gene regulation that control processes such as actin cytoskeletal integrity, proliferation, differentiation, cell adhesion, apoptosis, and cell migration. Mutations result in a constitutive activation of Ras and the entire signaling pathway. This activation results in the transduction of growth promoting signals to the nucleus, which institutes genetic programs promoting neoplastic transformation. Despite the detailed knowledge about the Ras-signaling pathway that communicates the signal to the nucleus, the exact nature of the genome-wide changes are only now beginning to be elucidated.

Recent evidence suggests that oncogenes such as *KRAS* are able to direct specific epigenetic alterations that are crucial for their ability to transform cells. In H-Ras-transformed rat fibroblasts, specific genes are epigenetically silenced in a methylation-dependent manner. These genes include *Clu* (clusterin), *Mmp2* (matrix metalloproteinase 2), *Timp2*, *Thbs1*, and *Sdc4* (syndecan4) (Lund et al. 2006). Both the DNMT inhibitor 5-aza-deoxycytidine (5′-aza) and the MEK inhibitor UO126 upregulate the expression of these genes in the Ras-transformed cells. Interestingly, Rouleau et al. showed that the Ras-signaling pathway can directly regulate DNA methylation by activation of the *DNMT1* promoter (Rouleau et al. 1995). In Y1 adrenocortical tumor cells, expression of GAP120, a down regulator of Ras activity, reverts the transformed phenotype of the cells and results in a concomitant drop in DNMT1 mRNA and DNA methylation. Introduction of an oncogenic H-ras allele into the GAP transfectants results in a reversion to the transformed state and a simultaneous elevation of DNMT1 activity and DNA methylation.

Constitutive Ras activation has been shown to promote resistance to apoptosis. H-ras downregulates the cell death-inducing protein FAS and renders cells resistant to FAS ligand-induced apoptosis. In Ras-transformed cells, FAS expression is undetectable and silencing of the gene is dependent on DNA methylation (Peli et al. 1999). The mechanistic basis of Ras-mediated hypermethylation was addressed by an intriguing study by Michael Green and colleagues. They performed a genome-wide RNA interference (RNAi) screen to identify genes that are required for Ras-mediated silencing of FAS by methylation. Interestingly, they showed that an elaborate pathway involving at least 28 genes is required for the inactivation of FAS by Ras. These genes included *DNMT1*, known transcriptional regulators (*CTCF*, *EID1*, *E2F1*, and *RCOR2*), three histone methyltransferases (*EZH2*, *DOT1L*, and *SMYD1*), the histone deacetylase *HDCA9*, and several Polycomb proteins (*BMI1*, *EED*). Nine of the effectors of Ras-induced epigenetic silencing were found to be directly associated with the FAS promoter in K-Ras-transformed cells but not in untransformed cells. Knockdown of any one of the 28 effectors resulted in a failure to recruit DNMT1 to the FAS promoter, loss of FAS hypermethylation, and a de-repression of FAS expression. These effectors were functionally important as hypermethylation and silencing of a number of the genes was required to maintain the Ras-transformed phenotype. Moreover, the effectors were required for the specific silencing of a number of other genes by hypermethylation, including the pro-apoptotic gene *PAR4* and the Wnt antagonist *SFRP1* (Gazin et al. 2007). The observation that Ras-induced transformation results in distinct epigenetic events that are required to establish and maintain the transformed phenotype highlights the close interplay between oncogenic signaling and epigenetic regulation. In the past, it was thought that gene silencing occurs simply by random acquisition of epigenetic marks that confer a selective growth advantage. From the data discussed above, it is evident now that at least in some circumstances, cancer-specific epigenetic lesions can be initiated by oncogenes through specific pathways. Furthermore, because methylation of these genes are required for the transformed phenotype and inhibitors of the pathway can reverse this methylation, the detection of the epigenetic state of these genes may be used as biomarkers for treatment efficacy by agents that target these pathways.

A second example that highlights the close association between oncogenic signaling pathways and epigenetic alterations involves the oncogenic tyrosine kinase NPM1-ALK. In non-Hodgkin's lymphomas, chromosomal translocations can cause the *ALK* gene to become fused with various partners, most notably the nucleophosmin gene (*NPM*) (Morris et al. 1994; Wasik 2002). The NPM1-ALK gene product is constitutively activated through autophosphorylation and mediates malignant cell transformation both in vitro and in vivo by activating downstream effectors such as STAT3. Wasik and colleagues showed in a series of experiments that NPM1-ALK induces epigenetic silencing of the *STAT5A* gene via hypermethylation. STAT5A can act as a tumor suppressor by inhibiting NPM1-ALK expression and its inhibition helps promote NPM1-ALK-mediated transformation. Furthermore, this silencing is functionally important because the loss of STAT5A expression is critical for NPM1-ALK-mediated oncogenesis as it permits uninterrupted NPM1-ALK transcription. Taken together, these observations show that there is a "double-feedback" loop in which the oncogenic tyrosine kinase NPM1-ALK becomes persistently expressed by inhibiting the expression of a transcriptional inhibitor targeted to its gene. These findings have substantial therapeutic implications for NPM1-ALK expressing malignancies and possibly for other cancers with chimeric tyrosine kinases. For these tumors, current efforts have concentrated on inhibition of the kinase activity, and in many cases, this approach is itself not curative and over time leads to drug resistance. Suppression of the expression of such kinases, in addition to inhibiting their enzymatic activity, may prove clinically beneficial. 5'-aza has already been shown to be effective in some patients and may offer a complementary, perhaps synergistic, approach to induce the expression of epigenetically silenced genes that are required for the maintenance of the cancerous state.

The finding that stable epigenetic alterations, in part, constitute the nuclear changes that occur in response to oncogenic signaling has important implications for the development of predictive biomarkers for targeted agents. This is especially important for evaluating the efficacy of new targeted agents. Are agents currently in trials not successful because the test drug is not delivered to the intended target efficiently, because the level of inhibition achieved is not sufficient, or because inhibition of the targeted pathway is not sufficient to induce a clinical response despite adequate target inhibition? Answering these fundamental questions will be crucial if we are to achieve the ability to use targeted agents in a judicious manner. Current approaches for developing biomarkers of response to targeted compounds, such as the PI3 kinase inhibitors, involves querying the phosphorylation status of downstream target proteins in the signaling cascade. This approach is frequently fraught with difficulty as the dynamic range of phosphorylation states is very variable, difficult to measure, and not always reflective of clinical response. The development of a methylation marker that is predictive of response to PI3 kinase pathway inhibition would provide distinctive advantages. These advantages include the ability to use DNA, which is a relatively stable material compared to phospho-proteins, the ability to use paraffin-embedded materials, and the availability of highly-quantitative assays to measure DNA methylation.

8 Future Perspectives

In this chapter, we have shown that epigenetic alterations, as well as genetic abnormalities, contribute to mechanisms underlying the stages of tumorigenesis. This recognition is providing the oncology community with new strategies for developing very potent biomarkers for molecular staging of cancer, for monitoring tumor behavior (including prediction and assessing the effects of therapies), and for tumor detection. The need to validate all of these approaches has been pointed out and will constitute a significant direction for clinical cancer research over years to come. In addition, it is apparent that ongoing efforts to screen cancer genomes for all abnormalities that contribute to cancer pathobiology must include strategies to chronicle epigenetic, as well as genetic, alterations. These efforts will not only further unravel the mechanisms underlying tumor initiation and progression, but will define many more biomarkers to weave into current strategies for refining our approaches to cancer management.

References

Abdel-Wahab O, Mullally A, Hedvat C, Garcia-Manero G, Patel J, Wadleigh M, Malinge S, Yao J, Kilpivaara O, Bhat R, Huberman K, Thomas S, Dolgalev I, Heguy A, Paietta E, Le Beau MM, Beran M, Tallman MS, Ebert BL, Kantarjian HM, Stone RM, Gilliland DG, Crispino JD, Levine RL (2009) Genetic characterization of TET1, TET2, and TET3 alterations in myeloid malignancies. Blood 114:144–147

Aggerholm A, Holm MS, Guldberg P, Olesen LH, Hokland P (2006) Promoter hypermethylation of p15INK4B, HIC1, CDH1, and ER is frequent in myelodysplastic syndrome and predicts poor prognosis in early-stage patients. Eur J Haematol 76:23–32

Ahluwalia A, Hurteau JA, Bigsby RM, Nephew KP (2001) DNA methylation in ovarian cancer II. Expression of DNA methyltransferases in ovarian cancer cell lines and normal ovarian epithelial cells. Gynecol Oncol 82:299–304

Antequera F, Bird A (1993) CpG islands. EXS 64:169–185

Antequera F, Bird A (1994) Predicting the total number of human genes. Nat Genet 8:114

Antequera F, Bird A (1999) CpG islands as genomic footprints of promoters that are associated with replication origins. Curr Biol 9:R661–R667

Bannister AJ, Schneider R, Myers FA, Thorne AW, Crane-Robinson C, Kouzarides T (2005) Spatial distribution of di- and tri-methyl lysine 36 of histone H3 at active genes. J Biol Chem 280:17732–17736

Baylin SB, Ohm JE (2006) Epigenetic gene silencing in cancer—a mechanism for early oncogenic pathway addiction? Nat Rev Cancer 6:107–116

Bell AC, Felsenfeld G (2000) Methylation of a CTCF-dependent boundary controls imprinted expression of the Igf2 gene. Nature 405:482–485

Bestor TH, Tycko B (1996) Creation of genomic methylation patterns. Nat Genet 12:363–367

Bird AP, Wolffe AP (1999) Methylation-induced repression–belts, braces, and chromatin. Cell 99:451–454

Bodey B, Siegel SE, Kaiser HE (2002) MAGE-1, a cancer/testis-antigen, expression in childhood astrocytomas as an indicator of tumor progression. In Vivo 16:583–588

Brock MV, Hooker CM, Ota-Machida E, Han Y, Guo M, Ames S, Glockner S, Piantadosi S, Gabrielson E, Pridham G, Pelosky K, Belinsky SA, Yang SC, Baylin SB, Herman JG (2008)

DNA methylation markers and early recurrence in stage I lung cancer. N Engl J Med 358:1118–1128

Chan TA, Glockner S, Yi JM, Chen W, Van Neste L, Cope L, Herman JG, Velculescu V, Schuebel KE, Ahuja N, Baylin SB (2008) Convergence of mutation and epigenetic alterations identifies common genes in cancer that predict for poor prognosis. PLoS Med 5:e114

Chaudhry P, Srinivasan R, Patel FD (2009) Utility of gene promoter methylation in prediction of response to platinum-based chemotherapy in epithelial ovarian cancer (EOC). Cancer Invest 27:877–884

Criniere E, Kaloshi G, Laigle-Donadey F, Lejeune J, Auger N, Benouaich-Amiel A, Everhard S, Mokhtari K, Polivka M, Delattre JY, Hoang-Xuan K, Thillet J, Sanson M (2007) MGMT prognostic impact on glioblastoma is dependent on therapeutic modalities. J Neurooncol 83:173–179

Cross SH, Meehan RR, Nan X, Bird A (1997) A component of the transcriptional repressor MeCP1 shares a motif with DNA methyltransferase and HRX proteins. Nat Genet 16:256–259

Deiss LP, Feinstein E, Berissi H, Cohen O, Kimchi A (1995) Identification of a novel serine/ threonine kinase and a novel 15-kD protein as potential mediators of the gamma interferon-induced cell death. Genes Dev 9:15–30

Delhommeau F, Dupont S, Della Valle V, James C, Trannoy S, Masse A, Kosmider O, Le Couedic JP, Robert F, Alberdi A, Lecluse Y, Plo I, Dreyfus FJ, Marzac C, Casadevall N, Lacombe C, Romana SP, Dessen P, Soulier J, Viguie F, Fontenay M, Vainchenker W, Bernard OA (2009) Mutation in TET2 in myeloid cancers. N Engl J Med 360:2289–2301

Diaz-Meyer N, Yang Y, Sait SN, Maher ER, Higgins MJ (2005) Alternative mechanisms associated with silencing of CDKN1C in Beckwith-Wiedemann syndrome. J Med Genet 42:648–655

Eads CA, Danenberg KD, Kawakami K, Saltz LB, Blake C, Shibata D, Danenberg PV, Laird PW (2000) MethyLight: a high-throughput assay to measure DNA methylation. Nucleic Acids Res 28:E32

Ehrich M, Nelson MR, Stanssens P, Zabeau M, Liloglou T, Xinarianos G, Cantor CR, Field JK, van den Boom D (2005) Quantitative high-throughput analysis of DNA methylation patterns by base-specific cleavage and mass spectrometry. Proc Natl Acad Sci U S A 102: 15785–15790

Ehrlich M, Gama-Sosa MA, Huang LH, Midgett RM, Kuo KC, McCune RA, Gehrke C (1982) Amount and distribution of 5-methylcytosine in human DNA from different types of tissues of cells. Nucleic Acids Res 10:2709–2721

Esteller M (2007) Cancer epigenomics: DNA methylomes and histone-modification maps. Nat Rev Genet 8:286–298

Esteller M (2008) Epigenetics in cancer. N Engl J Med 358:1148–1159

Esteller M, Garcia-Foncillas J, Andion E, Goodman SN, Hidalgo OF, Vanaclocha V, Baylin SB, Herman JG (2000a) Inactivation of the DNA-repair gene MGMT and the clinical response of gliomas to alkylating agents. N Engl J Med 343:1350–1354

Esteller M, Silva JM, Dominguez G, Bonilla F, Matias-Guiu X, Lerma E, Bussaglia E, Prat J, Harkes IC, Repasky EA, Gabrielson E, Schutte M, Baylin SB, Herman JG (2000b) Promoter hypermethylation and BRCA1 inactivation in sporadic breast and ovarian tumors. J Natl Cancer Inst 92:564–569

Esteller M, Corn PG, Baylin SB, Herman JG (2001) A gene hypermethylation profile of human cancer. Cancer Res 61:3225–3229

Fang F, Turcan S, Rimner A, Kaufman A, Giri D, Morris LG, Shen R, Seshan V, Mo Q, Heguy A, Baylin SB, Ahuja N, Viale A, Massague J, Norton L, Vahdat LT, Moynahan ME, Chan TA (2011) Breast cancer methylomes establish an epigenomic foundation for metastasis. Sci Trans Med 3:75ra25

Feinberg AP, Vogelstein B (1983) Hypomethylation distinguishes genes of some human cancers from their normal counterparts. Nature 301:89–92

Feinberg AP, Ohlsson R, Henikoff S (2006) The epigenetic progenitor origin of human cancer. Nat Rev Genet 7:21–33

Fraga MF, Esteller M (2002) DNA methylation: a profile of methods and applications. Biotechniques 33:632, 634, 636–649

Fraga MF, Ballestar E, Villar-Garea A, Boix-Chornet M, Espada J, Schotta G, Bonaldi T, Haydon C, Ropero S, Petrie K, Iyer NG, Perez-Rosado A, Calvo E, Lopez JA, Cano A, Calasanz MJ, Colomer D, Piris MA, Ahn N, Imhof A, Caldas C, Jenuwein T, Esteller M (2005) Loss of acetylation at Lys16 and trimethylation at Lys20 of histone H4 is a common hallmark of human cancer. Nat Genet 37:391–400

Gaudet F, Hodgson JG, Eden A, Jackson-Grusby L, Dausman J, Gray JW, Leonhardt H, Jaenisch R (2003) Induction of tumors in mice by genomic hypomethylation. Science 300:489–492

Gazin C, Wajapeyee N, Gobeil S, Virbasius CM, Green MR (2007) An elaborate pathway required for Ras-mediated epigenetic silencing. Nature 449:1073–1077

Girault I, Tozlu S, Lidereau R, Bieche I (2003) Expression analysis of DNA methyltransferases 1, 3A, and 3B in sporadic breast carcinomas. Clin Cancer Res 9:4415–4422

Goel A, Nagasaka T, Arnold CN, Inoue T, Hamilton C, Niedzwiecki D, Compton C, Mayer RJ, Goldberg R, Bertagnolli MM, Boland CR (2007) The CpG island methylator phenotype and chromosomal instability are inversely correlated in sporadic colorectal cancer. Gastroenterology 132:127–138

Greger V, Passarge E, Hopping W, Messmer E, Horsthemke B (1989) Epigenetic changes may contribute to the formation and spontaneous regression of retinoblastoma. Hum Genet 83:155–158

Gu M, Kim D, Bae Y, Choi J, Kim S, Song S (2009) Analysis of microsatellite instability, protein expression and methylation status of hMLH1 and hMSH2 genes in gastric carcinomas. Hepatogastroenterology 56:899–904

Hark AT, Schoenherr CJ, Katz DJ, Ingram RS, Levorse JM, Tilghman SM (2000) CTCF mediates methylation-sensitive enhancer-blocking activity at the H19/Igf2 locus. Nature 405:486–489

Hegi ME, Diserens AC, Gorlia T, Hamou MF, de Tribolet N, Weller M, Kros JM, Hainfellner JA, Mason W, Mariani L, Bromberg JE, Hau P, Mirimanoff RO, Cairncross JG, Janzer RC, Stupp R (2005) MGMT gene silencing and benefit from temozolomide in glioblastoma. N Engl J Med 352:997–1003

Herman JG, Baylin SB (2003) Gene silencing in cancer in association with promoter hypermethylation. N Engl J Med 349:2042–2054

Herman JG, Latif F, Weng Y, Lerman MI, Zbar B, Liu S, Samid D, Duan DS, Gnarra JR, Linehan WM et al (1994) Silencing of the VHL tumor-suppressor gene by DNA methylation in renal carcinoma. Proc Natl Acad Sci U S A 91:9700–9704

Herman JG, Graff JR, Myohanen S, Nelkin BD, Baylin SB (1996) Methylation-specific PCR: a novel PCR assay for methylation status of CpG islands. Proc Natl Acad Sci U S A 93: 9821–9826

Hirose Y, Kreklau EL, Erickson LC, Berger MS, Pieper RO (2003) Delayed repletion of O6-methylguanine-DNA methyltransferase resulting in failure to protect the human glioblastoma cell line SF767 from temozolomide-induced cytotoxicity. J Neurosurg 98:591–598

Hoffmann MJ, Schulz WA (2005) Causes and consequences of DNA hypomethylation in human cancer. Biochem Cell Biol 83:296–321

Hoque MO, Kim MS, Ostrow KL, Liu J, Wisman GB, Park HL, Poeta ML, Jeronimo C, Henrique R, Lendvai A, Schuuring E, Begum S, Rosenbaum E, Ongenaert M, Yamashita K, Califano J, Westra W, van der Zee AG, Van Criekinge W, Sidransky D (2008) Genome-wide promoter analysis uncovers portions of the cancer methylome. Cancer Res 68:2661–2670

Horsthemke B, Buiting K (2006) Imprinting defects on human chromosome 15. Cytogenet Genome Res 113:292–299

Howard G, Eiges R, Gaudet F, Jaenisch R, Eden A (2008) Activation and transposition of endogenous retroviral elements in hypomethylation induced tumors in mice. Oncogene 27:404–408

Huang Y, Greene E, Murray Stewart T, Goodwin AC, Baylin SB, Woster PM, Casero RA Jr (2007) Inhibition of lysine-specific demethylase 1 by polyamine analogues results in reexpression of aberrantly silenced genes. Proc Natl Acad Sci U S A 104:8023–8028

Huang Y, Stewart TM, Wu Y, Baylin SB, Marton LJ, Perkins B, Jones RJ, Woster PM, Casero RA Jr (2009) Novel oligoamine analogues inhibit lysine-specific demethylase 1 and induce reexpression of epigenetically silenced genes. Clin Cancer Res 15:7217–7228

Iliopoulos D, Oikonomou P, Messinis I, Tsezou A (2009) Correlation of promoter hypermethylation in hTERT, DAPK and MGMT genes with cervical oncogenesis progression. Oncol Rep 22:199–204

Inbal B, Shani G, Cohen O, Kissil JL, Kimchi A (2000) Death-associated protein kinase-related protein 1, a novel serine/threonine kinase involved in apoptosis. Mol Cell Biol 20:1044–1054

Issa JP (2008) Colon cancer: it's CIN or CIMP. Clin Cancer Res 14:5939–5940

Jacinto FV, Esteller M (2007) Mutator pathways unleashed by epigenetic silencing in human cancer. Mutagenesis 22:247–253

Jaenisch R, Young R (2008) Stem cells, the molecular circuitry of pluripotency and nuclear reprogramming. Cell 132:567–582

Jarmalaite S, Jankevicius F, Kurgonaite K, Suziedelis K, Mutanen P, Husgafvel-Pursiainen K (2008) Promoter hypermethylation in tumour suppressor genes shows association with stage, grade and invasiveness of bladder cancer. Oncology 75:145–151

Jones PA, Baylin SB (2007) The epigenomics of cancer. Cell 128:683–692

Jones PA, Laird PW (1999) Cancer epigenetics comes of age. Nat Genet 21:163–167

Jones PL, Veenstra GJ, Wade PA, Vermaak D, Kass SU, Landsberger N, Strouboulis J, Wolffe AP (1998) Methylated DNA and MeCP2 recruit histone deacetylase to repress transcription. Nat Genet 19:187–191

Kaina B, Christmann M, Naumann S, Roos WP (2007) MGMT: key node in the battle against genotoxicity, carcinogenicity and apoptosis induced by alkylating agents. DNA Repair (Amst) 6:1079–1099

Kakar S, Deng G, Cun L, Sahai V, Kim YS (2008) CpG island methylation is frequently present in tubulovillous and villous adenomas and correlates with size, site, and villous component. Hum Pathol 39:30–36

Kane MF, Loda M, Gaida GM, Lipman J, Mishra R, Goldman H, Jessup JM, Kolodner R (1997) Methylation of the hMLH1 promoter correlates with lack of expression of hMLH1 in sporadic colon tumors and mismatch repair-defective human tumor cell lines. Cancer Res 57:808–811

Karapetis CS, Khambata-Ford S, Jonker DJ, O'Callaghan CJ, Tu D, Tebbutt NC, Simes RJ, Chalchal H, Shapiro JD, Robitaille S, Price TJ, Shepherd L, Au HJ, Langer C, Moore MJ, Zalcberg JR (2008) K-ras mutations and benefit from cetuximab in advanced colorectal cancer. N Engl J Med 359:1757–1765

Keshet I, Schlesinger Y, Farkash S, Rand E, Hecht M, Segal E, Pikarski E, Young RA, Niveleau A, Cedar H, Simon I (2006) Evidence for an instructive mechanism of de novo methylation in cancer cells. Nat Genet 38:149–153

Kidani K, Osaki M, Tamura T, Yamaga K, Shomori K, Ryoke K, Ito H (2009) High expression of EZH2 is associated with tumor proliferation and prognosis in human oral squamous cell carcinomas. Oral Oncol 45:39–46

Kinzler KW, Vogelstein B (1996) Lessons from hereditary colorectal cancer. Cell 87:159–170

Kinzler KW, Vogelstein B (1997) Cancer-susceptibility genes. Gatekeepers and caretakers. Nature 386:761–763

Kleer CG, Cao Q, Varambally S, Shen R, Ota I, Tomlins SA, Ghosh D, Sewalt RG, Otte AP, Hayes DF, Sabel MS, Livant D, Weiss SJ, Rubin MA, Chinnaiyan AM (2003) EZH2 is a marker of aggressive breast cancer and promotes neoplastic transformation of breast epithelial cells. Proc Natl Acad Sci U S A 100:11606–11611

Kouzarides T (2007) Chromatin modifications and their function. Cell 128:693–705

Laird PW (1997) Oncogenic mechanisms mediated by DNA methylation. Mol Med Today 3:223–229

Langemeijer SM, Kuiper RP, Berends M, Knops R, Aslanyan MG, Massop M, Stevens-Linders E, van Hoogen P, van Kessel AG, Raymakers RA, Kamping EJ, Verhoef GE, Verburgh E, Hagemeijer A, Vandenberghe P, de Witte T, van der Reijden BA, Jansen JH (2009) Acquired mutations in TET2 are common in myelodysplastic syndromes. Nat Genet 41:838–842

Ley TJ, Ding L, Walter MJ, McLellan MD, Lamprecht T, Larson DE, Kandoth C, Payton JE, Baty J, Welch J, Harris CC, Lichti CF, Townsend RR, Fulton RS, Dooling DJ, Koboldt DC, Schmidt H, Zhang Q, Osborne JR, Lin L, O'Laughlin M, McMichael JF, Delehaunty KD, McGrath SD, Fulton LA, Magrini VJ, Vickery TL, Hundal J, Cook LL, Conyers JJ, Swift GW, Reed JP, Alldredge PA, Wylie T, Walker J, Kalicki J, Watson MA, Heath S, Shannon WD, Varghese N, Nagarajan R, Westervelt P, Tomasson MH, Link DC, Graubert TA, DiPersio JF, Mardis ER, Wilson RK (2010) DNMT3A mutations in acute myeloid leukemia. N Engl J Med 363:2424–2433

Li E, Beard C, Jaenisch R (1993) Role for DNA methylation in genomic imprinting. Nature 366:362–365

Liang G, Lin JC, Wei V, Yoo C, Cheng JC, Nguyen CT, Weisenberger DJ, Egger G, Takai D, Gonzales FA, Jones PA (2004) Distinct localization of histone H3 acetylation and H3-K4 methylation to the transcription start sites in the human genome. Proc Natl Acad Sci U S A 101:7357–7362

Lin YW, Chung MT, Lai HC, De Yan M, Shih YL, Chang CC, Yu MH (2009) Methylation analysis of SFRP genes family in cervical adenocarcinoma. J Cancer Res Clin Oncol 135:1665–1674

Lister R, Pelizzola M, Dowen RH, Hawkins RD, Hon G, Tonti-Filippini J, Nery JR, Lee L, Ye Z, Ngo QM, Edsall L, Antosiewicz-Bourget J, Stewart R, Ruotti V, Millar AH, Thomson JA, Ren B, Ecker JR (2009) Human DNA methylomes at base resolution show widespread epigenomic differences. Nature 462:315–322

Lopez-Serra L, Ballestar E, Fraga MF, Alaminos M, Setien F, Esteller M (2006) A profile of methyl-CpG binding domain protein occupancy of hypermethylated promoter CpG islands of tumor suppressor genes in human cancer. Cancer Res 66:8342–8346

Loriot A, Boon T, De Smet C (2003) Five new human cancer-germline genes identified among 12 genes expressed in spermatogonia. Int J Cancer 105:371–376

Lund P, Weisshaupt K, Mikeska T, Jammas D, Chen X, Kuban RJ, Ungethum U, Krapfenbauer U, Herzel HP, Schafer R, Walter J, Sers C (2006) Oncogenic HRAS suppresses clusterin expression through promoter hypermethylation. Oncogene 25:4890–4903

Mager J, Bartolomei MS (2005) Strategies for dissecting epigenetic mechanisms in the mouse. Nat Genet 37:1194–1200

Merlo A, Herman JG, Mao L, Lee DJ, Gabrielson E, Burger PC, Baylin SB, Sidransky D (1995) 5' CpG island methylation is associated with transcriptional silencing of the tumour suppressor p16/CDKN2/MTS1 in human cancers. Nat Med 1:686–692

Morin PJ, Sparks AB, Korinek V, Barker N, Clevers H, Vogelstein B, Kinzler KW (1997) Activation of beta-catenin-Tcf signaling in colon cancer by mutations in beta-catenin or APC. Science 275:1787–1790

Morin RD, Johnson NA, Severson TM, Mungall AJ, An J, Goya R, Paul JE, Boyle M, Woolcock BW, Kuchenbauer F, Yap D, Humphries RK, Griffith OL, Shah S, Zhu H, Kimbara M, Shashkin P, Charlot JF, Tcherpakov M, Corbett R, Tam A, Varhol R, Smailus D, Moksa M, Zhao Y, Delaney A, Qian H, Birol I, Schein J, Moore R, Holt R, Horsman DE, Connors JM, Jones S, Aparicio S, Hirst M, Gascoyne RD, Marra MA (2010) Somatic mutations altering EZH2 (Tyr641) in follicular and diffuse large B-cell lymphomas of germinal-center origin. Nat Genet 42:181–185

Morris SW, Kirstein MN, Valentine MB, Dittmer KG, Shapiro DN, Saltman DL, Look AT (1994) Fusion of a kinase gene, ALK, to a nucleolar protein gene, NPM, in non-Hodgkin's lymphoma. Science 263:1281–1284

Nan X, Meehan RR, Bird A (1993) Dissection of the methyl-CpG binding domain from the chromosomal protein MeCP2. Nucleic Acids Res 21:4886–4892

Epigenetic Biomarkers 213

Nan X, Ng HH, Johnson CA, Laherty CD, Turner BM, Eisenman RN, Bird A (1998) Transcriptional repression by the methyl-CpG-binding protein MeCP2 involves a histone deacetylase complex. Nature 393:386–389

Ng HH, Bird A (1999) DNA methylation and chromatin modification. Curr Opin Genet Dev 9:158–163

Ng HH, Ciccone DN, Morshead KB, Oettinger MA, Struhl K (2003) Lysine-79 of histone H3 is hypomethylated at silenced loci in yeast and mammalian cells: a potential mechanism for position-effect variegation. Proc Natl Acad Sci U S A 100:1820–1825

Noushmehr H, Weisenberger DJ, Diefes K, Phillips HS, Pujara K, Berman BP, Pan F, Pelloski CE, Sulman EP, Bhat KP, Verhaak RG, Hoadley KA, Hayes DN, Perou CM, Schmidt HK, Ding L, Wilson RK, Van Den Berg D, Shen H, Bengtsson H, Neuvial P, Cope LM, Buckley J, Herman JG, Baylin SB, Laird PW, Aldape K (2010) Identification of a CpG island methylator phenotype that defines a distinct subgroup of glioma. Cancer Cell 17:510–522

Ogino S, Meyerhardt JA, Kawasaki T, Clark JW, Ryan DP, Kulke MH, Enzinger PC, Wolpin BM, Loda M, Fuchs CS (2007) CpG island methylation, response to combination chemotherapy, and patient survival in advanced microsatellite stable colorectal carcinoma. Virchows Arch 450:529–537

Ogino S, Nosho K, Kirkner GJ, Kawasaki T, Meyerhardt JA, Loda M, Giovannucci EL, Fuchs CS (2009) CpG island methylator phenotype, microsatellite instability, BRAF mutation and clinical outcome in colon cancer. Gut 58:90–96

Ohlsson R, Nystrom A, Pfeifer-Ohlsson S, Tohonen V, Hedborg F, Schofield P, Flam F, Ekstrom TJ (1993) IGF2 is parentally imprinted during human embryogenesis and in the Beckwith-Wiedemann syndrome. Nat Genet 4:94–97

Ohm JE, McGarvey KM, Yu X, Cheng L, Schuebel KE, Cope L, Mohammad HP, Chen W, Daniel VC, Yu W, Berman DM, Jenuwein T, Pruitt K, Sharkis SJ, Watkins DN, Herman JG, Baylin SB (2007) A stem cell-like chromatin pattern may predispose tumor suppressor genes to DNA hypermethylation and heritable silencing. Nat Genet 39:237–242

Oshimo Y, Nakayama H, Ito R, Kitadai Y, Yoshida K, Chayama K, Yasui W (2003) Promoter methylation of cyclin D2 gene in gastric carcinoma. Int J Oncol 23:1663–1670

Oue N, Motoshita J, Yokozaki H, Hayashi K, Tahara E, Taniyama K, Matsusaki K, Yasui W (2002) Distinct promoter hypermethylation of p16INK4a, CDH1, and RAR-beta in intestinal, diffuse-adherent, and diffuse-scattered type gastric carcinomas. J Pathol 198:55–59

Park SJ, Rashid A, Lee JH, Kim SG, Hamilton SR, Wu TT (2003) Frequent CpG island methylation in serrated adenomas of the colorectum. Am J Pathol 162:815–822

Peli J, Schroter M, Rudaz C, Hahne M, Meyer C, Reichmann E, Tschopp J (1999) Oncogenic Ras inhibits Fas ligand-mediated apoptosis by downregulating the expression of Fas. Embo J 18:1824–1831

Peters AH, Mermoud JE, O'Carroll D, Pagani M, Schweizer D, Brockdorff N, Jenuwein T (2002) Histone H3 lysine 9 methylation is an epigenetic imprint of facultative heterochromatin. Nat Genet 30:77–80

Peters AH, Kubicek S, Mechtler K, O'Sullivan RJ, Derijck AA, Perez-Burgos L, Kohlmaier A, Opravil S, Tachibana M, Shinkai Y, Martens JH, Jenuwein T (2003) Partitioning and plasticity of repressive histone methylation states in mammalian chromatin. Mol Cell 12:1577–1589

Rashid A, Shen L, Morris JS, Issa JP, Hamilton SR (2001) CpG island methylation in colorectal adenomas. Am J Pathol 159:1129–1135

Reik W, Lewis A (2005) Co-evolution of X-chromosome inactivation and imprinting in mammals. Nat Rev Genet 6:403–410

Reik W, Dean W, Walter J (2001) Epigenetic reprogramming in mammalian development. Science 293:1089–1093

Rice JC, Ozcelik H, Maxeiner P, Andrulis I, Futscher BW (2000) Methylation of the BRCA1 promoter is associated with decreased BRCA1 mRNA levels in clinical breast cancer specimens. Carcinogenesis 21:1761–1765

Rouleau J, MacLeod AR, Szyf M (1995) Regulation of the DNA methyltransferase by the Ras-AP-1 signaling pathway. J Biol Chem 270:1595–1601

Schuebel KE, Chen WE, Cope L, Glockner S, Suzuki H, Yi JM, Chan TA, Van Neste L, Van Criekinge W, van den Bosch S, van Engeland M, Ting AH, Jair K, Yu W, Toyota M, Imai K, Ahuja N, Herman JG, Baylin SB (2007) Comparing the DNA hypermethalome with gene mutations in human colorectal cancer. PLoS Genetics doi:10.1371/journal.pgen.0030157.eor

Sharma G, Mirza S, Yang YH, Parshad R, Hazrah P, Datta Gupta S, Ralhan R (2009) Prognostic relevance of promoter hypermethylation of multiple genes in breast cancer patients. Cell Oncol 31:487–500

Shen L, Toyota M, Kondo Y, Lin E, Zhang L, Guo Y, Hernandez NS, Chen X, Ahmed S, Konishi K, Hamilton SR, Issa JP (2007) Integrated genetic and epigenetic analysis identifies three different subclasses of colon cancer. Proc Natl Acad Sci U S A 104:18654–18659

Shi Y, Lan F, Matson C, Mulligan P, Whetstine JR, Cole PA, Casero RA (2004) Histone demethylation mediated by the nuclear amine oxidase homolog LSD1. Cell 119:941–953

Sims JK, Houston SI, Magazinnik T, Rice JC (2006) A trans-tail histone code defined by monomethylated H4 Lys-20 and H3 Lys-9 demarcates distinct regions of silent chromatin. J Biol Chem 281:12760–12766

Singer MS, Kahana A, Wolf AJ, Meisinger LL, Peterson SE, Goggin C, Mahowald M, Gottschling DE (1998) Identification of high-copy disruptors of telomeric silencing in Saccharomyces cerevisiae. Genetics 150:613–632

Steinmann K, Sandner A, Schagdarsurengin U, Dammann RH (2009) Frequent promoter hypermethylation of tumor-related genes in head and neck squamous cell carcinoma. Oncol Rep 22:1519–1526

Sterner DE, Berger SL (2000) Acetylation of histones and transcription-related factors. Microbiol Mol Biol Rev 64:435–459

Stupp R, Mason WP, van den Bent MJ, Weller M, Fisher B, Taphoorn MJ, Belanger K, Brandes AA, Marosi C, Bogdahn U, Curschmann J, Janzer RC, Ludwin SK, Gorlia T, Allgeier A, Lacombe D, Cairncross JG, Eisenhauer E, Mirimanoff RO (2005) Radiotherapy plus concomitant and adjuvant temozolomide for glioblastoma. N Engl J Med 352:987–996

Suzuki H, Gabrielson E, Chen W, Anbazhagan R, van Engeland M, Weijenberg MP, Herman JG, Baylin SB (2002) A genomic screen for genes upregulated by demethylation and histone deacetylase inhibition in human colorectal cancer. Nat Genet 31:141–149

Suzuki H, Watkins DN, Jair KW, Schuebel KE, Markowitz SD, Chen WD, Pretlow TP, Yang B, Akiyama Y, Van Engeland M, Toyota M, Tokino T, Hinoda Y, Imai K, Herman JG, Baylin SB (2004) Epigenetic inactivation of SFRP genes allows constitutive WNT signaling in colorectal cancer. Nat Genet 36:417–422

Suzuki H, Toyota M, Carraway H, Gabrielson E, Ohmura T, Fujikane T, Nishikawa N, Sogabe Y, Nojima M, Sonoda T, Mori M, Hirata K, Imai K, Shinomura Y, Baylin SB, Tokino T (2008) Frequent epigenetic inactivation of Wnt antagonist genes in breast cancer. Br J Cancer 98:1147–1156

Szpakowski S, Sun X, Lage JM, Dyer A, Rubinstein J, Kowalski D, Sasaki C, Costa J, Lizardi PM (2009) Loss of epigenetic silencing in tumors preferentially affects primate-specific retroelements. Gene doi:S0378-1119(09)00437-5 [pii]10.1016/j.gene.2009.08.006

TCGA (2008) Comprehensive genomic characterization defines human glioblastoma genes and core pathways (Cancer Genome Atlas Network). Nature 455:1061–1068

Thibodeau SN, Bren G, Schaid D (1993) Microsatellite instability in cancer of the proximal colon. Science 260:816–819

Toyota M, Ahuja N, Ohe-Toyota M, Herman JG, Baylin SB, Issa JP (1999) CpG island methylator phenotype in colorectal cancer. Proc Natl Acad Sci U S A 96:8681–8686

Toyota M, Ohe-Toyota M, Ahuja N, Issa JP (2000) Distinct genetic profiles in colorectal tumors with or without the CpG island methylator phenotype. Proc Natl Acad Sci U S A 97:710–715

Uhlmann K, Brinckmann A, Toliat MR, Ritter H, Nurnberg P (2002) Evaluation of a potential epigenetic biomarker by quantitative methyl-single nucleotide polymorphism analysis. Electrophoresis 23:4072–4079

Urakami S, Shiina H, Enokida H, Hirata H, Kawamoto K, Kawakami T, Kikuno N, Tanaka Y, Majid S, Nakagawa M, Igawa M, Dahiya R (2006) Wnt antagonist family genes as biomarkers for diagnosis, staging, and prognosis of renal cell carcinoma using tumor and serum DNA. Clin Cancer Res 12:6989–6997

van den Bent MJ, Dubbink HJ, Sanson M, van der Lee-Haarloo CR, Hegi M, Jeuken JW, Ibdaih A, Brandes AA, Taphoorn MJ, Frenay M, Lacombe D, Gorlia T, Dinjens WN, Kros JM (2009) MGMT promoter methylation is prognostic but not predictive for outcome to adjuvant PCV chemotherapy in anaplastic oligodendroglial tumors: a report from EORTC Brain Tumor Group Study 26951. J Clin Oncol 27:5881–5886

van Haaften G, Dalgliesh GL, Davies H, Chen L, Bignell G, Greenman C, Edkins S, Hardy C, O'Meara S, Teague J, Butler A, Hinton J, Latimer C, Andrews J, Barthorpe S, Beare D, Buck G, Campbell PJ, Cole J, Forbes S, Jia M, Jones D, Kok CY, Leroy C, Lin ML, McBride DJ, Maddison M, Maquire S, McLay K, Menzies A, Mironenko T, Mulderrig L, Mudie L, Pleasance E, Shepherd R, Smith R, Stebbings L, Stephens P, Tang G, Tarpey PS, Turner R, Turrell K, Varian J, West S, Widaa S, Wray P, Collins VP, Ichimura K, Law S, Wong J, Yuen ST, Leung SY, Tonon G, DePinho RA, Tai YT, Anderson KC, Kahnoski RJ, Massie A, Khoo SK, Teh BT, Stratton MR, Futreal PA (2009) Somatic mutations of the histone H3K27 demethylase gene UTX in human cancer. Nat Genet 41:521–523

van Rijnsoever M, Grieu F, Elsaleh H, Joseph D, Iacopetta B (2002) Characterisation of colorectal cancers showing hypermethylation at multiple CpG islands. Gut 51:797–802

Varambally S, Dhanasekaran SM, Zhou M, Barrette TR, Kumar-Sinha C, Sanda MG, Ghosh D, Pienta KJ, Sewalt RG, Otte AP, Rubin MA, Chinnaiyan AM (2002) The polycomb group protein EZH2 is involved in progression of prostate cancer. Nature 419:624–629

Veeck J, Geisler C, Noetzel E, Alkaya S, Hartmann A, Knuchel R, Dahl E (2008) Epigenetic inactivation of the secreted frizzled-related protein-5 (SFRP5) gene in human breast cancer is associated with unfavorable prognosis. Carcinogenesis 29:991–998

Wajed SA, Laird PW, DeMeester TR (2001) DNA methylation: an alternative pathway to cancer. Ann Surg 234:10–20

Walsh CP, Chaillet JR, Bestor TH (1998) Transcription of IAP endogenous retroviruses is constrained by cytosine methylation. Nat Genet 20:116–117

Wang Y, Zhang H, Chen Y, Sun Y, Yang F, Yu W, Liang J, Sun L, Yang X, Shi L, Li R, Li Y, Zhang Y, Li Q, Yi X, Shang Y (2009) LSD1 is a subunit of the NuRD complex and targets the metastasis programs in breast cancer. Cell 138:660–672

Wasik MA (2002) Expression of anaplastic lymphoma kinase in non-Hodgkin's lymphomas and other malignant neoplasms. Biological, diagnostic, and clinical implications. Am J Clin Pathol 118(Suppl):S81–S92

Weber M, Davies JJ, Wittig D, Oakeley EJ, Haase M, Lam WL, Schubeler D (2005) Chromosome-wide and promoter-specific analyses identify sites of differential DNA methylation in normal and transformed human cells. Nat Genet 37:853–862

Weisenberger DJ, Siegmund KD, Campan M, Young J, Long TI, Faasse MA, Kang GH, Widschwendter M, Weener D, Buchanan D, Koh H, Simms L, Barker M, Leggett B, Levine J, Kim M, French AJ, Thibodeau SN, Jass J, Haile R, Laird PW (2006) CpG island methylator phenotype underlies sporadic microsatellite instability and is tightly associated with BRAF mutation in colorectal cancer. Nat Genet 38:787–793

Weksberg R, Shen DR, Fei YL, Song QL, Squire J (1993) Disruption of insulin-like growth factor 2 imprinting in Beckwith-Wiedemann syndrome. Nat Genet 5:143–150

Wilson AS, Power BE, Molloy PL (2007) DNA hypomethylation and human diseases. Biochim Biophys Acta 1775:138–162

Wissmann M, Yin N, Muller JM, Greschik H, Fodor BD, Jenuwein T, Vogler C, Schneider R, Gunther T, Buettner R, Metzger E, Schule R (2007) Cooperative demethylation by JMJD2C and LSD1 promotes androgen receptor-dependent gene expression. Nat Cell Biol 9:347–353

Wolf SF, Migeon BR (1982) Studies of X chromosome DNA methylation in normal human cells. Nature 295:667–671

Wu H, Chen Y, Liang J, Shi B, Wu G, Zhang Y, Wang D, Li R, Yi X, Zhang H, Sun L, Shang Y (2005) Hypomethylation-linked activation of PAX2 mediates tamoxifen-stimulated endometrial carcinogenesis. Nature 438:981–987

Yamane K, Toumazou C, Tsukada Y, Erdjument-Bromage H, Tempst P, Wong J, Zhang Y (2006) JHDM2A, a JmjC-containing H3K9 demethylase, facilitates transcription activation by androgen receptor. Cell 125:483–495

Yoder JA, Walsh CP, Bestor TH (1997) Cytosine methylation and the ecology of intragenomic parasites. Trends Genet 13:335–340

Yu J, Yu J, Rhodes DR, Tomlins SA, Cao X, Chen G, Mehra R, Wang X, Ghosh D, Shah RB, Varambally S, Pienta KJ, Chinnaiyan AM (2007) A polycomb repression signature in metastatic prostate cancer predicts cancer outcome. Cancer Res 67:10657–10663

Adjuvant Trials of Targeted Agents: The Newest Battleground in the War on Cancer

Robert L. Cohen

Abstract Two of the great successes in the many decades-long 'war on cancer' are the emergence of adjuvant chemotherapy regimens with lifesaving potential and the subsequent wave of 'targeted' therapies addressing the unique vulnerabilities of particular tumor types. The first intersection of adjuvant treatment and targeted treatment resulted in a spectacularly positive outcome as the addition of the anti-HER2 humanized monoclonal antibody trastuzumab to the standard adjuvant chemotherapy essentially halved the relapse rate among women with HER2+ tumors. Subsequent studies of adjuvant trastuzumab have confirmed its dramatic efficacy in a variety of chemotherapeutic contexts and have been instructive in elucidating some of the challenges ahead for newer targeted agents. The recent negative experience with bevacizumab in the adjuvant colon cancer setting suggests pitfalls and limitations of the current approach to developing adjuvant regimens. A change in thinking may be required to gain the substantial benefits implied by the trastuzumab experience in the broader context of targeted treatments. The case for a revitalized industry/academia/government partnership to address these challenges is compelling, with the potential for enormous patient and societal benefit. In order to bring potentially lifesaving benefits of this new generation of cancer drugs to patients more rapidly, changes to our 'war strategy' appear necessary.

Contents

1 Introduction.. 218
2 The Trastuzumab Experience... 220
3 The Bevacizumab Experience... 223

R. L. Cohen (✉)
Genentech Inc, 1 DNA Way, South San Francisco, CA 94080, USA
e-mail: cohen.robert@gene.com

Current Topics in Microbiology and Immunology (2012) 355: 217–232
DOI: 10.1007/82_2011_166
© Springer-Verlag Berlin Heidelberg 2011
Published Online: 5 August 2011

4 Imperatives for Successful Adjuvant Studies.. 225
5 Future Perspective 228
References.. 229

1 Introduction

Perhaps the greatest success of adult clinical oncology research over the past 40 years has been the demonstration that adjuvant treatment can be genuinely lifesaving in certain prevalent cancers such as those of the breast and colon. Adjuvant treatment regimens are generally administered to patients without evidence of residual disease, often following surgery for a high-risk primary tumor. It is essential to recognize that adjuvant trials are very different from trials in patients with measurable disease because *no patient in an adjuvant trial is evaluable for a specific treatment benefit.* Instead, large numbers of patients must be gathered, treated, and followed until sufficient numbers of clinical relapses have occurred so that meaningful comparisons can be made and hazard ratios calculated. The inability to read out clinically beneficial responses in individual patients makes adjuvant studies fundamentally inefficient despite their obvious importance.

Much of the apparatus that proved necessary to perform these complex trials was a direct result of the US National Cancer Institute's expanded management and control of cooperative groups following Richard Nixon's 'war on cancer' declaration in 1971. In fact, the chemotherapy pioneer Vincent DeVita and his colleague Edward Chu have called the 1970s 'the age of adjuvant chemotherapy' (DeVita and Chu 2008). In the US, adjuvant studies of combination chemotherapy were conceived and managed collaboratively by cooperative groups and NCI, beginning with pioneering work in breast cancer by NSABP and the Instituto Tumori in Italy. Initial successful trial results involving hundreds of patients were published in 1975 and 1976, respectively (Fisher et al. 1975; Bonadonna et al. 1976). Over subsequent years, new successful regimens emerged and were compared in sequential studies. As the efficacy of adjuvant treatment in breast and colon cancer became established, later studies necessarily involved active control arms, creating the need for ever-larger patient numbers to demonstrate significant benefits [see Fig. 1; reviewed in Gianni et al. (2009)].

The approach taken, although meticulous and careful, was very slow and limited in the number and extent of clinical questions that could be asked. As an example, initial demonstration of tamoxifen's activity in adjuvant treatment of breast cancer in the 1980s was an important success (Fisher et al. 1981, 1983; Mouridsen et al. 1988), but 15 more years and numerous additional studies were necessary to show definitively that the optimal single-agent tamoxifen schedule involved a treatment period of 2–5 years for patients with high-risk disease,

Table 1. Trials Comparing Adjuvant Anthracycline-Based Regimens With Anthracycline Plus Taxane-Based Regimens

Study	Design	No. of Patients (total)	HR	P
USON 9735[18,19]	4 × AC v 4 × DC	1,016	0.6	.015
CALGB9344/INT 0148[5]	4 AC v 4 AC→P	3,121	0.83	.006
NSABP B-28[20]	4 AC v 4 AC→4 P	3,060	0.83	.006
M. D. Anderson[21]	8 FAC v 4 P→4 FAC	524	0.66	.09
ECTO I[22]	4 A→4 CMF v 4 AP→4 CMF	904	0.66	.01
BCIRG 001[23]	6 FAC v 6 DAC	1,491	0.72	.001
PACS 01[24]	6 FEC v 3 FEC→3 D	1,999	0.83	.041
TAXIT 216[25]	4 E→4 CMF v 4 E→4 D→4 CMF	972	0.78	.05
BIG 2-98[26]	4 A→3 CMF v 4AC→3 CMF v 3A→3D→3 CMF v 4 AD→3 CMF	2,887	0.86 (D v non-D)	.051 (D v non-D)
NCIC CTG MA21[27]	4 AC→4 P (arm A) v 6 CEF (arm B) v (dd) 6 EC→4 P (arm C)	2,104	1.49 (arm A v B); 1.68 (arm A v C); 0.89 (arm C v B)	.005 (arm A v B); .0006 (arm A v C); .46 (arm C v B)
GEICAM 9906[28]	4 FEC→8 wP v 6 FEC	1,246	0.74	.006
HeCOG 10/97[29]	(dd) 4 E→4 CMF v (dd) 3 E→3 P→3 CMF	604	1.16	.31

Abbreviations: HR, hazard ratio; USON, US Oncology; A, doxorubicin; C, cyclophosphamide; D, docetaxel; CALGB, Cancer and Leukemia Group B; INT, Intergroup; NSABP, National Surgical Adjuvant Breast and Bowel Project; P, paclitaxel; F, fluorouracil; ECTO, European Cooperative Trial in Operable Breast Cancer; M, methotrexate; BCIRG, Breast Cancer International Research Group; PACS, Protocol Adjuvant dans le Cancer du Sein; E, epirubicin; BIG, Breast International Group; NCIC CTG, National Cancer Institute of Canada Clinical Trials Group; dd, dose dense; GEICAM, Spanish Group for the Investigation of Breast Cancer; wP, weekly paclitaxel; HeCOG, Hellenic Cooperative Oncology Group.

Fig. 1 Comparing adjuvant regimens typically requires thousands of patients followed for a period of years (Gianni et al. 2009). Reprinted with permission from American Society of Clinical Oncology, © 2009

regardless of nodal status, and that such treatment was most appropriate for post-menopausal patients whose tumors were estrogen receptor-positive (ER+) (Fisher et al. 2001; Wickerham 2002; Early Breast Cancer Trialists' Collaborative Group 1992a, b). An important side benefit of these trials was the recognition that ER and other analytes capable of predicting response to therapy needed to be measured consistently and accurately, and that this need could be met by central laboratories performing all assays across large studies (Bardou et al. 2003).

2 The Trastuzumab Experience

The development of trastuzumab is an outstanding example of the rapid translation of key laboratory insights about cancer to improve outcomes for patients. Little more than a decade after the identification of the first mammalian oncogene (Stehelin et al. 1976), Slamon and collaborators described examples of genomic amplification of the HER2 oncogene in a fraction of women with breast tumors and correlated these findings with adverse clinical outcomes (Slamon et al. 1987, 1989). A humanized anti-HER2 antibody designed for therapeutic purposes was described in Carter et al. (1992). Clinical trials were in progress by 1994 (Pegram et al. 1998). By 1998, an anti-HER2 humanized antibody, trastuzumab, was approved as a single agent and in combination with chemotherapy for the treatment of the fraction of metastatic breast cancers in which the HER2 protein was overexpressed (Cobleigh et al. 1999; Slamon et al. 2001).

The successful early experience with tamoxifen and subsequent focus on ER+ patients paved the way for evaluation of targeted agents such as trastuzumab in the adjuvant setting. The cooperative group mechanism proved equal to the complex task of conducting the critical initial studies, including performing central pathology reviews of tissue-based HER2 assessments. Ultimately, two independently-conducted cooperative group studies were analyzed together to bring forward compelling efficacy results that would have required years of additional follow-up if the studies had been analyzed separately (Romond et al. 2005). Academic and government investigators conceived this approach and worked to make it a reality, providing an outstanding example of effective industry/academic/ government collaboration in clinical cancer research. These initial adjuvant results with trastuzumab for HER2+ breast cancer were accompanied by other strongly positive data from a company-sponsored trial (HERA) in which trastuzumab was given, following a variety of adjuvant chemotherapy regimens (Piccart-Gebhart et al. 2005).

The cooperative groups also designed and performed informative interim analyses to determine whether important trastuzumab safety risks, such as cardiotoxicity, were within the acceptable limits for a relatively healthy adjuvant population. A newer cooperative group, BCIRG, took a different tack. Reacting to the known risk of cardiotoxicity from trastuzumab-anthracycline combinations (originally observed in pivotal studies of patients with metastatic disease and the basis for a 'black-box warning' in the product labeling), the BCIRG conceived and executed a large randomized adjuvant trial (BCIRG-006) in which a novel platinum-based regimen was assessed. The results, reported in abstract form (Robert et al. 2007), and described in product labeling (Herceptin 2009) confirmed the benefit of adding trastuzumab to standard treatment and demonstrated similar efficacy with the new regimen (docetaxel, carboplatin, and trastuzumab) compared to more traditional anthracycline-based combinations. The incidence of cardiotoxicity was substantially lower with the new regimen, suggesting that it might serve as an effective alternative for patients at increased risk of cardiotoxicity.

The challenges and ethical concerns faced by the BCIRG in conducting BCIRG-006 illustrate the complexities that future targeted treatments will face, in trying to move rapidly to adjuvant indications. The non-standard platinum-containing chemotherapy regimen was clearly active, based on Phase II studies in patients with metastatic disease (Pegram et al. 2004), but many investigators questioned whether the level of activity justified randomization of adjuvant patients away from 'standard' chemotherapy with its proven survival benefit. Perhaps fortunately, the view of standard adjuvant chemotherapy in Europe and in the rest of the world was somewhat less ossified than in the US, making the proposed randomization acceptable to many. In addition, trastuzumab was not yet generally available in many countries for this indication, providing a unique opportunity for some patients with HER2+ tumors to receive adjuvant trastuzumab.

In all, nearly 10,000 patients have been randomized in the initial wave of adjuvant trastuzumab studies, similar to the prior experience with tamoxifen [Fig. 2; (Jahanzeb 2008)]. This effort has required dedicated collaboration among the industry, academia, government, and patient advocates. What has been learned from this huge investment of time, effort, and money? Clearly, the most important lesson is that newer targeted therapies have powerful curative potential in combination with chemotherapy in the adjuvant setting, at least in some clinical situations. However, as we anticipate the coming wave of newer targeted therapies with potential adjuvant applications, a question looms concerning the scalability of this type of resource-intensive trial mechanism.

Finally, the successful adjuvant trials involving trastuzumab also created a new lens through which the pharmacoeconomic benefits of potentially costly new agents can be viewed. Estimates of the incremental cost-effectiveness ratio (ICER) for trastuzumab-based adjuvant treatment are in the range of $20,000–40,000/ quality-adjusted life-year saved (Garrison and Veenstra 2009; Liberato et al. 2007; Kurian et al. 2007). In fact, studies suggest that the ICER, expressed as $/quality-adjusted life-year saved ($/(QALY), is approximately threefold lower in the adjuvant setting compared to treatment in the metastatic setting [Fig. 3; (Garrison and Veenstra 2009)]. These investigators also found that the likely migration of patients to effective adjuvant therapy over the life cycle of trastuzumab would result in an overall ICER of approximately $35,000/QALY. This important analysis highlights the societal value of achieving adjuvant success rapidly.

Table 1 Summary of Adjuvant Trial Efficacy Data

Trial	Number of Patients	Study Design	Median Follow-up	Disease-Free Survival, Percent Event Free	Overall Survival
NSABP B-31 and NCCTG N9831 (Perez et al, 2007; Rastogi et al, 2007)	3351	Arm 1/A: AC followed by T (control); Arm 2/C: AC followed by T + H × 52 weeks	2.9 Years	Control arm: 73.1% H arm: 85.9% HR, 0.48 $P = 3 \times 10^{-12}$	Control arm: 89.4% H arm: 92.6% HR, 0.65 $P = .0007$
HERA (Smith et al, 2007; Suter et al, 2007)	3401*	Arm 1: 4 cycles of CT (control); Arm 2: CT followed by H × 52 weeks	23.5 Months	Control arm: 74.3% H arm: 80.6% HR, 0.64 $P < .0001$	Control arm: 89.7% H arm: 92.4% HR, 0.66 $P = .0115$
BCIRG 006 (Slamon et al, 2006)	3222	Arm 1: AC followed by Docetaxel (control); Arm 2: AC followed by Docetaxel + H × 52 weeks (AC → Docetaxel/H); Arm 3: Docetaxel + Carboplatin + H (Docetaxel CH)	36 Months	Control arm: 77% AC → Docetaxel/H arm: 83% HR, 0.61 $P < .0001$ Docetaxel CH arm: 82% HR, 0.67 $P = .0003$	Control arm: 86% AC → Docetaxel/H arm: 92% HR, 0.59 $P = .004$ Docetaxel CT arm: 91% HR, 0.66 $P = .017$

*Does not include the 1694 patients enrolled in the 2-year trastuzumab arm.
Abbreviations: AC = doxorubicin/cyclophosphamide; BCIRG = Breast Cancer International Research Group; CT = chemotherapy; H = trastuzumab; HERA = Herceptin Adjuvant trial; HR = hazard ratio; NSABP = National Surgical Adjuvant Breast and Bowel Project; NCCTG = North Central Cancer Treatment Group; T = paclitaxel

Fig. 2 Adjuvant trials of trastuzumab including patient numbers and median follow-up (Jahanzeb 2008). Reprinted with permission from Cancer Information Group, © 2008

Adjuvant Trials of Targeted Agents

Table 2 Assumptions regarding the cost-effectiveness of trastuzumab in metastatic and early breast cancer

Inputs*	Costs and outcomes of treatment for early breast cancer[†]	Costs and outcomes of treatment for metastatic breast cancer[‡]
Total costs—no trastuzumab	$28,749	$40,000
Total costs with trastuzumab	$73,672	$87,728
QALY: no trastuzumab	10.08	0.70
QALY: trastuzumab	11.78	1.26
Difference		
Cost	$44,923	$47,728
QALYS	1.70	0.56
Incremental cost/QALY gained (ICER)	$26,417	$85,676

*All costs and outcomes discounted at 3% annual rate.
[†]Garrison et al. [9].
[‡]Based on current drug costs, survival estimates from Hornberger et al. [8] and utility weights from Elkin et al. [7].
QALY, quality-adjusted life years; ICER, incremental cost-effectiveness ratio.

Fig. 3 Cost-effectiveness of trastuzumab is much greater in the adjuvant setting than in the metastatic setting (Garrison and Veenstra 2009). Reprinted with permission from Blackwell Publishing Group, © 2009

3 The Bevacizumab Experience

While the success of the trastuzumab adjuvant trials set a very high standard for future adjuvant trials of targeted agents, the recent less positive experience with bevacizumab in colon cancer indicates the daunting complexities ahead and suggests the need for new approaches to maximize the chances for successful outcomes of key clinical studies. In contrast to trastuzumab, bevacizumab's molecular target, vascular endothelial growth factor (VEGF), contributes to malignant behavior in a remarkably broad range of tumors including non-small cell lung cancer, colorectal cancer, breast cancer, glioblastoma, melanoma, and others [reviewed in Ferrara (2004)]. Consistent with VEGF expression across a variety of tumor types, bevacizumab has shown clinical benefit and been approved for use in metastatic tumors of the breast, colon, and lung in combination with chemotherapy, in advanced renal cell cancer in combination with interferon, and as a single agent in glioblastoma (Avastin 2009; see Chapter entitled "Toxin-induced Apoptosis"). Clinical development in many other tumor types is ongoing.

Bevacizumab's mechanism of action (inhibiting angiogenesis) would seem particularly well suited to adjuvant applications in which the goal is ostensibly to prevent previously seeded metastatic cells from developing into gross tumor masses. In view of the safety and activity demonstrated in multiple clinical studies together with the appealing mechanism of action, hopes for bevacizumab adjuvant success were extremely high. The first test of bevacizumab in the adjuvant setting was the C-08 trial led by NSABP in which the effect of the new drug added to standard chemotherapy was assessed (Allegra et al. 2009). The trial was initiated based on the improvement in the overall survival observed in patients with metastatic colorectal cancer patients treated with a regimen including bevacizumab plus the chemotherapeutic agents, irinotecan and 5-fluorouracil (Hurwitz et al. 2004). As in the trastuzumab adjuvant trials, the decision was made to combine bevacizumab with the best chemotherapy regimen for adjuvant colon cancer based on the available clinical data. The chemotherapy regimen chosen, mFOLFOX6, was based on the successful MOSAIC and C-07 trials that evaluated slightly different regimens of oxaliplatin, 5-FU, and leucovorin [reviewed and compared in Sharif et al. (2008)]. Since no biomarker with the potential to predict response had emerged from key studies in the metastatic setting (Hurwitz et al. 2004), a relatively unselected patient population was chosen for the adjuvant trials.

In the experimental arm of C-08, bevacizumab was given together with mFOLFOX6 for the first six months following surgery and then continued after the completion of chemotherapy for an additional six months for a total of one year of treatment (Hurwitz et al. 2004). It is important to point out the paucity of clinical data upon which the bevacizumab treatment duration was based. In the absence of preclinical models to assess optimal treatment duration in the adjuvant setting, one year of bevacizumab essentially reflected a balance between a desire for long-term suppression of angiogenesis in micrometastases and the desire to avoid potentially toxic treatment for excessive amounts of time, given the uncertain clinical benefits.

As reported in abstract form at ASCO 2009 (Wolmark et al. 2009) the results of this study are remarkable, with significant implications for future efforts. The primary end point was disease-free survival (DFS), a standard measure which takes into account relapse events and all causes of mortality. More than 2700 patients were randomized into one of two arms as described above. An interim safety analysis on an initial cohort of patients revealed no unexpected or unmanageable safety concerns, including cardiovascular toxicity, and the trial was continued until a sufficient number of events occurred to allow a robust read-out of efficacy (Sharif et al. 2008). The overall efficacy results showed no significant difference in three year DFS. Strikingly, however, there appeared to be a time-dependent effect of bevacizumab such that the hazard ratio for DFS was reported to be 0.6 in favor of the bevacizumab-containing arm one year from randomization, a result which was highly significant. Following cessation of bevacizumab, however, the effect appeared to diminish progressively over the next two years of follow-up, resulting in a negative study overall (Wolmark et al. 2009).

An obvious suggestion is that the treatment period with bevacizumab might have been too short for sustained efficacy to be observed. Those who are attracted to the apparent protection from relapse in the first year wonder whether the effect would have continued or even increased if the bevacizumab treatment had been continued longer. However, longer treatment duration, even if successful, would likely result in higher societal costs as reflected by measures of pharmacoeconomic benefit such as ICERs and perhaps more significant risks to patients. At present, there is no consensus on whether such studies should be considered.

The failure of the C-08 trial stands in stark contrast to the dramatic success of the trastuzumab adjuvant trials. Most frustrating, perhaps, is the sense that embedded within the negative C-08 result is a potentially important signal of bevacizumab activity that the clinical study, as designed, failed to capture as meaningful patient benefit. In light of the costly failure and unanswered questions, one wonders whether the community of cancer researchers needs to rethink its approach to adjuvant studies in the era of effective targeted therapies.

4 Imperatives for Successful Adjuvant Studies

Given the dramatic results achieved when early stage cancer is treated with active adjuvant regimens, it is critical to reconcile the difficulty of these studies with their potential importance. A clear goal of modern cancer drug development must be the creation of genuinely effective treatments for patients with a variety of early stage, but high risk, tumors. The availability of a new generation of targeted agents together with the relatively recent understanding that identifiable subsets of tumors may be critically dependent on particular pathways makes even more urgent the need to embrace a more rigorous approach to hypothesis-driven adjuvant studies (Di Cosimo and Baselga 2008).

I believe that there are four basic imperatives to enable success in this critical battleground in the war on cancer and discuss each below. Implementing appropriate tactics will require a concerted effort among academic, industry, and government researchers.

1. *Know Your Enemy*: Over the past decades we have learned that cancer is a collection of related, but heterogeneous, disorders. Going further, molecularly based disease classification will be increasingly important. In the near future, an oncologist sending a biopsy to the pathologist will need more than a description of the tissue received and a diagnosis of malignancy. He or she will want to know much more information that might bear on the choice of treatment. Increasingly, this information will take the form of a classification based on driving mutations and pathway alterations. Knowing, for example that a tumor is HER2-amplified, KRAS mutant, or rearranged for ALK will have dramatic treatment implications. And this will be true regardless of the stage of disease—such information will be essential for the management of patients in both metastatic and adjuvant settings. The newer generation of adjuvant trials will need to reflect this new reality, with careful attention paid to inclusion/exclusion criterion and patient stratification based on molecular profiling.

There has been a tendency to expect that such information will become available in the form of 'companion diagnostics', each purpose-built to support a particular therapeutic (Papadopoulos et al. 2006). This is demonstrably not the case. Mutations in the K-ras oncogene have been shown to be potent predictors of response to several EGFR-targeted treatments and are now considered an essential piece of diagnostic information when considering such treatments in several clinical situations [reviewed in Linn and Van't Veer (2009); Linardou et al. (2008)]. Development of diagnostics for critical markers like K-ras should not be left to chance (see "Predictive Genomic Biomarkers"). A more reasonable approach would be a concerted effort, perhaps led by pathologists, to develop more modern disease classification approaches that would indicate in a much more direct and intuitive way, the attractiveness of particular targeted treatments. Such an approach would lessen the complexity enforced on the treating physicians by 'companion diagnostics' and enable comparisons across studies that may be impossible with current approaches to diagnostics-based patient inclusion. Standards are urgently needed in many cases. Even in the relatively simple clinically validated case of HER2, diagnostic discrepancies still plague the field and continue to cloud interpretation of clinical data (Paik et al. 2008; Dowsett et al. 2009). The recent emergence of PARP inhibitors potentially active in refractory 'triple-negative' breast cancer underscores the critical need for reproducible molecular classification. Encouragingly, such cases seem to cluster within a population that can be recognized by routine transcriptional analysis (Linn and Van't Veer 2009; Sørlie et al. 2001).

2. *Develop Better Intelligence*: Each patient destined to relapse in adjuvant studies (and perhaps most or all adjuvant patients) harbors residual cancer cells at a time when he or she shows no evidence of disease via commonly available assessments. Demonstrating and tracking such minimal residual disease would allow clinical correlations and might provide a means by which many more adjuvant patients become evaluable for drug response. This information would ultimately allow enhanced ability to predict beneficial (or deleterious) treatment effect much sooner and perhaps with fewer patients than cumbersome clinical endpoints currently allow. Some progress has been made already via determination of circulating tumor cells [reviewed in Pantel et al. (2009)] and imaging correlates of response (Neves and Brindle 2006), but predicting clinical responses to targeted agents has been elusive (Ma et al. 2009). Biomarkers capable of identifying meaningful activity in extremely high risk patients could be remarkably useful in enhancing the power of event-driven adjuvant studies (Simon et al. 2009).

3. *Learn on the Battlefield*: Treatment of measurable, fully evaluable human cancer provides the clearest view of safety and efficacy of particular regimens and the potential predictors of any responses observed. Inevitably, it is on this battlefield that lessons critical to winning the war on cancer must be learned. As a community of investigators we must be looking to extract more information from clinical studies of such patients. Experience has taught that many agents which prove lifesaving in the adjuvant setting can be identified by their activity in more advanced stages of disease. Effective translation from studies of patients with metastatic disease into studies in the adjuvant indication is critical if the clinical and societal benefits of new treatments are to be fully realized.

Recognizing the many challenges implicit in trying to assess drug activity in the metastatic setting, some investigators have begun exploiting particular clinical situations that offer high potential for translational approaches. For example,

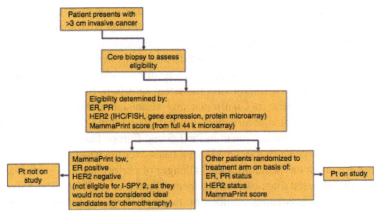

Fig. 4 Example of clinical trial design to facilitate rapid translation. I-SPY 2 assigns different experimental treatments based on tissue assessment. The neoadjuvant setting allows rapid assessment and characterization of tumor response following treatment (Barker et al. 2009). Reprinted with permission from Mosby, Inc., © 2009

Esserman and colleagues are pursuing an innovative adaptive trial design in the neoadjuvant breast cancer setting (Fig. 4; Barker et al. 2009). Tissue-based and other diagnostics are used to match patients to targeted treatment regimens. 'Efficacy' assessments are based on biomarkers in subsequently resected tumor tissue and clinical measurements. The adaptive design is meant to focus trial resources quickly on active regimens, potentially accelerating the introduction of newer targeted regimens for testing in the adjuvant setting.

Choosing the regimens with the greatest chance of success in adjuvant trials must include meaningful evaluation of the results obtained with targeted agents in more advanced patient populations. In effect, investigators must be in a 'think forward' mode with regard to development of adjuvant regimens via initial clinical experience in patients with more advanced disease and should strive to collect all essential information. The bevacizumab example illustrates the pitfalls associated with inadequate information about the optimum duration of adjuvant treatment in light of the potential trade-offs among duration of treatment, benefit, and safety risk. Many bevacizumab-containing regimens were shown to be active in advanced-stage patients during the development of this new agent [reviewed in Grothey and Galanis (2009)]. It seems plausible that efforts to characterize the direct cytotoxic potential of these regimens might have informed the design of critical adjuvant trials. For example, comparative time-to-response evaluation might have been useful information to consider in the development of limited-duration adjuvant regimens. In any event, the limitations of simply adding a targeted treatment to a proven adjuvant chemotherapy regimen are now clear. We must learn and adapt.

4. *Command and Control*: Effective coordination lies at the heart of any successful military campaign. By analogy, the many complexities inherent in adjuvant trials of targeted agents demand a comprehensive, flexible approach to preparing and managing the battlefield. As suggested above, preparing the battlefield involves a systematic approach to disease classification to facilitate a pathway-based approach to adjuvant treatment selection. Efforts are underway in breast cancer [reviewed in Cianfrocca and Gradishar (2009)] and other major tumor types, but national-level leadership will be required to ensure consistency. The cooperative group mechanism in the US and Europe has proven itself capable of organizing and executing large adjuvant trials over the past several decades. The groups have taken on the additional challenges of performing and quality-assuring essential tissue-based diagnostic assessments (Simon et al. 2009). The industry has provided an unprecedented number of targeted drug candidates against well-credentialed cancer targets. The regulatory authorities have proven competent and responsive in approving adjuvant treatment regimens, including those involving diagnostically-defined subsets. What seems to be necessary now is a more rigorous and parsimonious approach to developing, prioritizing, and executing key adjuvant efficacy trials based on molecular classification.

In the recent years, increasing attention has been paid to the design of oncology therapeutic trials. Recommendations on improvements to Phase I and II trials have been made by several high-level task forces (Booth et al. 2008a, b), with the general goal of increasing the efficiency of the process by which active drugs and improved regimens are identified. Strikingly, much less attention has been paid to improving the approach to adjuvant trials. For example, a recent report from the US Institute of Medicine analyzed the current state of the NCI Cooperative Group Program with the broad aim of identifying key areas for improvement (Nass et al. 2010). While the report explicitly embraced the goal of incorporating innovative science and trial design into cancer clinical trials, no specific recommendations pertain to adjuvant studies. Given the potential of such trials to have major effects on cancer outcomes, optimizing the conduct of adjuvant trials is an increasingly urgent priority. Of note, the committee recommended that NCI implement a 'grand-challenge' grant competition with the aim of dramatically increasing the efficiency and innovation of critical cancer clinical trials. In this regard, a specific focus on adjuvant trials seems warranted at this point.

5 Future Perspective

The compelling demonstration of the role of oncogenes in causing and promoting particular malignancies initiated a revolution in our understanding of cancer and therapeutic approach beginning in the mid-1990s (Weinberg 1994). Based on these insights, the targeted era of cancer treatment is now in full bloom. Even allowing for historical levels of attrition, a large number of appealing targeted approaches will likely succeed in demonstrating substantial activity in selected patients with advanced disease. Examples based on currently promising programs include agents targeting raf, hedgehog, PI3 kinase, mTOR, EGFR, alk, PARP, and others. Many of these agents will present near-term opportunities for testing in adjuvant trials.

Can the best regimens be extracted from trials in more advanced patients and evaluated in an ethically defensible way in adjuvant studies? Experience suggests good reasons for optimism. Tactics such as interim safety evaluations and adaptive trial designs are now standard items in the clinical science toolbox and will certainly prove useful. More needs to be done, however, to ensure greater participation in clinical trials. Availability of a larger number of patients will have direct positive effects on the time and cost of developing new adjuvant treatments. The US healthcare reform may offer opportunities to improve trials participation. Lingering concerns related to the ethics of randomizing patients to relatively untested adjuvant regimens need to be addressed and broad-based consensus gained. Concerns over intellectual property ownership arising from the results of cooperative group trials need to be addressed in ways that are mutually satisfactory to the industry, academic, and government investigators. NCI and other large funding agencies must take the lead to ensure a free flow of important information bearing on targeted approaches to adjuvant treatment. New information must be sought where it is lacking. The need for animal models of adjuvant treatment to provide validation of potential new treatment approaches is particularly acute and might be an appropriate topic on which granting agencies could solicit proposals. A critical question that remains to be answered is whether the basic biology of the early metastatic process targeted by adjuvant treatments is fundamentally different from the biology involving gross tumors (Hanahan and Weinberg 2000).

The next phase in the war on cancer will be far more complex than the last, necessarily fragmented by new ways of interrogating and classifying tumors, and fueled by a plethora of new targeted agents. A new and re-invigorated approach to adjuvant trials will help ensure success.

References

Allegra CJ, Yothers G, O'Connell MJ et al (2009) Initial safety report of NSABP C-08: a randomized phase III study of modified FOLFOX6 with or without bevacizumab for the adjuvant treatment of patients with stage II or III colon cancer. J Clin Oncol 27(20): 3385–3390 Epub 2009 May 4

Avastin [package insert] (2009) Genentech, Inc., South San Francisco, CA

Bardou VJ, Arpino G, Elledge RM, Osborne CK, Clark GM (2003) Progesterone receptor status significantly improves outcome prediction over estrogen receptor status alone for adjuvant endocrine therapy in two large breast cancer databases. J Clin Oncol 21(10):1973–1979

Barker AD, Sigman CC, Kelloff GJ, Hylton NM, Berry DA, Esserman LJ (2009) I-SPY 2: an adaptive breast cancer trial design in the setting of neoadjuvant chemotherapy. Clin Pharmacol Ther 86(1):97–100 Epub 2009 May 13

Bonadonna G, Brusamolino E, Valagussa P et al (1976) Combination chemotherapy as an adjuvant treatment in operable breast cancer. N Engl J Med 294(8):405–410

Booth CM, Calvert AH, Giaccone G, Lobbezoo MW, Seymour LK, Eisenhauer EA (2008a) Endpoints and other considerations in phase I studies of targeted anticancer therapy: recommendations from the task force on methodology for the development of innovative cancer therapies (MDICT). Eur J Cancer 44(1):19–24 Epub 2007 Sep 2

Booth CM, Calvert AH, Giaccone G, Lobbezoo MW, Eisenhauer EA, Seymour LK (2008b) Design and conduct of phase II studies of targeted anticancer therapy: recommendations from the task force on methodology for the development of innovative cancer therapies (MDICT). Eur J Cancer 44(1):25–29 Epub 2007 Sep 12

Carter P, Presta L, Gorman CM et al (1992) Humanization of an anti-p185HER2 antibody for human cancer therapy. Proc Natl Acad Sci U S A 89(10):4285–4289

Cianfrocca M, Gradishar W (2009) New molecular classifications of breast cancer. CA Cancer J Clin 59(5):303–313

Cobleigh MA, Vogel CL, Tripathy D et al (1999) Multinational study of the efficacy and safety of humanized anti-HER2 monoclonal antibody in women who have HER2-overexpressing metastatic breast cancer that has progressed after chemotherapy for metastatic disease. J Clin Oncol 17(9):2639–2648

DeVita VT Jr, Chu E (2008) A history of cancer chemotherapy. Cancer Res 68(21):8643–8653

Di Cosimo S, Baselga J (2008) Targeted therapies in breast cancer: Where are we now? Eur J Cancer 44(18):2781–2790 Epub 2008 Nov 14

Dowsett M, Procter M, McCaskill-Stevens W et al (2009) Disease-free survival according to degree of HER2 amplification for patients treated with adjuvant chemotherapy with or without 1 year of trastuzumab: the HERA Trial. J Clin Oncol 27(18):2962–2969 Epub 2009 Apr 13

Early Breast Cancer Trialists' Collaborative Group (1992a) Systemic treatment of early breast cancer by hormonal, cytotoxic, or immune therapy. 133 randomised trials involving 31,000 recurrences and 24,000 deaths among 75,000 women. Lancet 339(8784):1–15 (Jan 4)

Early Breast Cancer Trialists' Collaborative Group (1992b) Systemic treatment of early breast cancer by hormonal, cytotoxic, or immune therapy. 133 randomised trials involving 31,000 recurrences and 24,000 deaths among 75,000 women. Lancet 339(8785):71–85 (Jan 11)

Ferrara N (2004) Vascular endothelial growth factor: basic science and clinical progress. Endocr Rev 25(4):581–611

Fisher B, Carbone P, Economou SG et al (1975) 1-Phenylalanine mustard (L-PAM) in the management of primary breast cancer. A report of early findings. N Engl J Med 292(3):117–122

Fisher B, Redmond C, Brown A et al (1981) Treatment of primary breast cancer with chemotherapy and tamoxifen. N Engl J Med 305(1):1–6

Fisher B, Redmond C, Brown A et al (1983) Influence of tumor estrogen and progesterone receptor levels on the response to tamoxifen and chemotherapy in primary breast cancer. J Clin Oncol 1(4):227–241

Fisher B, Dignam J, Bryant J, Wolmark N (2001) Five versus more than five years of tamoxifen for lymph node-negative breast cancer: updated findings from the National Surgical Adjuvant Breast and Bowel Project B-14 randomized trial. J Natl Cancer Inst 93(9):684–690

Garrison LP Jr, Veenstra DL (2009) The economic value of innovative treatments over the product life cycle: the case of targeted trastuzumab therapy for breast cancer. Value Health 12(8):1118–1123 Epub 2009 Jul 14

Gianni L, Norton L, Wolmark N et al (2009) Role of anthracyclines in the treatment of early breast cancer. J Clin Oncol 27(28):4798–4808 Epub 2009 Aug 17

Grothey A, Galanis E (2009) Targeting angiogenesis: progress with anti-VEGF treatment with large molecules. Nat Rev Clin Oncol 6(9):507–518 Epub 2009 Jul 28

Hanahan D, Weinberg RA (2000) The hallmarks of cancer. Cell 100(1):57–70

Herceptin [package insert] (2009) Genentech, Inc., South San Francisco, CA

Hurwitz H, Fehrenbacher L, Novotny W et al (2004) Bevacizumab plus irinotecan, fluorouracil, and leucovorin for metastatic colorectal cancer. N Engl J Med 350(23):2335–2342

Jahanzeb M (2008) Adjuvant trastuzumab therapy for HER2-positive breast cancer. Clin Breast Cancer 8(4):324–333

Kurian AW, Thompson RN, Gaw AF, Arai S, Ortiz R, Garber AM (2007) A cost-effectiveness analysis of adjuvant trastuzumab regimens in early HER2/neu-positive breast cancer. J Clin Oncol 25(6):634–641

Liberato NL, Marchetti M, Barosi G (2007) Cost effectiveness of adjuvant trastuzumab in human epidermal growth factor receptor 2-positive breast cancer. J Clin Oncol 25(6):625–633

Linardou H, Dahabreh IJ, Kanaloupiti D (2008) Assessment of somatic k-RAS mutations as a mechanism associated with resistance to EGFR-targeted agents: a systematic review and meta-analysis of studies in advanced non-small-cell lung cancer and metastatic colorectal cancer. Lancet Oncol 9(10):962–972 Epub 2008 Sep 17

Linn SC Van't Veer LJ (2009) Clinical relevance of the triple-negative breast cancer concept: genetic basis and clinical utility of the concept. Eur J Cancer 45(Suppl 1):11–26

Ma WW, Jacene H, Song D et al (2009) [18F]fluorodeoxyglucose positron emission tomography correlates with Akt pathway activity but is not predictive of clinical outcome during mTOR inhibitor therapy. J Clin Oncol 27(16):2697–2704 Epub 2009 Apr 20

Mouridsen HT, Rose C, Overgaard M et al (1988) Adjuvant treatment of postmenopausal patients with high risk primary breast cancer. Results from the danish adjuvant trials DBCG 77 C and DBCG 82 C. Acta Oncol 27(6A):699–705

Nass SJ et al (eds) (2010) A national cancer clinical trials system for the 21st century. The national academies press, Washington, DC

Neves AA, Brindle KM (2006) Assessing responses to cancer therapy using molecular imaging. Biochim Biophys Acta 1766(2):242–261 Epub 2006 Oct 24

Paik S, Kim C, Wolmark N (2008) HER2 status and benefit from adjuvant trastuzumab in breast cancer. N Engl J Med 358(13):1409–1411

Pantel K, Alix-Panabières C, Riethdorf S (2009) Cancer micrometastases. Nat Rev Clin Oncol 6(6):339–351

Papadopoulos N, Kinzler KW, Vogelstein B (2006) The role of companion diagnostics in the development and use of mutation-targeted cancer therapies. Nat Biotechnol 24(8):985–995

Pegram MD, Lipton A, Hayes DF et al (1998) Phase II study of receptor-enhanced chemosensitivity using recombinant humanized anti-p185HER2/neu monoclonal antibody plus cisplatin in patients with HER2/neu-overexpressing metastatic breast cancer refractory to chemotherapy treatment. J Clin Oncol 16(8):2659–2671

Pegram MD, Pienkowski T, Northfelt DW et al (2004) Results of two open-label, multicenter phase II studies of docetaxel, platinum salts, and trastuzumab in HER2-positive advanced breast cancer. J Natl Cancer Inst 96(10):759–769

Piccart-Gebhart MJ, Procter M, Leyland-Jones B et al (2005) Trastuzumab after adjuvant chemotherapy in HER2-positive breast cancer. N Engl J Med 353(16):1659–1672

Robert NJ, Eiermann W, Pienkowski T et al (2007) BCIRG 006: docetaxel and trastuzumab-based regimens improve DFS and OS over AC-T in node positive and high risk node negative HER2 positive early breast cancer patients: quality of life (QOL) at 36 months follow-up. 2007 ASCO annual meeting proceedings (post-meeting edition), 25(18S):19647 (June 20 Supplement)

Romond EH, Perez EA, Bryant J et al (2005) Trastuzumab plus adjuvant chemotherapy for operable HER2-positive breast cancer. N Engl J Med 353(16):1673–1684

Sharif S, O'Connell MJ, Yothers G, Lopa S, Wolmark N (2008) FOLFOX and FLOX regimens for the adjuvant treatment of resected stage II and III colon cancer. Cancer Invest 26(9): 956–963

Simon RM, Paik S, Hayes DF (2009) Use of archived specimens in evaluation of prognostic and predictive biomarkers. J Natl Cancer Inst 101:1446–1452 8 Oct 2009 (Epub ahead of print)

Slamon DJ, Clark GM, Wong SG, Levin WJ, Ullrich A, McGuire WL (1987) Human breast cancer: correlation of relapse and survival with amplification of the HER-2/neu oncogene. Science 235(4785):177–182

Slamon DJ, Godolphin W, Jones LA et al (1989) Studies of the HER-2/neu proto-oncogene in human breast and ovarian cancer. Science 244(4905):707–712

Slamon DJ, Leyland-Jones B, Shak S et al (2001) Use of chemotherapy plus a monoclonal antibody against HER2 for metastatic breast cancer that overexpresses HER2. N Engl J Med 344(11):783–792

Sørlie T, Perou CM, Tibshirani R et al (2001) Gene expression patterns of breast carcinomas distinguish tumor subclasses with clinical implications. Proc Natl Acad Sci USA 98(19): 10869–10874

Stehelin D, Varmus HE, Bishop JM, Vogt PK (1976) DNA related to the transforming gene(s) of avian sarcoma viruses is present in normal avian DNA. Nature 260(5547):170–173

Weinberg RA (1994) Oncogenes and tumor suppressor genes. CA Cancer J Clin 44(3):160–170

Wickerham L (2002) Tamoxifen—an update on current data and where it can now be used. Breast Cancer Res Treat 75(Suppl 1):S7–S12 discussion S33-35

Wolmark N, Yothers G, O'Connell MJ et al (2009) A phase III trial comparing mFOLFOX6 to mFOLFOX6 plus bevacizumab in stage II or III carcinoma of the colon: results of NSABP protocol C-08. J Clin Oncol 27:18s (suppl; abstr LBA4)

Index

A
Acral melanomas, 103
Adjuvant regimens, 219
Adjuvant, 219
AKT, 111
Attrition, 20
AZD6244, 107

B
Bevacizumab, 219
Biomarker, 155, 191–210, 175–176, 179–181,
183–185
BRAF, 83–93

C
Cancer therapy, 161
Cancer, 191, 192, 194–205, 207–210
CDK4, 103
CDK4 and 6, 108
CDKN2A, 103, 109
Chromatin, 191–193, 195, 196, 198, 203, 204
CINK4, 109
Cyclin D1, 109
Cytokines, 122, 131

D
Drug development, 4, 9, 12, 13, 19, 20, 22,
24–25, 140, 152, 154–155, 157
Drug discovery, 4
Drug resistance, 88, 91, 92
DTIC, Dacar, 102

E
EGFR mutations, 62–64, 66, 67, 72
EGFR, 59–68, 70, 72, 109,
176, 179–186
Epigenetic, 191–194, 196–205,
207–210
ErbB-2, 177, 178
ErbB-3, 109
ErbB-4, 109
ErbB4, 110
Erlotinib, 61–68, 70, 72
Ex vivo, 30

F
Fibroblast growth factor, 113
Flavopiridol, 109

G
Gastrointestinal stromal tumor (GIST),
41–54
Gefitinib, 61–64, 66–70, 72
Genetically engineered mouse models, 19, 23
Glioma, 137–155, 157
GNA11, 106
GNAQ, 106

H
Hepatocyte growth factor, 112
HER2, 109
HER2+ tumors, 219
HRAS, 106

Index

I

Imatinib, 104
In vitro, 19–21, 30–31
In vivo, 21, 22, 24, 30–31
Incidence of melanoma, 102
Interferon-a 2B, 102
Interleukin-2, 102

J

JAK inhibitors, 128, 130–131
JAK-STAT signaling, 121, 127, 129, 130

K

kinase inhibitors, 19, 26, 33
Kinases, 140, 144, 146–147, 150
KIT, 4, 41–46, 48–49, 51–54, 104
KRAS mutation, 179–181
KRAS, 106, 179–181, 185–186

L

Lung cancer, 59, 60, 62, 65–68, 72

M

MEK inhibitors, 87–89, 91–92, 107
Melanocortin receptor 1, 102
Melanocytic nevi, 102
Melanoma, 83–93
Met, 112
mTOR, 111
Mucosal melanoma, 103
Mutation, 176, 179–185
Myeloproliferative disease, 130, 132

N

Neural crest, 103
NRAS, 106

O

Oncomouse, 32

P

p16, 108
PD-0332991, 109
PDK1, 111
Pharmacology, 21
PI3-kinase, 111
Platelet-derived growth factor receptor
   (PDGFR), 41–46, 52, 53
Preclinical models, 20
Progression, 191, 192, 194, 196, 199–200, 203,
   210

R

RAF inhibitors, 89, 91–93
Raf inhibitors, 4

S

S6 kinase, 111
Skin rash, 107
Spitz nevi, 106
Subtypes, 103
Succinate dehydrogenase B (SDHB), 45, 46

T

Tanning response, 103
Targeted treatments, 219
Trastuzumab, 219

U

UCN-01, 109
Uveal melanoma, 104

V

Vascular endothelial growth factor receptor
   (VEGFR), 41, 53

X

XL184, 113

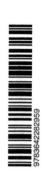